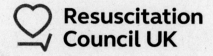

Day 2

8.00	15 min	Tea / coffee and mentor groups			
08:15		**Peri-arrest workshops** *(continued after tea/coffee break)*			
		Tachycardia, cardioversion and drugs		**Bradycardia, pacing and drugs**	
08:15	45 min	Group 1	Group 2	Group 3	Group 4
09:00	45 min	Group 3	Group 4	Group 1	Group 2
09:45	15 min	*Tea / coffee break*			
		Arterial blood gas analysis			
10:00	45 min	Group 2	Group 4	Group 3	Group 1
10:45		**Special Circumstances workshops**			
		Special Circs 1		**Special Circs 2**	
10:45	30 min	Group 1	Group 2	Group 3	Group 4
11.15	30 min	Group 4	Group 3	Group 2	Group 1
		Special Circs 3			
11.45	30 min	Group 1	Group 2	Group 3	Group 4
12.15	45 min	*Lunch*			
		CASTeach 4			
13.00	45 min	Group 1	Group 2	Group 3	Group 4
		CASTeach 5			
13:45	45 min	Group 1	Group 2	Group 3	Group 4
14:30	15 min	*Tea / coffee break*			
14:45	120 min	**CASTest and MCQ**			
17:30	15 min	**Faculty meeting**			
18:00		**Candidate feedback in mentor groups**			
		End of course			

Please note that 18.00 hrs is an ESTIMATED time to finish and to make sure you arrange your travel home accordingly

Dec 2014
ALS Provider Course
Course programme

Resuscitation Council (UK)
Tel: (020) 7388 4678 | Fax: (020) 7383 0773
ALS@resus.org.uk | www.resus.org.uk

Page 2 of 2

Resuscitation Council UK

 ALS

Advanced Life Support Provider Course Programme

Post Graduate Centre – County Hospital, Stafford, ST16 3SA

Day 1

Time	Duration	Session			
8.00 – 8.30		*Faculty Meeting and Candidate Registration*			
08.30 - 08.45		*Welcome & Introductions*			
08:45	10 min	**Lecture:** ALS in Perspective			
08:55	25 min	**Lecture**: Causes and Prevention of Cardiac Arrest			
09:20	20 min	**Lecture:** Acute Coronary Syndromes			
09:40	60 min	**Demonstration/lecture**			
		• CASDemo (including non-technical skills) • ALS Algorithm			
10:40	15 min	*Tea / coffee break*			
10:55		**Skill stations and workshops:**			
		• Associated Resuscitation Skills • The Deteriorating Patient • Rhythm Recognition (RR) and 12-Lead ECG • High quality CPR and Defibrillation			
		Associated Resuscitation Skills			
10:55	50 min	Group 1	Group 2	Group 3	Group 4
		The Deteriorating Patient Inc. IO			
11.45	50 min	Group 1	Group 2	Group 3	Group 4
12:35	45 min	*Lunch break*			
13:20		**Skill stations and workshops** *continued*			
		RR and 12-lead ECG			
13:20	50 min	Group 1	Group 2	Group 3	Group 4
		CPR and Defibrillation			
14:10	50 min	Group 1	Group 2	Group 3	Group 4
15:00	25 min	**Lecture:** Post Resuscitation Care			
15:25	15 min	*Tea / coffee break*			
15:40		**Cardiac Arrest Simulations Teaching Sessions (CASTeach) 1-3**			
		CASTeach 1			
15:40	30 min	Group 1	Group 2	Group 3	Group 4
		CASTeach 2			
16:10	30 min	Group 1	Group 2	Group 3	Group 4
		CASTeach 3			
16:40	30 min	Group 1	Group 2	Group 3	Group 4
17:10	30 min	**Mentor feedback**			
17:40		**Faculty meeting**			

Dec 2014
ALS Provider Course
Course programme

Resuscitation Council (UK)
Tel: (020) 7388 4678 | Fax: (020) 7383 0773
ALS@resus.org.uk | www.resus.org.uk

Page 1 of 2

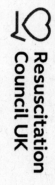

Resuscitation Council UK

ALS

ALS Provider Course - Continuous Assessment for High-Quality CPR & Defibrillation

Structure Skill description	Process Demonstration of competency during the skills practice	Desired skill outcome	Assessment (Please tick)	
			Achieved	Not achieved
Confirmation of cardiac arrest	Open airway, check for breathing and circulation simultaneously, call the resuscitation team and send for resuscitation equipment.	Confirms cardiac arrest and ensures help is called		
Delivery of high-quality chest compressions	Hand position, depth, rate and recoil of compressions. 30:2 ratio. Avoids unnecessary interruptions in chest compression.	Support of the circulation during cardiac arrest		
Task allocation and planning for defibrillation	Identifies competencies and allocates tasks accordingly: —√ communicated effectively the sequence to team members to minimise pre-shock pause —√ pads applied while chest compressions are ongoing —√ compressions stopped for rhythm check, < 5 s —√ clear instructions given to the person doing chest compressions to continue whilst the defibrillator is charged, and all other team members informed to stand clear and remove oxygen as appropriate —√ compressions stop, hands clear of the chest, and shock delivery immediate resumption of CPR.	Allocates tasks and plans actions of team to minimise pre-shock pause		
Safe and effective use of the defibrillator	Ensures delivery of planned actions by team: —√ correct diagnosis of a shockable rhythm —√ Selects the appropriate energy on the defibrillator —√ minimises pre-shock pause; warns the team to stand clear on the defibrillator —√ tells person delivering chest compressions to stand clear and ensures oxygen delivery device has been removed, as appropriate —√ shock safely delivered and immediate resumption of CPR —√ no pause or rhythm checks immediately post-shock —√ ensures the safety of self and team at all times.	Safe and effective defibrillation, minimal pre-shock pause		

Candidate name:

1st Instructor name:

2nd Instructor name:

Achieved assessment outcome: Yes ☐   No ☐   **Date:**

Comments: (Continue overleaf if required)

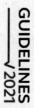

Advanced Life Support

8th Edition, May 2021

ALS

Advanced Life Support
8th Edition, May 2021

ISBN - 978-1-903812-35-8

Published by © Resuscitation Council UK
5th Floor, Tavistock House North, Tavistock Square, London WC1H 9HR
Tel: 020 7388 4678 email: enquiries@resus.org.uk www.resus.org.uk

Printed by All About Print
Tel: 020 7205 4022 email: hello@allaboutprint.co.uk www.allaboutprint.co.uk
Printed on responsibly sourced environmentally friendly paper made with elemental chlorine free fibre from legal and sustainably managed forests.

Photographs © Resuscitation Council UK
Photography by Ed Tyler, Ashley Prytherch and Mike Scott
Chain of Prevention © Gary Smith
ECGs © Oliver Meyer
Electrical conduction of the heart (Figure 8.6 and 10.1) © LifeART image (1989–2001) Wolters Kluwer Health, Inc.-Lippincott Williams & Wilkins. All rights reserved.

Design and artwork by Fruition London
www.fruitionlondon.com

The Resuscitation Council UK Guidelines are adapted from the European Resuscitation Council guidelines and have been developed using a process accredited by The National Institute for Health and Care Excellence. The UK guidelines are consistent with the European guidelines but include minor modifications to reflect the needs of the National Health Service.

This Advanced Life Support (ALS) manual is written by the Resuscitation Council UK ALS Subcommittee and forms part of the resources for the Resuscitation Council UK ALS course, which is delivered in accredited course centres throughout the UK.

Acknowledgements

We thank and acknowledge the members of the ERC 2021 Guidelines Writing Group who have contributed directly or indirectly to this ALS Manual: Abbas Khalifa, Sean Ainsworth, Annette Alfonzo, Hans-Richard Arntz, Helen Askitopoulou, Alessandro Barelli, Abdelouahab Bellou, Berthold Bein, Farzin Beygui, Dominique Biarent, Robert Bingham, Joost JLM Bierens, Marieke Blom, Bernd W Böttiger, Leo L Bossaert, Guttorm Brattebø, Jan Breckwoldt, Hermann Brugger, Jos Bruinenberg, Roman Burkart, Alain Cariou, Pierre Carli, Francesc Carmona, Pascal Cassan, Maaret Castrén, Athanasios F Chalkias, Diana Cimpoesu, Patricia Conaghan, Keith Couper, Tobias Cronberg, Charles D Deakin, Jana Djakow, Therresa Djarv, Emmy DJ De Buck, Patrick Druwé, Joel Dunning, Wiebe De Vries, Hege Ersdal, Thomas R Evans, Christoph Eich, Hans Friberg , Cornelia Genbrugge, Marios Georgiou, Violeta Gonzalez-Salvado, Jan-Thorsten Gräsnr, Robert Greif, Christina M Hafner, Anthony J Handley, Kirstie L Haywood, Johan Herlitz, Jochen Hinkelbein Silvija Hunyadi-Antlcevlc, Rudolph W Koster, Artem Kuzovlev, Anne Lippert, Freddy Lippert, Gisela Lilja, Ileana Lulic, David J Lockey, Andrew S Lockey, Jesús López-Herce, Carsten Lott, Ian K Maconochie, John Madar, Siobhan Masterson, Spyros D Mentzelopoulos, Daniel Meyran, Koenraad G Monsieurs, Colin Morley, Veronique RM Moulaert, Nikolaos I Nikolaou, Jerry Nolan, Theresa Olasveengen, Fernando Rosell-Ortiz, Peter Paal, Arjan tePas, Tommaso Pellis, Gavin D Perkins, Lucas Pflanzl-Knizacek, Thomas Rajka, Violetta I Raffay, Giuseppe Ristagno, Antonio Rodríguez-Núnez, Charles Christoph Roehr, Mario Rüdiger, Ferenc Sari, Federico Semeraro, Claudio Sandroni, Schunder-Tatzber, Salma Shammet, Eunice M Singletary, Christiane Skare, Markus B Skrifvars, Andrea Scapigliati, Joachim Schlieber, Sebastian Schnaubelt, Gary B Smith, Michael A Smyth, Jasmeet Soar, Hildigunner Svavarsdottir, Fabio Taccone, Karl-Christian Thies, Ingvild BM Tjelmeland, Daniele Trevisanuto, Anatolij Truhlár, Nigel Turner, Philippe G Vandekerckhove, Patrick Van de Voorde, Kjetil Sunde, Berndt Urlesberger, Volker Wenzel, Dominic Wilkinson, Jan Wnent, Jonathan Wyllie, Theodoros T Xanthos, Joyce Yeung, David A Zideman.

We thank the Nuffield Hospital, Guildford, for the use of their facilities, The Royal Sussex County Hospital NHS Foundation Trust, specifically the Resuscitation Department for their assistance with photography, Lifecast Body Simulation for the loan of manikins and all the Instructors who gave up their time to take part in the photography shoot.

We thank Oliver Meyer for digital preparation of the 12-lead ECGs and rhythm strips.

We thank Ed Tyler, Ashley Prytherch and Mike Scott for the photography taken and digitally prepared for the manual.

Hot Debrief, STOP-5 tool is reproduced with the permission of Dr Craig Walker on behalf of Edinburgh Emergency Medicine and The Scottish Centre for Simulation & Clinical Human Factors.

Editors

Jasmeet Soar
Adam Benson Clarke
Carl Gwinnutt
Isabelle Hamilton-Bower
Sue Hampshire
Andrew Lockey
Jerry Nolan
Gavin Perkins
David Pitcher

Contributors

Adam Benson Clarke
James Bolton
Sarah Cocker
Matthew Cordingly
Keith Couper
Ron Daniels
Robin Davies
Joseph De Bono
Charles Deakin
Sarah Dickie
Joel Dunning
Zoe Fritz
James Fullerton
David Gabbott
Paul Greig
Carl Gwinnutt
Michelle Hall
Isabelle Hamilton-Bower
Sue Hampshire
Tony Handley
Anil Hornis
Wayne Hurst
Andrew Lockey
Kevin Mackie
Oliver Meyer
Sian Moxham
Jerry Nolan
Gavin Perkins
Joe Phillips
David Pitcher
Susanna Price
Mike Scott
Gary Smith
Jasmeet Soar
Chris Thorne
Shahana Uddin
Andrew Wragg
Joyce Yeung

Contents

Glossary 7

01 **Advanced life support in perspective** 9
   The problem 9
   The Chain of Survival 10
   ALS algorithm 10
   Improving outcomes from cardiac arrest ... 12
   The ALS course 14
   Further reading 15

02 **Non-technical skills in resuscitation** 17
   Introduction 17
   Situational awareness 18
   Decision-making 18
   Team working, including team leadership ... 18
   Task management 19
   The importance of communication when managing
   a sick patient 20
   Resuscitation teams 22
   Further reading 23
   Acknowledgment 23

03 **Recognising deterioration and preventing
   cardiorespiratory arrest** 25
   Introduction 25
   Prevention of in-hospital cardiac arrest:
   the Chain of Prevention 26
   Recognising the deteriorating patient 27
   Response to critical illness 28
   Causes of deterioration and cardiac arrest ... 28
   The ABCDE approach 32
   Further reading 37

04 **Cardiac causes of cardiac arrest** 39
   Introduction 39
   Acute coronary syndromes 39
   Diagnosis of acute coronary syndromes ... 45
   Quantitative risk assessment scores: GRACE and CRUSADE ... 48
   Immediate treatment 49
   Subsequent management of patients with acute coronary
   syndromes 52
   Cardiac arrhythmia complicating acute coronary syndromes ... 54
   Other cardiac arrhythmia 54
   Other cardiac causes of cardiac arrest and sudden
   cardiac death 57
   Avoidance of cardiac arrest in people at risk ... 58
   Further reading 59

05 **In-hospital resuscitation** 61
   Introduction 61
   Features specific to in-hospital resuscitation ... 61
   Sequence for a collapsed patient in hospital ... 62
   Further reading 69

06 **Advanced life support algorithm** 71
   Introduction 71
   Shockable rhythms (VF/pVT) 72
   Non-shockable rhythms (PEA and asystole) ... 75

During CPR 75
End-tidal CO_2 during CPR 78
Identification and treatment of reversible causes ... 80
Ultrasound during advanced life support ... 81
The use of automated mechanical chest compression devices ... 81
Extracorporeal CPR 81
The duration of a resuscitation attempt 82
Diagnosing death after unsuccessful resuscitation ... 82
Post-event tasks 82
Further reading 83

07 **Airway management and ventilation** 85
   Introduction 85
   Causes of airway obstruction 85
   Recognition of airway obstruction 85
   Choking 86
   Basic techniques for opening the airway .. 88
   Oxygen 90
   Suction 91
   Ventilation 91
   Supraglottic airways 92
   Aids to intubation 96
   Cricothyroidotomy 96
   Further reading 97

08 **Rhythm recognition** 99
   Introduction 99
   Techniques for ECG monitoring 100
   Diagnosis from cardiac monitors 101
   Basic electrocardiography 102
   How to read a rhythm strip 103
   Cardiac arrest rhythms 106
   Peri-arrest arrhythmias 108
   The QT interval 110
   Further reading 111

09 **Defibrillation** 117
   Introduction 117
   The probability of successful defibrillation ... 117
   Mechanism of defibrillation 118
   Factors affecting defibrillation success ... 118
   CPR or defibrillation first? 119
   Shock sequence 119
   Witnessed and monitored VF/pVT cardiac arrest ... 119
   Shock energies 119
   Safety 120
   Automated external defibrillators 120
   Manual defibrillation 122
   Synchronised cardioversion 123
   Implanted electronic devices 123
   Internal defibrillation 124
   Further reading 125

10 **Cardiac pacing** 127
   Introduction 127

Contents

Formation and failure of the heart's electrical signal 127
Methods of pacing 128
Further reading 133

11 Peri-arrest arrhythmias 135
Introduction 135
Sequence of actions to take in all arrhythmias 135
Tachyarrhythmia 136
Bradyarrhythmia 140
Further reading 143

12 Resuscitation in special circumstances 145
Introduction 145
Life-threatening electrolyte disorders 146
Potassium 146
Hyperkalaemia 146
Hypokalaemia 148
Calcium and magnesium disorders 150
Dialysis 150
Sepsis 150
Toxins (poisoning) 151
Hypoxia 154
Asthma 154
Anaphylaxis 156
Pregnancy 162
Traumatic cardiorespiratory arrest 164
Tension pneumothorax 166
Perioperative cardiac arrest 166
Drowning 168
Accidental hypothermia 170
Hyperthermia 172
Obesity 174
Further reading 175

13 Post-resuscitation care 177
Introduction 177
Continued resuscitation 178
Optimising organ function 181
Prognostication 185
Rehabilitation 185
Organ donation 185
Cardiac arrest centres 185
Further reading 187

14 Pre-hospital cardiac arrest 189
Introduction 189
Resuscitation at scene versus transfer to hospital 189
Team approach 190
Pre-hospital airway management 190
Breathing 192
Circulation 192
Recognition of life extinct 193
Communication with relatives 194
Patient destination 195
Team handover and debriefing 196

Audit 196
Further reading 197

15 Blood gas analysis and pulse oximetry 199
Introduction 199
Interpreting blood gas values using the 6-step approach 199
Case studies 203
Pulse oximetry 207
Further reading 209

16 Making decisions about CPR 211
Introduction 211
Ethical and legal framework 212
Integrating recommendations relating to CPR into overarching emergency care and treatment plans 212
Shared decision-making 212
Communication: discussing recommendations with those close to the person 213
Communication: discussing recommendations when a person lacks capacity 213
Deciding whether or not to provide CPR 214
Recording emergency care and treatment plans (including CPR) 214
Communicating recommendations and the person's wishes 214
When it is reasonable not to attempt CPR 215
Decisions about implanted cardioverter-defibrillators 215
Defining 'success' and 'futility' 215
Predicting outcome 215
Avoiding discrimination 216
Deciding to stop CPR 216
Special considerations 216
Withdrawal of other treatment during the post-resuscitation period 216
Auditing cardiac arrests and decisions about CPR 216
Further reading 216

17 Supporting relatives and teams in resuscitation practice 219
Introduction 219
The involvement of relatives and friends 220
Caring for the recently bereaved 220
Early contact with one person 220
Provision of a suitable room 220
Breaking bad news and supporting the grief response 220
Arranging viewing of the body 221
Religious requirements, legal and practical arrangements 221
Staff support and debriefing 221
STOP-5 debrief tool 221
Further reading 222

Appendices
A Drugs used during the treatment of cardiac arrest 223
B Drugs used in the peri-arrest period 225
C Useful links 228

Notes

Glossary

Abbreviation	In full
A	amperes
AC	alternating current
ACEI	angiotensin converting enzyme inhibitor
ACS	acute coronary syndrome
ACVPU	alert, new confusion, voice, pain, unresponsive
AED	automated external defibrillator
AF	atrial fibrillation
ALS	advanced life support
AMI	acute myocardial infarction
AV	atrioventricular as in atrioventricular node
BLS	basic life support
BP	blood pressure
CABG	coronary artery bypass grafting
CCU	coronary care unit
CK	creatine kinase
CHB	complete heart block
CPR	cardiopulmonary resuscitation
CVP	central venous pressure
DC	direct current
DNACPR	do not attempt cardiopulmonary resuscitation
ECG	electrocardiogram
ED	emergency department
EMS	emergency medical services (e.g. ambulance service)
EWS	early warning score
GCS	Glasgow coma score
h	hour
HDU	high dependency unit
ICD	implantable cardioverter-defibrillator
ICU	intensive care unit
IHCA	in-hospital cardiac arrest
IM	intramuscular
IO	intraosseous

Abbreviation	In full
IV	intravenous
JVP	jugular venous pressure
LBBB	left bundle branch block
LMA	laryngeal mask airway
LT	laryngeal tube
LV	left ventricular
MET	medical emergency team
min	minute
NEWS	National Early Warning Score 2
NSTEMI	non-ST-elevation myocardial infarction
OHCA	out-of-hospital cardiac arrest
PCI	percutaneous coronary intervention
PPCI	primary percutaneous coronary intervention
PEA	pulseless electrical activity
ReSPECT	Recommended Summary Plan for Emergency Care and Treatment
ROSC	return of spontaneous circulation
RSVP	reason, story, vitals, plan
RV	right ventricular
s	second
SA	sino-atrial as in sino-atrial node
SBARD	situation, background, assessment, recommendation. decision
SBP	systolic blood pressure
SCD	sudden cardiac death
SGA	supraglottic airway
STEMI	ST-elevation myocardial infarction
SVT	supraventricular tachycardia
TDP	torsade de pointes
VT	ventricular tachycardia
VF/pVT	ventricular fibrillation/ pulseless VT
WPW	Wolff-Parkinson-White syndrome

Throughout this publication:

- The terms cardiorespiratory arrest and cardiac arrest have been used interchangeably.

- Adrenaline is the preferred term for adrenaline/epinephrine.

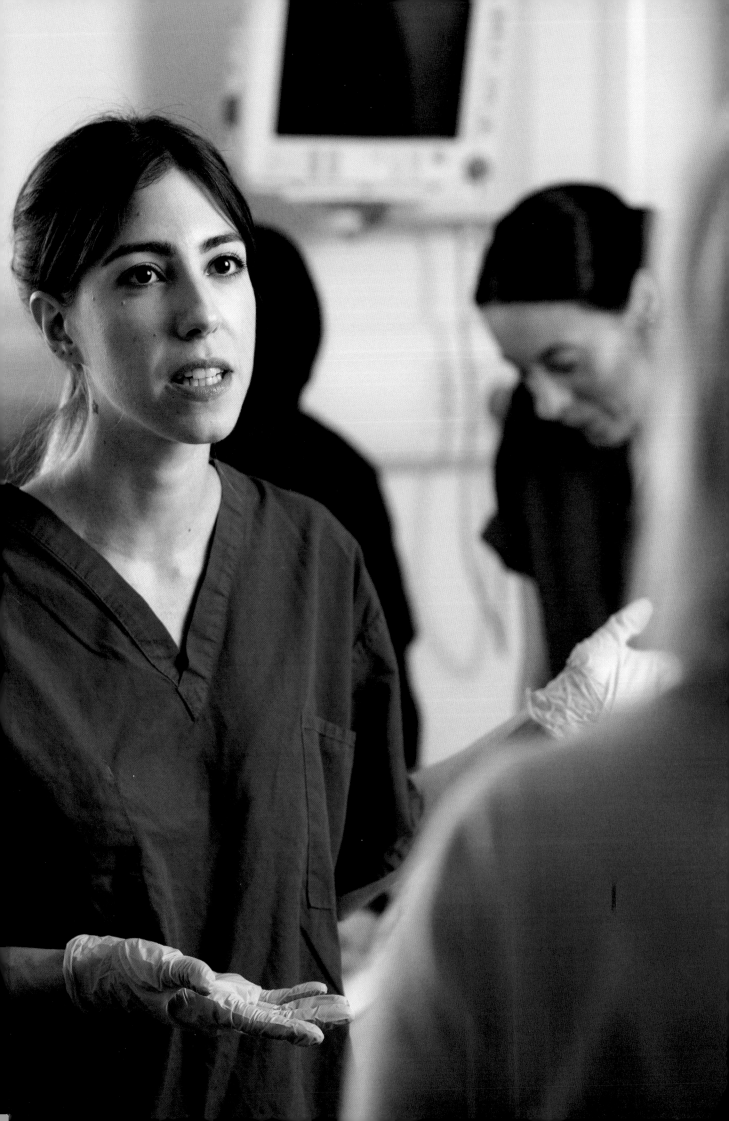

Advanced life support in perspective

The problem

Ischaemic heart disease (IHD) is the second biggest single cause of death in the UK, following dementia. In 2018, there were 40 214 male deaths and 23 662 female deaths from IHD. There are nearly half a million hospital admissions associated with IHD in the UK each year.

Out-of-hospital cardiac arrest

English ambulance services start cardiopulmonary resuscitation (CPR) on about 30 000 patients who sustain an out-of-hospital cardiac arrest each year. Most cardiac arrests occur in the home and are presumed to have a cardiac cause.

Around a half of cardiac arrests are witnessed by either a bystander or ambulance staff. The presenting rhythm is shockable (ventricular fibrillation/pulseless ventricular tachycardia (VF/pVT)) in about a quarter of cases and non-shockable in the remainder – asystole in about 50% and pulseless electrical activity (PEA) in about 25% of cases.

Amongst those in whom resuscitation is attempted, 30% initially achieve a return of spontaneous circulation (ROSC) but only 9.7% survive to go home from hospital.

In-hospital cardiac arrest

The incidence of in-hospital cardiac arrest is difficult to assess because it is influenced heavily by factors such as the criteria for hospital admission and implementation of do not attempt cardiopulmonary resuscitation (DNACPR) recommendations.

Data from 175 hospitals contributing to the UK National Cardiac Arrest Audit showed that during 2019–2020 the overall incidence of adult in-hospital cardiac arrest was about 1 per 1000 hospital admissions, and a reduction from 1.6 per 1000 hospital admissions in 2013. The incidence varied seasonally, peaking in winter. The overall survival to hospital discharge was 23.9%, which is also an improvement on 18.4% in 2013.

The trend in the UK is therefore one of improvement for in-hospital cardiac arrest and survival rates. This has occurred due to various factors such as improvements in guidelines and treatment options, as well as a greater understanding of which patients would not benefit from CPR. The role of training in cardiac arrest management is therefore vital.

The presenting rhythm was shockable (VF/pVT) in 18.1% and non-shockable (asystole or pulseless electrical activity) in 73.1% of cases, and rates of survival to hospital discharge associated with these rhythms were 50.6% and 14.4% respectively, but varied substantially across hospitals. All these individuals received chest compressions and/or defibrillation and were attended by the hospital resuscitation team in response to a 2222 call.

Many patients who have an in-hospital cardiac arrest have significant comorbidity, which influences the initial rhythm and, in these cases, strategies to prevent cardiac arrest are particularly important.

> Amongst those in whom resuscitation is attempted out-of-hospital, 9% survive to return home

> In 2019-20, the overall survival of adult in-hospital cardiac arrest to hospital discharge was 23.9%

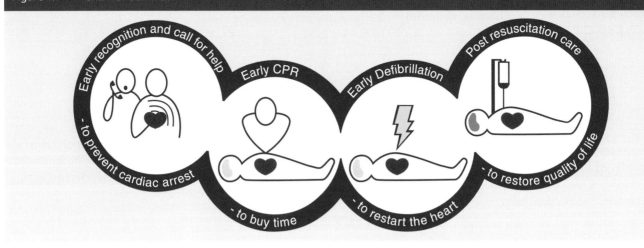

Figure 1.1   Chain of Survival

The Chain of Survival

The interventions that contribute to a successful outcome after a cardiac arrest can be conceptualised as a chain – the Chain of Survival (Figure 1.1).

The chain is only as strong as its weakest link; all four links of the Chain of Survival must be strong. They are:

- Early recognition and call for help
- Early cardiopulmonary resuscitation (CPR)
- Early defibrillation
- Post-resuscitation care.

Early recognition and call for help

Out-of-hospital, early recognition of the importance of chest pain will enable the person or a bystander to call the ambulance service so that the person can receive treatment that may prevent cardiac arrest. Once cardiac arrest has occurred, early recognition is critical to enable rapid activation of the ambulance service and prompt initiation of bystander CPR. In the UK, the ambulance service can be contacted by dialling 999.

In hospital, early recognition of the critically ill patient who is at risk of cardiac arrest and a call for the resuscitation team or medical emergency team (MET) will enable treatment to prevent cardiac arrest (Chapter 3). A universal number for calling the resuscitation team or MET should be adopted in all hospitals – in the UK this number is 2222. If cardiac arrest occurs, do not delay defibrillation until arrival of the resuscitation team – clinical staff should be trained to use a defibrillator.

Early CPR

Chest compressions and ventilation of the person's lungs will slow down the rate of deterioration of the brain and heart. After out-of-hospital cardiac arrest, bystander CPR extends the period in which resuscitation may be successful and at least doubles the chance of survival after VF/pVT cardiac arrest. Performing chest-compression-only CPR is better than giving no CPR at all. Bystander CPR rates in the UK have risen to over 60% following successful initiatives (e.g. Restart a Heart) to promote the benefits for this intervention.

After in-hospital cardiac arrest, chest compressions and ventilation must be undertaken immediately, but should not delay attempts to defibrillate those patients in VF/pVT. Interruptions to chest compressions must be minimised and should occur only very briefly during defibrillation attempts and rhythm checks.

Early defibrillation

Defibrillation within 3-5 min of collapse can produce survival rates as high as 50–70%. This can be achieved through public access defibrillation, when a bystander uses a nearby automated external defibrillator (AED) to deliver the first shock. Each minute of delay to defibrillation reduces the probability of survival to hospital discharge by 10–12%. In the UK, an AED is deployed in about 5% of out-of-hospital cardiac arrests (OHCA) before ambulance arrival. In hospitals, sufficient healthcare personnel should be trained and authorised to use a defibrillator to enable the first responder to a cardiac arrest to attempt defibrillation as rapidly as possible and certainly within 3 min.

Post-resuscitation care

Return of a spontaneous circulation is an important phase in the continuum of resuscitation; however, the ultimate goal is to return the patient to a state of normal cerebral function, a stable cardiac rhythm, and normal haemodynamic function, so that they can leave hospital in reasonable health at minimum risk of a further cardiac arrest.

The quality of treatment in the post-resuscitation period influences the patient's ultimate outcome. The post-resuscitation phase starts at the location where ROSC is achieved. The ALS provider must be capable of providing high-quality post-resuscitation care until the patient is transferred to an appropriate high-care area.

ALS algorithm

The ALS algorithm (Figure 1.2) is the centre point of the ALS course and is applicable to most CPR situations. Some modifications may be required when managing cardiac arrest in special circumstances (Chapter 12).

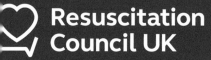
Adult advanced life support

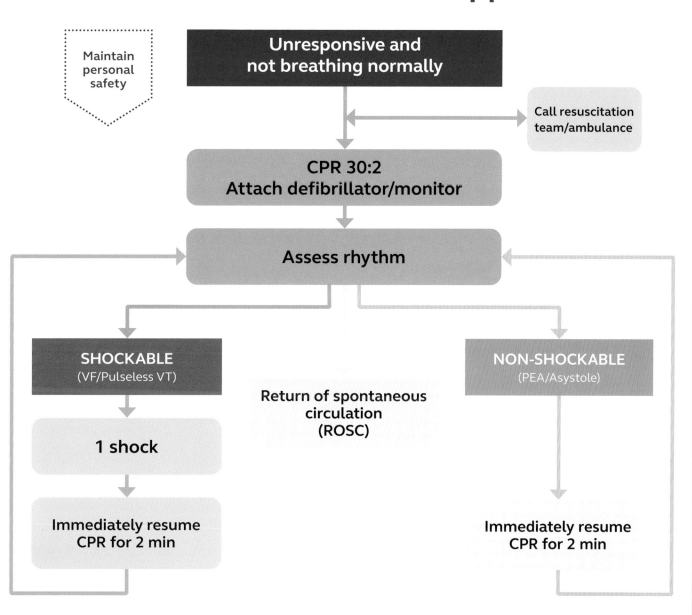

Maintain personal safety

Unresponsive and not breathing normally

Call resuscitation team/ambulance

CPR 30:2
Attach defibrillator/monitor

Assess rhythm

SHOCKABLE
(VF/Pulseless VT)

NON-SHOCKABLE
(PEA/Asystole)

Return of spontaneous circulation (ROSC)

1 shock

Immediately resume CPR for 2 min

Immediately resume CPR for 2 min

Give high-quality chest compressions, and:

- Give oxygen
- Use waveform capnography
- Continuous compressions if advanced airway
- Minimise interruptions to compressions
- Intravenous or intraosseous access
- Give adrenaline every 3–5 min
- Give amiodarone after 3 shocks
- Identify and treat reversible causes

Identify and treat reversible causes

- Hypoxia
- Hypovolaemia
- Hypo-/hyperkalaemia/ metabolic
- Hypo/hyperthermia
- Thrombosis – coronary or pulmonary
- Tension pneumothorax
- Tamponade – cardiac
- Toxins

Consider ultrasound imaging to identify reversible causes

Consider

- Coronary angiography/ percutaneous coronary intervention
- Mechanical chest compressions to facilitate transfer/treatment
- Extracorporeal CPR

After ROSC

- Use an ABCDE approach
- Aim for SpO$_2$ of 94–98% and normal PaCO$_2$
- 12-lead ECG
- Identify and treat cause
- Targeted temperature management

Figure 1.2   Adult Advanced Life Support algorithm   11

Improving outcomes from cardiac arrest

High-quality care is safe, effective, patient-centred, timely, efficient and equitable. Hospitals, resuscitation teams and ALS providers should ensure they deliver these aspects of quality to improve the care of the deteriorating patient and patients in cardiac arrest. We describe below some of the strategies to improve outcomes.

Evidence-based guidelines

Improving outcomes from cardiac arrest depends on the implementation of evidence-based guidelines. The contents of this ALS provider manual are consistent with the Resuscitation Council UK (RCUK) Guidelines. The process used to produce the Resuscitation Council UK Guidelines has been accredited by the National Institute for Health and Care Excellence (NICE). The guidelines process includes:

- Systematic reviews with grading of the quality of evidence and strength of recommendations. This led to the 2020 International Liaison Committee on Resuscitation (ILCOR) Consensus on Cardiopulmonary Resuscitation and Emergency Cardiovascular Care Science with Treatment Recommendations.
- The involvement of stakeholders from around the world including members of the public and cardiac arrest survivors.
- Collaboration with the European Resuscitation Council, and adapting its guidelines for use in the UK using a NICE accredited process.

The current Resuscitation Council UK Guidelines for cardiopulmonary resuscitation can be found at www.resus.org.uk

Quality Standards

Healthcare organisations have an obligation to provide a high-quality resuscitation service, and to ensure that staff are trained and updated regularly and with appropriate frequency to a level of proficiency appropriate to each individual's expected role. The same core standards apply to all healthcare settings:

- The deteriorating patient is recognised early and there is an effective system to summon help in order to prevent cardiorespiratory arrest.
- Cardiorespiratory arrest is recognised early and CPR is started immediately.
- Emergency assistance is summoned immediately, as soon as cardiorespiratory arrest is recognised, if help has not been summoned already.
- Defibrillation, if appropriate, is attempted within 3 min of identifying cardiorespiratory arrest.
- Appropriate post-cardiorespiratory-arrest care is received by those who are resuscitated successfully. This includes safe transfer.
- Implementation of standards is measured continually and processes are in place to deal with any problems identified.
- Staff receive at least annual training and updates in CPR, based on their expected roles.
- Staff have an understanding of decisions relating to CPR.
- Appropriate equipment is immediately available for resuscitation.

The Resuscitation Council UK Quality standards for cardiopulmonary resuscitation practice and training provide further detailed information.

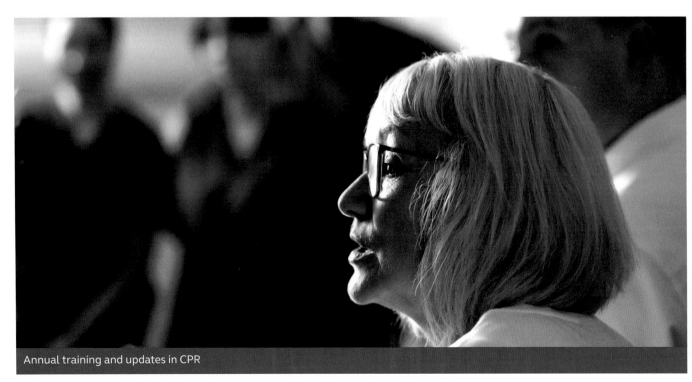

Annual training and updates in CPR

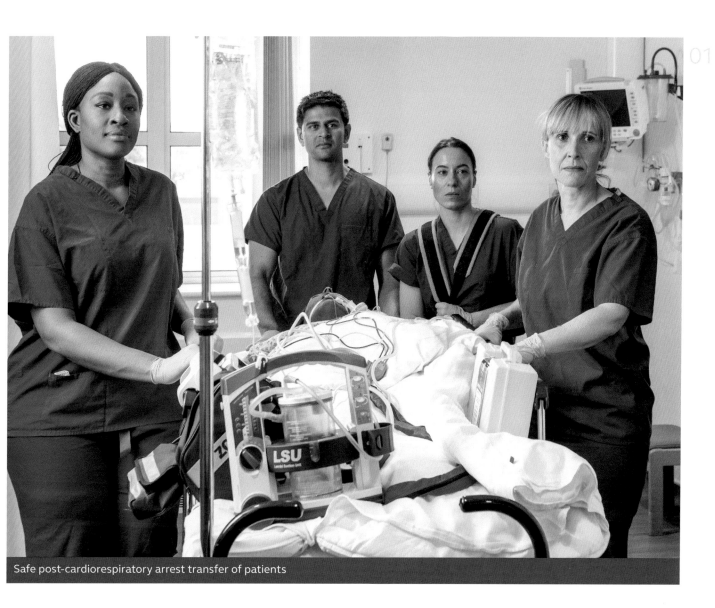
Safe post-cardiorespiratory arrest transfer of patients

Measuring patient outcomes

Continuous measurement of compliance with processes and patient outcomes at a national and local level provides information on the impact of changes in practice, identifies areas for improvement, and also enables comparison in outcomes between different organisations. Uniform definitions for collecting data for cardiac arrest exist.

The National Out-of-Hospital Cardiac Arrest Outcomes project measures patient, process and outcome variables from out-of-hospital-cardiac arrest in the UK. The project is run in collaboration with the National Ambulance Service Medical Directors Group with support from the British Heart Foundation, Resuscitation Council UK and University of Warwick. The project is designed to measure the epidemiology and outcomes of cardiac arrest and to serve as a national resource for continuous quality improvement initiatives for cardiac arrest.

The National Cardiac Arrest Audit (NCAA) is an ongoing, national, comparative outcome audit of in-hospital cardiac arrests. It is a joint initiative between Resuscitation Council UK and the Intensive Care National Audit & Research Centre (ICNARC) and is open to all acute hospitals in the UK and Ireland. The audit monitors and reports on the incidence of, and outcome from,

in-hospital cardiac arrest in order to inform practice and policy. It aims to identify and foster improvements in the prevention, care delivery and outcomes from cardiac arrest.

Data are collected according to standardised definitions and entered onto the NCAA secure web-based system. Once data are validated, hospitals are provided with activity reports and risk-adjusted comparative reports, allowing a comparison to be made not only within, but also between, hospitals locally, nationally and internationally.

Safety incident reporting

In England and Wales, hospitals can report patient safety incidents to the National Reporting and Learning System (NRLS) (https://improvement.nhs.uk/resources/learning-from-patient-safety-incidents/). A patient safety incident is defined as 'any unintended or unexpected incident that could have harmed or did lead to harm for one or more patients being cared for by the National Health Service (NHS)'. Resuscitation related incidents are associated with equipment problems, communication, delays in the resuscitation team attending, and failure to escalate treatment.

The ALS course

The Resuscitation Council UK ALS course provides a standardised approach to cardiopulmonary resuscitation in adults. It has been shown that the participation of one, or more, members of an in-hospital cardiac arrest team on an accredited advanced life support course is associated with improved patient outcomes.

The course is targeted at doctors, nurses, paramedics and other healthcare professionals who are expected to provide ALS in and out-of-hospital. The multidisciplinary nature of the course encourages efficient teamwork. By training together, all ALS providers are given the opportunity to gain experience as both resuscitation team members and team leaders. The ALS course teaches the knowledge and skills required to:

- recognise and treat the deteriorating patient using a structured ABCDE approach
- deliver standardised CPR in adults
- manage a cardiac arrest by working with a multidisciplinary team in an emergency situation
- use non-technical skills to facilitate strong team leadership and effective team membership.

Resuscitation Council UK offers the option for a two-day face-to-face ALS course, or the eALS course that consists of one day of e-learning that can be done in the participant's own time and one day of face-to-face teaching at an ALS course centre. A large multi-centre randomised-controlled trial showed that the learning outcomes were similar for these two courses, and equivalence between the two courses was confirmed with a subsequent descriptive analysis of over 27 000 participant outcomes.

The face-to-face component of both courses includes workshops, skill stations, cardiac arrest simulation (CAS) training, and lectures. Candidates' knowledge is assessed by means of a multiple-choice question paper. Practical skills in airway management and the initial approach to a collapsed patient (including defibrillation where appropriate) are assessed continuously. There is also assessment of a simulated cardiac arrest (CASTest). Candidates reaching the required standard receive a Resuscitation Council UK ALS Provider certificate.

Resuscitation knowledge and skills deteriorate with time and therefore recertification is required for those who have not recently undertaken the course to maintain ALS Provider status. Recertification provides the opportunity to refresh resuscitation skills and to be updated on resuscitation guidelines, and can be undertaken by attending a provider course or an accredited recertification course. All ALS providers have a responsibility to maintain their skills in resuscitation and to keep current with changes in guidelines and practice, and the requirement for recertification should be seen as an absolute minimum frequency of refreshing skills and knowledge.

Further reading

Lockey A, Lin Y, and Cheng A. Impact of adult advanced cardiac life support participation on patient outcomes – a systematic review and meta-analysis. Resuscitation 2018;129:48-54.

Perkins GD, Graesner JT, Semeraro F, Olasveengen T, Soar J, Lott C, Van de Voorde P, Madar J, Zideman D, Mentzelopoulos S, Bossaert L, Greif R, Monsieurs K, Svasvasdottir H and Nolan JP. European Resuscitation Council Guidelines 2021– Executive summary. Resuscitation. 2021;161.

National Confidential Enquiry into Patient Outcome and Death (NCEPOD): Inpatient Management of Out of Hospital Cardiac Arrests: https://www.ncepod.orq.uk/

Nolan J, Soar J, Eikeland H. The chain of survival. Resuscitation 2006;71:270-1.

Office for National Statistics: Leading causes for death, UK 2001-2018: https://www.ons.gov.uk/releases/leadingcausesofdeathuk

Olasveengen TM, Semeraro F, Ristagno G, Castren M, Handley A, Kuzovlev A, Monsieurs KG, Raffay V, Smyth M, Soar J, Svavarsdottir H and Perkins GD. European Resuscitation Council Guidelines 2021: Basic Life Support. Resuscitation. 2021;161.

Perkins GD, Kimani PK, Bullock I, et al. Improving the efficiency of advanced life support training: a randomized, controlled trial. Ann Intern Med. 2012;157(1):19-28.

Resuscitation Council UK. Quality standards for cardiopulmonary resuscitation and training: https://www.resus.org.uk/quality-standards/

Soar J, Berg KM, Andersen LW, Böttiger BW, Cacciola S, Callaway CW, et al; Adult Advanced Life Support Collaborators. Adult Advanced Life Support: 2020 International Consensus on Cardiopulmonary Resuscitation and Emergency Cardiovascular Care Science with Treatment Recommendations. Resuscitation. 2020;156:A80-A119.

Soar J, Böttiger BW, Carli P, Couper K, Deakin CD, Djärv T, Lott C, Olasveengen TM, Paal P, Pellis T, Perkins GD, Sandroni C, Nolan JP. European Resuscitation Council Guidelines 2021: Advanced Life Support. Resuscitation. 2021;161.

The UK Out-of-Hospital Cardiac Arrest Outcomes (OHCAO) Project: https://warwick.ac.uk/fac/sci/med/research/ctu/trials/ohcao/

The UK National Cardiac Arrest Audit: https://ncaa.icnarc.org/Home

Thorne CJ, Lockey A, Bullock I, Hampshire S, Begum-Ali S, and Perkins GD. E-learning in advanced life support – an evaluation by the Resuscitation Council (UK). Resuscitation 2015;90:79-84.

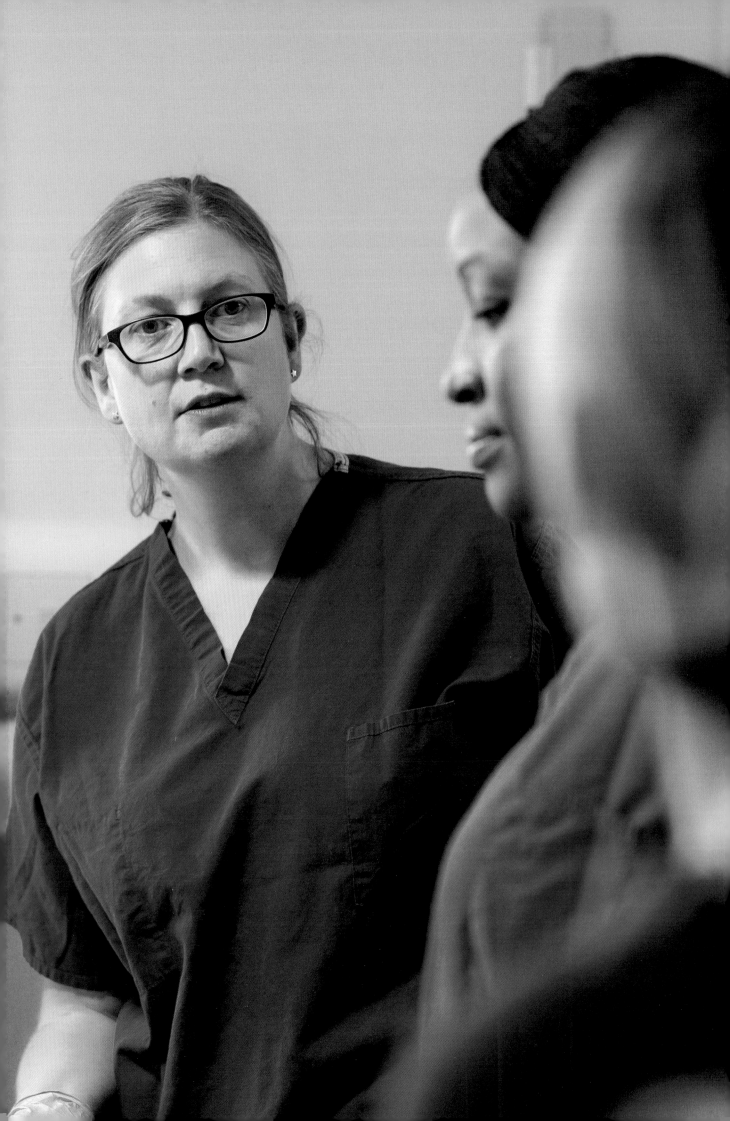

In this chapter

Non-technical skills

Situational awareness

Decision-making

Team working, including team leadership

Task management

The importance of communication

Resuscitation teams

The learning outcomes will enable you to:

Be an effective team leader and team member

Consider the role of non-technical skills during resuscitation

Effectively use structured communication tools such as SBARD and RSVP

Introduction

The skills of chest compressions, defibrillation, and rhythm recognition are important aspects of cardiac arrest management. These are all technical skills that are learnt from books, lectures, courses and peers. Although they are important for the successful resuscitation of a patient, there is another group of important skills called non-technical skills.

Non-technical skills can be defined as the cognitive, social and personal resource skills that complement technical skills and contribute to safe and efficient task performance. More simply, they are the things that affect our personal performance. Non-technical skills of leadership and teamwork have been identified as important contributory factors to technical skill performance in both simulated settings and poor clinical outcomes in acute medical settings.

The importance of non-technical skills in emergencies is now widely accepted across many acute clinical specialties including surgery, anaesthesia, critical care and acute medicine. Examples of poor non-technical skills include unwillingness to help, poor communication, poor leadership, poor decision-making, and no clear roles, all of which can lead to system errors. Episodes of cardiac arrest with documented system errors are associated with poor clinical outcomes such as decreased rates of return of spontaneous circulation (ROSC) and worse survival. In the context of advanced life support, which is fundamentally a team effort, the contribution of teamwork and leadership is therefore expected to make a significant contribution to patient outcome.

Previous research has shown that leadership behaviour is correlated with quality of CPR, with shorter hands-off time, pre-shock pauses and time to first shock. Understanding and improving non-technical skills may help to reduce human errors, creating more effective teams and improving patient safety. An effective team leader can help focus the team members, improve team commitment and act as a role model for the others.

The key non-technical skills are:

- situational awareness
- decision-making
- team working and leadership
- task management.

Non-technical skills can be defined as the cognitive, social and personal resource skills that contribute to safe and efficient task performance

Examples of poor non-technical skills include: unwillingness to help, poor communication, poor leadership, poor decision-making, and no clear roles

Situational awareness

This is an individual's awareness of the environment at the moment of an event and their analysis of this to understand how an individual's actions may impact on future events. This becomes particularly important when many events are happening simultaneously, for example, at a cardiac arrest. High information input with poor situational awareness may lead to poor decision-making and serious consequences. At a cardiac arrest, those participating will have varying degrees of situational awareness. In a well-functioning team, all members will have a common understanding of current events, or shared situational awareness. It is important that only the relevant information is shared, otherwise there is too much distraction or noise.

Situational awareness in cardiac arrest will include perception of environment and events taking place, comprehension of their meaning, and future projection:

Information gathering
What are the potential causes of cardiac arrest?
- location of arrest
- information from staff about events leading up to the arrest
- note the actions already initiated
- confirm who is present – names, skills, roles and who is leading.

Interpretation
What immediate steps are needed?
- confirm diagnosis
- checking that a monitor has been attached and interpreting what it shows
- determine immediate needs and necessary actions.

Future planning
What are the next steps?
- consider the impact of interventions
- plan for next steps.

Decision-making

This is defined as the cognitive process of choosing a specific course of action from several alternatives. At a cardiac arrest, the many decisions to be made usually fall to the team leader. The leader will assimilate information from the team members and from personal observation and will use this to determine appropriate interventions.

Typical decisions made at a cardiac arrest include:
- choice of shock energy to be used for defibrillation
- likely reversible causes of the cardiac arrest
- appropriate treatment such as drugs or airway management
- how long to continue resuscitation
- appropriate post-resuscitation care.

Once a decision has been made, clear unambiguous communication with the team members is essential to ensure that it is implemented.

Team working, including team leadership

This is one of the most important non-technical skills that contributes to successful management of critical situations. A team is a group of individuals working together with a common goal or purpose. In a team, the members usually have complementary skills and, through coordination of effort, work synergistically. Teams work best when everyone knows each other's name, when they are doing something they perceive to be important, and when their role is within their experience and competence. Optimal team function mandates a team leader.

There are several characteristics of a good resuscitation team member:

Competence – has the skills required at a cardiac arrest and performs them to the best of their ability.

Commitment – strives to achieve the best outcome for the patient.

Communicates openly – is able to articulate their findings and actions taken, raise concerns about clinical or safety issues, and listen to briefings and instructions.

Supportive – enables others to achieve their best.

Accountable – for their own and the team's actions.

Prepared to admit when help is needed.

Creative – suggests different ways of interpreting the situation.

Participates in providing feedback.

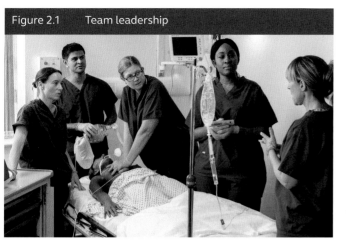

Figure 2.1   Team leadership

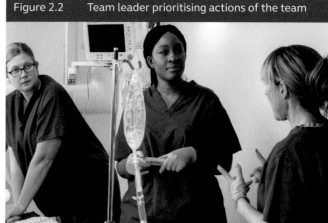

Figure 2.2   Team leader prioritising actions of the team

Team leadership

A team leader provides guidance, direction and instruction to the team members to enable successful completion of their stated objective (Figure 2.1). They lead by example and integrity. Team leaders need experience, not simply seniority. Team leadership can be considered a process; it is available to everyone with training and is not restricted to those with leadership traits. There are several attributes recognisable in a good team leader:

- knows everyone in the team by name and knows their capability
- accepts the leadership role
- is able to delegate tasks appropriately
- is knowledgeable and has sufficient credibility to influence the team through role modelling and professionalism
- recognises their own limitations and ask for support from the team
- is a good communicator – not just good at giving instructions, but is also a good listener and decisive in action
- stays calm, keeps everyone focused and controls distractions
- is empathetic towards the whole team
- is assertive and authoritative when required
- shows tolerance towards hesitancy or nervousness in the emergency setting
- has good situational awareness; able to constantly monitor the situation, with an up-to-date overview, listening and deciding on a course of action.

During a cardiac arrest, the role of team leader is not always immediately obvious. The leader should state early on that they are assuming the role of team leader. Specifically, at a cardiac arrest the leader should:

- follow current resuscitation guidelines or explain a reason for any significant deviation from standard protocols
- consult with the team or call for senior advice and assistance if unsure about an intervention
- play to the strengths of team members and allow them some autonomy if their skills are adequate

- allocate roles and tasks throughout the resuscitation and be specific – this limits the risks of nobody, or alternatively too many people, attempting the task
- use the two minute periods of chest compressions to plan tasks and safety aspects of the resuscitation attempt with the team
- thank the team at the end of the resuscitation attempt and ensure that staff and relatives are being supported (Chapter 17)
- complete all documentation and ensure an adequate handover.

Task management

During the resuscitation of a patient, either in full cardiac arrest or peri-arrest, there are numerous tasks to be carried out by the team members, either sequentially or simultaneously. Cognitive aids such as checklists or easy-access guidelines could be used as support but will need a dedicated team member to read and check. The coordination and control, or management, of these tasks is the responsibility of the team leader (Figure 2.2).

Tasks can include:

- planning and, where appropriate, briefing of the team (e.g. prior to arrival of the patient in the emergency department)
- identifying the resources required – ensuring that equipment is checked and specifics organised and delegated
- being inclusive of all team members
- being prepared for both the expected and the unexpected
- prioritising actions of the team
- watching out for fatigue, stress and distress amongst the team
- managing conflict
- communicating with relatives
- communicating with experts for safe handover both by telephone and in person
- debriefing the team
- reporting untoward incidents, particularly equipment or system failures
- participation in audit (Chapter 1).

To illustrate the importance of non-technical skills, a modified team performance tool, the Team Emergency Assessment Measure (TEAM) tool, is used during scenario teaching on the ALS Course. This tool is used as a teaching instrument and discussion point for both instructors and candidates throughout the face-to-face teaching and during teaching scenarios. (Table 2.1).

The importance of communication when managing a sick patient

Communication problems are a factor in up to 80% of adverse incidents or near-miss reports in hospitals. Failure of communication is also evident when a medical emergency occurs on a ward and a doctor or nurse summons senior help. The call for help is often suboptimal, with failure by the caller to communicate the seriousness of the situation and to convey information in a way that informs the recipient of the urgency of the situation. The poor-quality information heightens the anxiety of the person responding to the call, who is then uncertain of the nature of the problem they are about to face. A well-structured process that is simple, reliable and dependable, will enable the caller to convey the important facts and urgency, and will help the recipient to plan ahead. It was for similar reasons that the ABCDE approach was developed as an aide memoire of the key technical skills required to manage a cardiac arrest.

The use of the SBARD (Situation, Background, Assessment, Recommendation, Decisions) or RSVP (Reason, Story, Vital signs, Plan) tool enables effective, timely communication between individuals from different clinical backgrounds and hierarchies (Table 2.2).

Table 2.1 TEAM tool (Team Emergency Assessment Measure) Adapted and modified from Cooper et al.

Leadership		Not seen ✔	Observed ✔
1	The team leader let the team know what was expected of them through direction and command. Examples: Uses members' names, allocates tasks, makes clear decisions.		
2	The team leader maintained a global perspective. Examples: Monitors clinical procedures, checks safety, plans ahead, remains 'hands off'.		
Teamwork		Not seen ✔	Observed ✔
3	The team communicated effectively, using both verbal and non-verbal communication. Examples: relay findings, raise concerns, use names, appropriate body language.		
4	The team worked together to complete tasks in a timely manner. Examples: coordination of defibrillation, maintain chest compressions, assist each other.		
5	The team acted with composure and control. Examples: performed allocated roles, accept criticism.		
6	The team adapted to changing situations. Examples: Adapt to rhythm changes, patient deterioration, change of roles.		
7	The team monitored and reassessed the situation Examples: rhythm changes, ROSC, when to terminate resuscitation.		
8	The team anticipated potential actions. Examples: defibrillation, airway management, drug delivery.		
Task management		Not seen ✔	Observed ✔
9	The team prioritised tasks. Examples: continuous chest compressions, defibrillation, airway management, drug delivery.		
10	The team followed approved standards/guidelines.		
Comments			
Examples: What area was good? What area needs improvement?			

Table 2.2 SBARD (Situation, Background, Assessment, Recommendation, Decisions) **and RSVP** (Reason, Story, Vital signs, Plan)

SBARD	RSVP	Content	Example
Situation	**Reason**	Introduce yourself and check you are speaking to the correct person. Identify the patient you are calling about (who and where). Say what you think the current problem is, or appears to be. State what you need advice about. Useful phrases: • The problem appears to be cardiac/respiratory/neurological/sepsis. • I'm not sure what the problem is but the patient is deteriorating. • The patient is unstable, getting worse and I need help.	*Hi, I'm Dr Smith the medical F2.* *I am calling about Mr Brown on acute medical admissions who I think has a severe pneumonia and is septic.* *He has an oxygen saturation of 90% despite high-flow oxygen and I am very worried about him.*
Background	**Story**	Background information about the patient. Reason for admission. Relevant past medical history.	*He is 55 and previously fit and well.* *He has had fever and a cough for 2 days.* *He arrived 15 minutes ago by ambulance.*
Assessment	**Vital signs**	Include specific observations and vital sign values based on ABCDE approach. • Airway • Breathing • Circulation • Disability • Exposure • The NEWS2 score is…	*He looks very unwell and is tiring.* *Airway – he can say a few words.* *Breathing – his respiratory rate is 24, he has bronchial breathing on the left side. His oxygen saturation is 90% on high-flow oxygen. I am getting a blood gas and chest X-ray.* *Circulation – his pulse is 110, his blood pressure is 110/60.* *Disability – he is drowsy but can say a few words.* *Exposure – he has no rashes.*
Recommendation	**Plan**	State explicitly what you want the person you are calling to do. What by when? Useful phrases: • I am going to start the following treatment; is there anything else you can suggest? • I am going to do the following investigations; is there anything else you can suggest? • If they do not improve; when would you like to be called? • I don't think I can do anymore; I would like you to see the patient urgently.	*I am getting antibiotics ready and he is on IV fluids.* *I need help – please can you come and see him straight away.*
Decisions		Summarise what has been agreed. Confirm what has been discussed.	*We have agreed that you will come and review the patient straight away.* *In the meantime I will repeat the BP reading.*

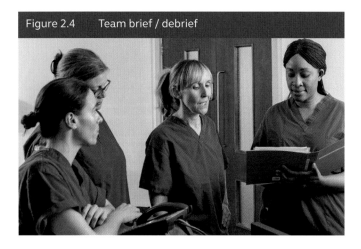

Figure 2.4   Team brief / debrief

Resuscitation teams

The resuscitation team may take the form of a traditional cardiac arrest team, which is called only when cardiac arrest is recognised. Alternatively, hospitals may have strategies to recognise patients at risk of cardiac arrest and to summon a team (e.g. medical emergency team) before cardiac arrest occurs (Chapter 3). The term resuscitation team reflects the range of response teams. As the team members may change daily or more frequently, as shift pattern working is introduced, members may not know each other or the skill mix of the team members. The team should therefore meet at the beginning of their period on duty to:

- Introduce themselves; communication is much easier and more effective if people can be referred to by their name.
- Identify everyone's skills and experience.
- Allocate the team leader. Skill and experience take precedence over seniority.
- Allocate responsibilities; if key skills are lacking (e.g. advanced airway management), work out how this deficit can be managed (Figure 2.4).
- Review any patients who have been identified as 'at risk' during the previous duty period.

Finally, every effort should be made to enable the team members to meet to debrief (e.g. difficulties or concerns about their performance, problems or concerns with equipment and submit incident reports). It may also be possible to carry out a formal handover to the incoming team.

02: Summary learning

Non-technical skills are important during resuscitation.

Use SBARD or RSVP for effective communication.

My key take-home messages from this chapter are:

Further reading

Andersen PO, Jensen MK, Lippert A, et al: Identifying non-technical skills and barriers for improvement of teamwork in cardiac arrest teams. Resuscitation 2010; 81:695–702.

Cooper S, Cant R, Porter J, et al: Rating medical emergency teamwork performance: Development of the Team Emergency Assessment Measure (TEAM). Resuscitation 2010; 81:446–452.

Featherstone P, Chalmers T, Smith GB. RSVP: a system for communication of deterioration in hospital patients. Br J Nurs 2008;17:860-64.

Flin R, O'Connor P, Crichton M. Safety at the Sharp End: a Guide to Non- Technical Skills. Aldershot: Ashgate, 2008.

Peltonen V, Peltonen LM, Salantera S et al. An observational study of technical and non-technical skills in advanced life support in the clinical setting. Resuscitation 2020; 53:162-168.

Yeung J, Ong G, Davies R, Gao F, Perkins GDP. Factors affecting team leadership skills and their relationship with quality of cardiopulmonary resuscitation. Crit Care Med 2012; 40:2617–2621.

Acknowledgment

TEAM tool adapted and modified from Cooper et al (2010) to be used in ALS training courses. See http://medicalemergencyteam.com/ for full details.

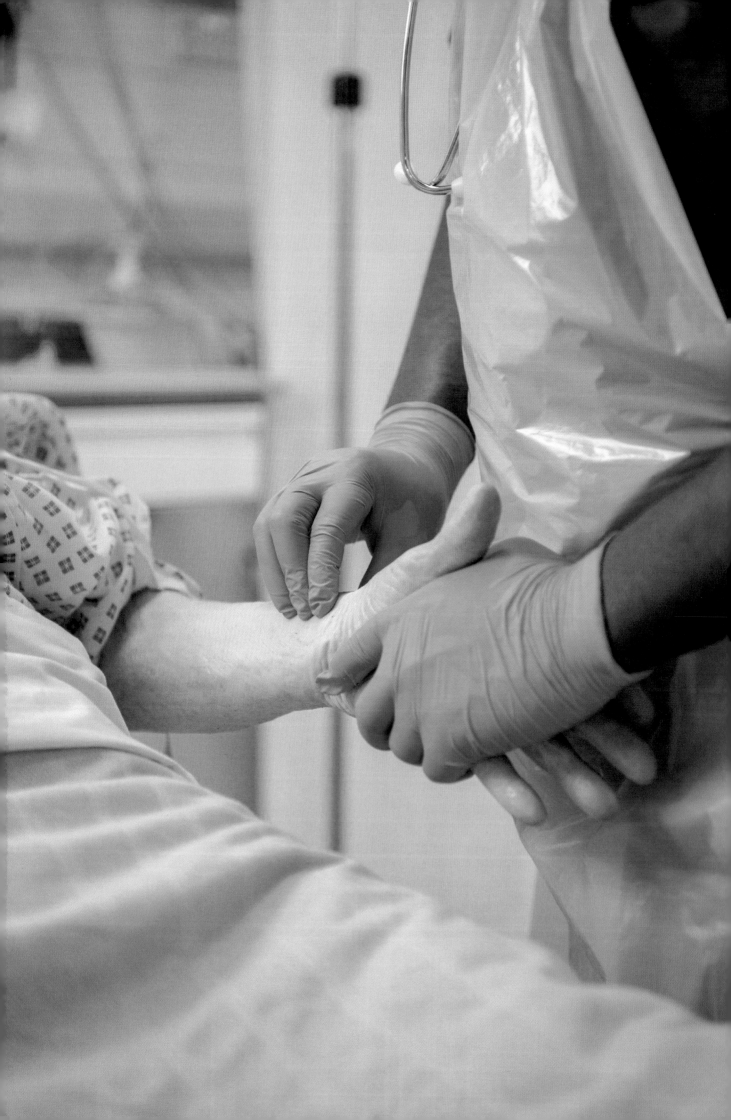

Recognising deterioration and preventing cardiorespiratory arrest

In this chapter

Prevention of in-hospital cardiac arrest: the Chain of Prevention

Recognising the deteriorating patient

Response to critical illness

Causes of deterioration and cardiac arrest

The ABCDE approach

The learning outcomes will enable you to:

Understand the importance of early recognition of the deteriorating patient

Consider the relevant causes of cardiac arrest in adults

Identify and treat patients at risk of cardiac arrest using the Airway, Breathing, Circulation, Disability, Exposure (ABCDE) approach

Introduction

Early recognition of the deteriorating patient and prevention of cardiac arrest is the first link in the Chain of Survival. About 24% of patients who have an in-hospital cardiac arrest will survive to go home. Prevention of in-hospital cardiac arrest requires staff education, monitoring of patients, recognition of patient deterioration, a system to call for help, and an effective response.

Survival after in-hospital cardiac arrest is more likely if the arrest is witnessed and monitored, the rhythm is ventricular fibrillation/pulseless ventricular tachycardia (VF/pVT), the primary cause is myocardial ischaemia, and the patient is successfully defibrillated immediately. Most cardiac arrests in hospital are not sudden or unpredictable events: in approximately 80% of cases there is deterioration in clinical signs during the few hours before cardiac arrest.

These patients often have slow and progressive physiological deterioration, particularly hypoxia and hypotension (i.e. Airway, Breathing, Circulation problems) that is unnoticed by staff, or is recognised but sub-optimally treated. The cardiac arrest rhythm in this group is usually non-shockable (pulseless electrical activity (PEA) or asystole) and the survival rate to hospital discharge is around 14%.

Early recognition and effective treatment of the deteriorating patient might prevent cardiac arrest, death or an unanticipated intensive care unit (ICU) admission. Hospitals with the lowest incidence of in-hospital cardiac arrest have the highest cardiac arrest survival, perhaps suggesting better selection of patients suitable for cardiopulmonary resuscitation (CPR) or better prevention of cardiac arrest. Closer attention to patients who have a false cardiac arrest (i.e. a cardiac arrest team call when the patient has not had a cardiac arrest) may also improve outcome, because up to one-third of these patients die during their in-hospital stay. Early recognition will also help to identify individuals for whom CPR is not appropriate or who do not wish to have resusciation attempted.

> About 24% of patients who have an in-hospital cardiac arrest will survive to go home

> In approximately 80% of cases there is deterioration in clinical signs during the few hours before cardiac arrest

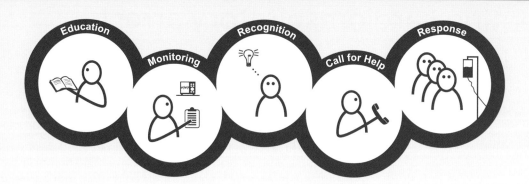

Prevention of in-hospital cardiac arrest: the Chain of Prevention

The Chain of Prevention can assist hospitals in structuring care processes to prevent and detect patient deterioration and cardiac arrest. The five rings of the chain represent: staff education; the monitoring of patients; the recognition of patient deterioration; a system to call for help; and an effective response (Figure 3.1).

Education

Education should include how to observe patients, and the interpretation of observed signs of deterioration, using the ABCDE approach. Healthcare practitioners should be confident to stabilise the patient using their skills, pending the arrival of more experienced help. Underpinning this is their knowledge of the rationale for a rapid response system used in healthcare settings.

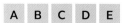

Monitoring

Monitoring and patient assessment requires the measurement and recording of vital signs and accurate documentation.

Recognition

Recognition encompasses the tools available to identify patients in need of additional monitoring or intervention, including suitably designed vital signs charts and sets of predetermined 'calling criteria' to 'flag' the need to escalate monitoring or to call for more expert help.

Call for help

Call for help protocols for summoning a response to a deteriorating patient should be universally known and understood, unambiguous and mandated. Healthcare professionals may find it difficult to ask for help or escalate treatment as they feel their clinical judgement may be criticised. Hospitals should ensure all staff are empowered to call for help. A structured communication tool such as SBARD (Situation, Background, Assessment, Recommendation, Decision) or RSVP (Reason, Story, Vital signs, Plan) should be used to call for help.

Response

Response to a deteriorating patient must be assured, of specified speed and by staff with appropriate acute or critical care skills, and experience.

Table 3.1   National Early Warning Score (NEWS2)

Physiological parameter		Score						
		3	2	1	0	1	2	3
A & B	Respiration rate (per minute)	≤ 8		9–11	12–20		21–24	≥ 25
	SpO₂ Scale 1 (%)	≤ 91	92–93	94–95	≥ 96			
	SpO₂ Scale 2 (%)*	≤ 83	84–85	86–87	88–92 ≥ 93 on air	93–94 on oxygen	95–96 on oxygen	≥ 97 on oxygen
	Air or oxygen?		Oxygen		Air			
C	Systolic blood pressure (mmHg)	≤ 90	91–100	101–110	111–219			≥ 220
	Pulse (per minute)	≤ 40		41–50	51–90	91–110	111–130	≥ 131
D	Consciousness**				Alert			Confusion VPU
E	Temperature (°C)	≤ 35.0		35.1–36.0	36.1–38.0	38.1–39.0	≥ 39.1	

* Use Scale 2 if target range is 88–92% (e.g. in hypercapnic respiratory failure).
** Score for new onset confusion, no score if chronic confusion.

Recognising the deteriorating patient

In general, the clinical signs of critical illness are similar whatever the underlying process because they reflect failing respiratory, cardiovascular, and neurological systems (i.e. ABCDE problems) (see below). Abnormal physiology is common on general wards, yet the measurement and recording of important physiological observations of acutely ill patients occurs less frequently than is desirable, especially at night. The assessment of very simple vital signs, such as respiratory rate, may help to predict cardiac arrest. To help early detection of critical illness, many hospitals use early warning scores (EWS) or calling criteria.

Early warning scoring systems allocate points to measurements of routine vital signs on the basis of their derangement from an arbitrarily agreed 'normal' range. The weighted score of one or more vital sign observations, or the total EWS, indicates the level of intervention required (e.g. increased frequency of vital signs monitoring, or the need to call ward doctors or resuscitation teams to the patient). In the UK, the National Early Warning Score 2 (NEWS2) is recommended (Table 3.1).

Early warning scores are dynamic and change over time and the frequency of observations should be increased to track improvement or deterioration in a patient's condition. If it is clear a patient is deteriorating, call for help early rather than waiting for the patient to reach a specific score.

An increased NEWS2 score indicates an increased risk of deterioration and death. There should be a graded response to scores according to local hospital protocols (Table 3.2).

Alternatively, systems incorporating calling criteria are based on routine observations, which activate a response when one or more variables reach an extremely abnormal value. Recent research suggests that EWS may be better discriminators of outcomes than calling criteria. Some hospitals combine elements of both systems.

Nurse concern may also be an important predictor of patient deterioration. Even when doctors are alerted to a patient's abnormal physiology, there is often a delay in attending to the patient or referring to higher levels of care.

Table 3.2   Escalation protocol based on early warning score

NEW score	Frequency of monitoring	Clinical response
0	Minimum 12 hourly	Continue routine NEWS monitoring.
Total 1–4	Minimum 4-6 hourly	Inform registered nurse, who must assess the patient. Registered nurse decides whether increased frequency of monitoring and/or escalation of care is required.
3 in single parameter	Minimum 1 hourly	Registered nurse to inform medical team caring for the patient, who will review and decide whether escalation of care is necessary.
Total 5 or 6: Urgent response threshold	Minimum 1 hourly	Registered nurse to immediately inform the medical team caring for the patient. Registered nurse to request urgent assessment by a clinician or team with core competencies in the care of acutely ill patients. Provide clinical care in an environment with monitoring facilities.
Total 7 or more: Emergency response threshold	Continuous monitoring of vital signs	Registered nurse to immediately inform the medical team caring for the patient – this should be at least at specialist registrar level. Emergency assessment by a team with critical care competencies, including practitioner(s) with advanced airway management skills. Consider transfer of care to a level 2 or 3 clinical care facility i.e. higher-dependency unit or ICU. Clinical care in an environment with monitoring facilities.

Response to critical illness

The traditional response to cardiac arrest is reactive: the name 'cardiac arrest team' implies that it will be called only after cardiac arrest has occurred. In many hospitals the role of the cardiac arrest team is incorporated into that of other rapid response systems (e.g. rapid response team, critical care outreach team, medical emergency team (MET)). These teams are usually activated according to the patient's EWS (see above) or according to specific calling criteria. For example, the MET usually comprises medical and nursing staff from intensive care and acute medicine and responds to specific calling criteria (Table 3.3). Any member of the healthcare team, and in some cases the patient or their relatives, can initiate a MET call. Early involvement of the MET may reduce cardiac arrests, deaths and unanticipated ICU admissions, and may facilitate decisions about limitation of treatment (e.g. do not attempt cardiopulmonary resuscitation (DNACPR) decisions).

Rapid response systems are recommended by the Institute for Healthcare Improvement and other national patient safety initiatives around the world. Hospitals should consider the introduction of a rapid response system to reduce the incidence of in-hospital cardiac arrest (IHCA) and in-hospital mortality.

In the UK, a system of pre-emptive ward care known as critical care outreach has developed. Outreach services exist in many forms ranging from a single nurse to a 24-hour, seven days per week multi-professional team. An outreach team or system may reduce ward deaths, postoperative adverse events, ICU admissions and readmissions, and increase survival. Rapid response teams, such as outreach teams or METs, play a role in educating and improving acute care skills of ward personnel.

All critically ill patients should be admitted to a clinical area that can provide an appropriate level of organ support and nursing care. This is usually in a critical care area (e.g. ICU, high dependency unit (HDU), or resuscitation room). These areas should be staffed by doctors and nurses experienced in advanced resuscitation and critical care skills.

Hospital staffing tends to be at its lowest during the night and at weekends. This influences patient monitoring, treatment and outcomes. Admission to general wards in the evening, or to hospital at weekends is associated with increased mortality. Studies have shown that in-hospital cardiac arrests occurring in the late afternoon, at night or at weekends are more often non-witnessed and have a lower survival rate. Patients discharged at night from ICUs to general wards have an increased risk of ICU readmission and in-hospital death compared with those discharged during the day and those discharged to HDUs.

Table 3.3 Medical emergency team (MET) calling criteria

CALL MEDICAL EMERGENCY TEAM IF		
Acute change in:		Physiology:
A	Airway	Threatened
B	Breathing	All respiratory arrests
		Respiratory rate < 5 min^{-1}
		Respiratory rate > 36 min^{-1}
C	Circulation	All cardiac arrests
		Pulse rate < 40 min^{-1}
		Pulse rate > 140 min^{-1}
		Systolic blood pressure < 90 mmHg
D	Disability – neurology	Sudden decrease in level of consciousness
		Decrease in GCS of > 2 points
		Repeated or prolonged seizures
E	Exposure – other	Any patient causing concern who does not fit the above criteria

Causes of deterioration and cardiac arrest

Deterioration and cardiac arrest can be caused by primary airway and/or breathing and/or cardiovascular problems.

A = Airway obstruction

For a detailed review of airway management see Chapter 7.

Causes

Airway obstruction can be complete or partial. Complete airway obstruction rapidly leads to cardiac arrest. Partial obstruction often precedes complete obstruction. Partial airway obstruction can cause cerebral or pulmonary oedema, exhaustion, secondary apnoea, hypoxic brain injury and, eventually cardiac arrest.

Central nervous system depression may cause loss of airway patency and protective reflexes. Causes include head injury and intracerebral disease, hypercapnia, the depressant effect of metabolic disorders (e.g. diabetes mellitus), and drugs, including alcohol, opioids and general anaesthetics. Laryngospasm can occur with upper airway stimulation in a semi-conscious patient whose airway reflexes remain intact.

Causes of airway obstruction

- central nervous system depression
- blood
- vomitus
- foreign body (e.g. tooth, food)
- direct trauma to face or throat
- epiglottitis
- pharyngeal swelling (e.g. infection, oedema)
- laryngospasm
- bronchospasm – causes narrowing of the small airways in the lung
- bronchial secretions
- blocked tracheostomy.

In some people, the upper airway can become obstructed when asleep (obstructive sleep apnoea). This is more common in obese patients and obstruction can be worsened in the presence of other factors (e.g. sedative drugs).

Recognition

Assess the patency of the airway in anyone at risk of obstruction. A conscious patient will complain of difficulty in breathing, may be choking, and will be distressed. With partial airway obstruction, efforts at breathing will be noisy. Complete airway obstruction is silent and there is no air movement at the patient's mouth. Any respiratory movements are usually strenuous. The accessory muscles of respiration will be involved, causing a 'see-saw' or 'rocking-horse' pattern of chest and abdominal movement: the chest is drawn in and the abdomen expands on inspiration, and the opposite occurs on expiration.

Treatment

The priority is to ensure that the airway remains patent. Treat any problem that places the airway at risk; for example, suck blood and gastric contents from the airway and, unless contraindicated, turn the patient on their side. Give oxygen as soon as possible to achieve an arterial blood oxygen saturation by pulse oximetry (SpO_2) in the range of 94–98%. Assume actual or impending airway obstruction in anyone with a depressed level of consciousness, regardless of cause. Take steps to safeguard the airway and prevent further complications such as aspiration of gastric contents. This may involve nursing the patient on their side or with a head-up tilt. Simple airway opening manoeuvres (head tilt/chin lift or jaw thrust), insertion of an oropharyngeal or nasopharyngeal airway, elective tracheal intubation or tracheostomy may be required. Consider insertion of a nasogastric tube to empty the stomach.

B = Breathing problems

Causes

Breathing inadequacy may be acute or chronic. It may be continuous or intermittent, and severe enough to cause apnoea (respiratory arrest), which will rapidly cause cardiac arrest. Respiratory arrest often occurs because of a combination of factors; for example, in a patient with chronic respiratory inadequacy, a chest infection, muscle weakness or fractured ribs can lead to exhaustion, further depressing respiratory function. If breathing is insufficient to oxygenate the blood adequately (hypoxaemia), a cardiac arrest will occur eventually.

Respiratory drive

Central nervous system depression may decrease or abolish respiratory drive. The causes are the same as those for airway obstruction from central nervous system depression.

Respiratory effort

The main respiratory muscles are the diaphragm and intercostal muscles. The latter are innervated at the level of their respective ribs and may be paralysed by a spinal cord lesion above this level. The innervation of the diaphragm is at the level of the third, fourth and fifth segment of the cervical cord. Spontaneous breathing cannot occur with severe cervical cord damage above this level.

Inadequate respiratory effort, caused by muscle weakness or nerve damage, occurs with many diseases (e.g. myasthenia gravis, Guillain-Barré syndrome, and multiple sclerosis). Chronic malnourishment and severe long-term illness may also contribute to generalised weakness.

Breathing can also be impaired with restrictive chest wall abnormalities such as kyphoscoliosis. Pain from fractured ribs or sternum will prevent deep breaths and coughing.

Lung disorders

Lung function is impaired by a pneumothorax or haemothorax. A tension pneumothorax causes a rapid failure of gas exchange, a reduction of venous return to the heart, and a fall in cardiac output. Severe lung disease will impair gas exchange. Causes include infection, aspiration, exacerbation of chronic obstructive pulmonary disease (COPD), asthma, pulmonary embolus, lung contusion, acute respiratory distress syndrome (ARDS) and pulmonary oedema.

Recognition

A conscious patient will complain of shortness of breath and be distressed. The history and examination will usually indicate the underlying cause. Hypoxaemia and hypercapnia can cause irritability, confusion, lethargy and a decrease in the level of consciousness. Cyanosis may be visible but is a late sign.

A fast respiratory rate (> 25 min^{-1}) is a useful, simple indicator of breathing problems.

Pulse oximetry is an easy, non-invasive measure of the adequacy of oxygenation (Chapter 15). However, it is not a reliable indicator of ventilation and an arterial blood gas sample is necessary to obtain values for arterial carbon dioxide tension ($PaCO_2$) and pH.

A rising $PaCO_2$ and a decrease in pH are often late signs in a patient with severe respiratory problems.

Treatment

Give oxygen to all acutely ill hypoxaemic patients and treat the underlying cause. Give oxygen initially at 15 L min^{-1} using a high-concentration reservoir mask.

In most emergency situations, oxygen is given to patients immediately without a formal prescription or drug order. The lack of a prescription should never preclude oxygen being given when needed in an emergency situation. However, a subsequent written record must be made of what oxygen therapy has been given to every patient in a similar manner to the recording of all other emergency treatment.

Once SpO_2 can be reliably recorded, aim for a SpO_2 in the range of 94–98%, or 88-92% in hypercapnic respiratory failure.

For example, suspect a tension pneumothorax from a history of chest trauma and confirm by clinical signs and symptoms. Early needle decompression (thoracocentesis), or thoracostomy, followed by chest drain insertion is needed (Chapter 12).

Patients who are having difficulty breathing or are becoming tired will need respiratory support. Non-invasive ventilation using a face mask or a hood can be useful and may prevent the need for tracheal intubation and ventilation.

For patients who cannot breathe adequately, sedation, tracheal intubation and controlled ventilation is needed.

C = Circulation problems

Causes

For a detailed review of cardiac causes of cardiac arrest see Chapter 4.

Circulation problems may be caused by primary heart disease or by heart abnormalities secondary to other problems. Most often, circulation problems in acutely ill patients are due to hypovolaemia. The heart may stop suddenly or may produce an inadequate cardiac output for a period of time before stopping.

Primary heart problems

The commonest cause of sudden cardiac death (SCD) is an arrhythmia caused by either ischaemia or myocardial infarction. Cardiac arrest can also be caused by an arrhythmia due to other forms of heart disease, by heart block, electrocution and some drugs.

Sudden cardiac arrest may also occur with for example cardiac failure, cardiac tamponade, cardiac rupture, myocarditis and hypertrophic cardiomyopathy.

Causes of ventricular fibrillation

- acute coronary syndromes (Chapter 4)
- hypertensive heart disease
- valve disease
- drugs (e.g. antiarrhythmic drugs, tricyclic antidepressants, digoxin)
- inherited cardiac diseases (e.g. long QT syndromes)
- acidosis
- abnormal electrolyte concentration (e.g. potassium, magnesium, calcium)
- hypothermia
- electrocution.

Secondary heart problems

The heart is affected by changes elsewhere in the body. For example, cardiac arrest will occur rapidly following asphyxia from airway obstruction or apnoea, tension pneumothorax, or acute severe blood loss. Severe hypoxia and anaemia, hypothermia, oligaemia and severe septic shock will also impair cardiac function, and this may lead to cardiac arrest.

Recognition

The signs and symptoms of cardiac disease include chest pain, shortness of breath, syncope, tachycardia, bradycardia, tachypnoea, hypotension, poor peripheral perfusion (prolonged capillary refill time), altered mental state, and oliguria.

Although the risk of SCD is greater for patients with known severe cardiac disease, most SCDs occur in people with unrecognised disease. Asymptomatic or silent cardiac disease may include hypertensive heart disease, aortic valve disease, cardiomyopathy, myocarditis, and coronary disease.

Recognition of risk of sudden cardiac death out-of-hospital

Coronary artery disease is the commonest cause of SCD. Non-ischaemic cardiomyopathy and valvular disease account for some other SCD events. A small percentage of SCDs are caused by inherited abnormalities (e.g. long and short QT syndromes, Brugada syndrome, hypertrophic cardiomyopathy, arrhythmogenic right ventricular cardiomyopathy), and by congenital heart disease.

In patients with a known diagnosis of cardiac disease, syncope (with or without prodrome – particularly recent or recurrent) is as an independent risk factor for increased risk of death. Apparently healthy children and young adults who have SCD may also have had symptoms and signs (e.g. syncope/pre-syncope, chest pain, palpitation, heart murmur) that should alert healthcare professionals to seek expert help to prevent cardiac arrest.

Features that indicate a high probability of arrhythmic syncope include:

- syncope in the supine position
- syncope occurring during or after exercise (although syncope after exercise is often vasovagal)
- syncope with no or only brief prodromal symptoms
- repeated episodes of unexplained syncope
- syncope in individuals with a family history of sudden death or inherited cardiac condition.

Assessment in a clinic specialising in the care of those at risk for SCD is recommended in family members of young cases of SCD or those with a known cardiac disorder resulting in an increased risk of SCD.

Treatment

Treat the underlying cause of circulatory failure. In many sick patients, this means giving intravenous fluids to treat hypovolaemia. Assess patients with chest pain for an acute coronary syndrome (ACS). A comprehensive description of the management of ACS is given in Chapter 4. Most patients with cardiac ischaemic pain will be more comfortable sitting up. In some instances, lying flat may provoke or worsen the pain.

Survivors of an episode of VF are likely to have a further episode unless preventative treatment is given. These patients may need percutaneous coronary intervention, coronary artery bypass grafting, or an implantable defibrillator.

Treating the underlying cause should prevent many secondary cardiac arrests. Cardiovascular support includes correction of underlying electrolyte or acid-base disturbances, and treatment to achieve a desirable cardiac rate, rhythm and output. Advanced cardiovascular monitoring and echocardiography may be indicated. Appropriate manipulation of cardiac filling may require fluid therapy and vasoactive drugs. Inotropic drugs and vasoconstrictors may be indicated to support cardiac output and blood pressure.

The A B C D E approach

Underlying principles

The approach to all deteriorating or critically ill patients is the same. The underlying principles are:

1. Use the Airway, Breathing, Circulation, Disability, Exposure (ABCDE) approach to assess and treat the patient.

2. Do a complete initial assessment and re-assess regularly.

3. Treat life-threatening problems before moving to the next part of assessment.

4. Assess the effects of treatment.

5. Recognise when you will need extra help. Call for appropriate help early.

6. Use all members of the team. This enables interventions (e.g. assessment, attaching monitors, intravenous access), to be undertaken simultaneously.

7. Communicate effectively – use the SBARD or RSVP approach (Chapter 2).

8. The aim of the initial treatment is to keep the patient alive and achieve some clinical improvement. This will buy time for further treatment and making a diagnosis.

9. Remember – it can take a few minutes for treatments to work, so wait a short while before reassessing the patient after an intervention.

First steps

1. **Ensure personal safety.** Wear personable protective equipment as appropriate and check for and avoid any hazards to your safety.

2. **First look at the patient** in general to see if the patient appears unwell (Figure 3.1).

3. **If the patient is awake**, ask "How are you?". If the patient appears unconscious or has collapsed, shake them and ask "Are you alright?". If they respond normally then they are breathing and have a patent airway, and have brain perfusion. If they speak only in short sentences, they may have breathing problems. Failure of the patient to respond is a clear marker of critical illness.

4. **This first rapid 'Look, Listen and Feel'** of the patient should take about 30 s and will often indicate that a patient is critically ill and there is a need for urgent help. Ask a colleague to ensure appropriate help is coming.

5. **If the patient is unconscious, unresponsive and is not breathing normally** (occasional gasps are not normal) start CPR according to the guidance in Chapter 5. If you are confident and trained to do so, feel for a pulse to determine if the patient has a respiratory arrest. If there are any doubts about the presence of a pulse, start CPR.

6. **Monitor vital signs early.** Attach a pulse oximeter, ECG monitor and a non-invasive blood pressure monitor to all critically ill patients as soon as possible.

7. **Insert an intravenous cannula as soon as possible.** Take blood for investigation when inserting the intravenous cannula. Consider inserting an intraosseous needle if there is failure to gain intravenous access.

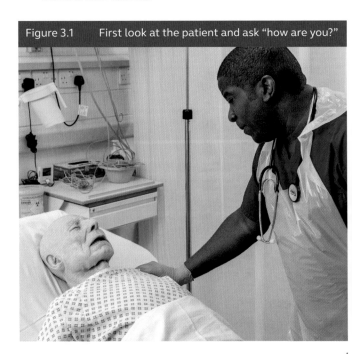

Figure 3.1   First look at the patient and ask "how are you?"

A = Airway

Airway obstruction is an emergency. Get expert help immediately. Untreated, airway obstruction causes hypoxia and risks damage to the brain, kidneys and heart, cardiac arrest, and death.

1. Look for the signs of airway obstruction.
Airway obstruction causes paradoxical chest and abdominal movements ('see-saw' respirations) and the use of the accessory muscles of respiration. Central cyanosis is a late sign of airway obstruction. In complete airway obstruction, there are no breath sounds at the mouth or nose. In partial obstruction, air entry is diminished and often noisy

In the critically ill patient, depressed consciousness often leads to airway obstruction.

2. Treat airway obstruction as a medical emergency.
Obtain expert help immediately. Untreated, airway obstruction causes hypoxaemia (low PaO_2) with the risk of hypoxic injury to the brain, kidneys and heart, cardiac arrest, and even death.

In most cases, only simple methods of airway clearance are required (e.g. airway opening manoeuvres, airway suction, insertion of an oropharyngeal or nasopharyngeal airway). Tracheal intubation may be required when these fail.

3. Give oxygen at high concentration.
Provide high-concentration oxygen using a non-rebreather mask with oxygen reservoir. Ensure that the oxygen flow is sufficient (usually 15 L min^{-1}) to prevent collapse of the reservoir during inspiration. In acute respiratory failure, aim to maintain an oxygen saturation of 94–98%. In patients at risk of hypercapnic respiratory failure (see below) aim for an oxygen saturation of 88–92%.

B = Breathing

During the immediate assessment of breathing, it is vital to diagnose and treat immediately life-threatening conditions (e.g. acute severe asthma, pulmonary oedema, tension pneumothorax, and massive haemothorax).

1. Look, listen and feel for the general signs of respiratory distress.
Sweating, central cyanosis, use of the accessory muscles of respiration, and abdominal breathing.

2. Count the respiratory rate.
The normal rate is 12–20 breaths min^{-1}. A high (> 25 min^{-1}) or increasing respiratory rate is a marker of illness and a warning that the patient may deteriorate suddenly.

3. Assess the depth of each breath, the pattern (rhythm) of respiration and whether chest expansion is equal on both sides.

4. Note any chest deformity (this may increase the risk of deterioration in the ability to breathe normally); look for a raised jugular venous pulse (JVP) (e.g. in acute severe asthma or a tension pneumothorax); note the presence and patency of any chest drains; remember that abdominal distension may limit diaphragmatic movement, thereby worsening respiratory distress.

5. Record the inspired oxygen concentration (%) and the SpO_2 reading of the pulse oximeter.
The pulse oximeter does not detect hypercapnia. If the patient is receiving supplemental oxygen, the SpO_2 may be normal in the presence of a very high $PaCO_2$.

6. Listen to the patient's breath sounds a short distance from their face.
Rattling airway noises indicate the presence of airway secretions, usually caused by the inability of the patient to cough sufficiently or to take a deep breath. Stridor or wheeze suggests partial, but significant, airway obstruction.

7. Percuss the chest.
Hyper-resonance may indicate a pneumothorax; dullness may suggest consolidation or pleural fluid.

8. Auscultate the chest.
Abnormal breath sounds such as bronchial breathing may indicate lung consolidation with patent airways; absent or reduced sounds may suggest a pneumothorax or pleural fluid or lung consolidation caused by complete obstruction.

9. Check the position of the trachea in the suprasternal notch.
Deviation to one side indicates mediastinal shift (e.g. pneumothorax, lung fibrosis or pleural fluid).

10. Feel the chest wall to detect surgical emphysema or crepitus (suggesting a pneumothorax until proven otherwise).

11. The specific treatment of respiratory disorders depends upon the cause.
Nevertheless, all critically ill patients should be given oxygen. In a subgroup of patients with COPD, high concentrations of oxygen may depress breathing (i.e. they are at risk of hypercapnic respiratory failure – often referred to as type 2 respiratory failure). Nevertheless, these patients will also sustain end-organ damage or cardiac arrest if their blood oxygen tensions are allowed to decrease. In this group, aim for a lower than normal PaO_2 and oxygen saturation. Give oxygen via a Venturi mask at 24% or 28% initially and reassess. Aim for a target SpO_2 range of 88–92% in most COPD patients, but evaluate the target for each patient based on the patient's arterial blood gas measurements during previous exacer-bations (if available). Some patients with chronic lung disease carry an oxygen alert card (that documents their target saturation) and their own appropriate Venturi mask.

12. If the patient's depth or rate of breathing is judged to be inadequate or absent, use bag-mask ventilation to improve oxygenation and ventilation, whilst calling immediately for expert help.
In cooperative patients who do not have airway obstruction consider the use of non-invasive ventilation (NIV). In patients with an acute exacerbation of COPD, the use of NIV is often helpful and may prevent the need for tracheal intubation and invasive ventilation.

C = Circulation

In almost all medical and surgical emergencies, consider hypovolaemia as the likely cause of shock, until proven otherwise. Unless there are obvious signs of a cardiac cause, give intravenous fluid to any patient with cool peripheries and a fast heart rate. In surgical patients, rapidly exclude haemorrhage (overt or hidden). Remember that breathing problems, such as a tension pneumothorax, can also compromise a patient's circulatory state. This should have been treated earlier on in the assessment.

1. Look at the colour of the hands and digits.
Are they blue, pink, pale or mottled?

2. Assess the limb temperature by feeling the patient's hands. Are they cool or warm?

3. Measure the capillary refill time (CRT).
Apply cutaneous pressure for 5 s with enough pressure to cause blanching. Press on the sternum for central CRT or on a fingertip held at heart level for peripheral CRT. Time how long it takes for the skin to return to the colour of the surrounding skin after releasing the pressure. The normal value for CRT is usually < 2 s. A prolonged CRT suggests poor perfusion. Other factors can hinder CRT interpretation (e.g. cold surroundings, poor lighting, old age can prolong CRT).

4. Assess the state of the veins. They may be under-filled or collapsed when hypovolaemia is present.

5. Palpate peripheral and central pulses, assessing for presence, rate, quality, regularity and equality of volume. Barely palpable central pulses suggest a low cardiac output, whilst a bounding pulse may indicate sepsis.

6. Measure the patient's blood pressure.
Even in shock, the blood pressure may be normal, because compensatory mechanisms increase peripheral resistance in response to reduced cardiac output. A low diastolic blood pressure suggests arterial vasodilation (as in anaphylaxis or sepsis). A narrow pulse pressure (difference between systolic and diastolic pressures; normally 35–45 mmHg) suggests arterial vasoconstriction (cardiogenic shock or hypovolaemia) and may occur with rapid tachyarrhythmia.

7. Auscultate the heart. This may allow detection of a murmur, a pericardial rub or abnormal (e.g. muffled) heart sounds or reveal that the heart rate is much faster than the palpable pulse rate.

8. Look for other signs of a low cardiac output, such as reduced conscious level and, if the patient has a urinary catheter, oliguria (urine volume < 0.5 mL kg^{-1} h^{-1}).

9. Look thoroughly for external haemorrhage from wounds or drains for evidence of concealed haemorrhage (e.g. thoracic, intra-peritoneal, retroperitoneal or into gut). Intra-thoracic, intra-abdominal or pelvic blood loss may be significant, even if drains are empty.

10. The specific treatment of cardiovascular collapse depends on the cause, but should be directed at fluid replacement, haemorrhage control and restoration of tissue perfusion. Seek the signs of conditions that are immediately life-threatening (e.g. cardiac tamponade, massive or continuing haemorrhage, septicaemic shock) and treat them urgently.

11. Insert one or more large (14 or 16 G) intravenous cannulae. Use short, wide bore cannulae, because they enable the highest flow. Consider inserting an intraosseous needle if failure to gain intravenous access.

12. Take blood from the cannula for routine haematological, biochemical, coagulation and microbiological investigations, and cross-matching, before infusing intravenous fluid.

13. Give a bolus of 500 mL of warmed crystalloid solution (e.g. Hartmann's solution or 0.9% sodium chloride) over less than 15 min if the patient is hypotensive. Use smaller volumes (e.g. 250 mL) for patients with known cardiac failure or trauma and use closer monitoring (listen to the chest for crackles after each bolus).

14. Reassess the heart rate and BP regularly (every 5 min), aiming for the patient's normal BP or, if this is unknown, a target > 100 mmHg systolic.

15. If the patient does not improve, repeat the fluid challenge. Seek expert help if there is a lack of response to repeated fluid boluses.

16. If there are symptoms and signs of cardiac failure (dyspnoea, increased heart rate, raised JVP, a third heart sound and pulmonary crackles on auscultation) occur, decrease the fluid infusion rate or stop the fluids altogether. Seek alternative means of improving tissue perfusion (e.g. inotropes or vasopressors).

17. If the patient has primary chest pain and a suspected ACS, record a 12-lead ECG early.

18. Immediate general treatment for ACS includes:
- aspirin 300 mg, orally, crushed or chewed, as soon as possible
- nitroglycerine, as sublingual glyceryl trinitrate (tablet or spray)
- oxygen: only give oxygen if the patient's SpO$_2$ is less than 94%
- morphine (or diamorphine) IV, titrated to avoid sedation and respiratory depression.

D = Disability

Common causes of unconsciousness include profound hypoxia, hypercapnia, cerebral hypoperfusion, or the recent administration of sedatives or analgesic drugs.

1. Review and treat the ABCs. Exclude or treat hypoxia and hypotension.

2. Check the patient's drug chart for reversible drug-induced causes of depressed consciousness. Give an antagonist where appropriate (e.g. naloxone for opioid toxicity).

3. Examine the pupils (size, equality and reaction to light).

4. Make a rapid initial assessment of the patient's conscious level using the ACVPU method. Alert, new confusion, responds to Vocal stimuli, responds to Painful stimuli or Unresponsive (ACVPU) to all stimuli. Alternatively, use the Glasgow Coma Scale (GCS) score. A painful stimulus can be given by applying trapezium squeeze.

5. Measure the blood glucose to check for hypoglycaemia using a rapid finger-prick bedside testing method.
In a peri-arrest patient use a venous or arterial blood sample for glucose measurement as finger-prick sample glucose measurements can be unreliable in sick patients. Follow local protocols for management of hypoglycaemia. For example, if the blood glucose is less than 4.0 mmol L^{-1} in an unconscious patient, give an initial dose of 50 mL of 10% glucose solution intravenously. If necessary, give further doses of intravenous 10% glucose every minute until the patient has fully regained consciousness, or a total of 250 mL of 10% glucose has been given. Repeat blood glucose measurements to monitor the effects of treatment. If there is no improvement consider further doses of 10% glucose. Specific national guidance exists for the management of hypoglycaemia in adults with diabetes mellitus.

6. Nurse unconscious patients in the lateral position if their airway is not protected.

E = Exposure

To examine the patient properly full exposure of the body may be necessary. Respect the patient's dignity and minimise heat loss (Figure 3.2).

Additional information

- Take a full clinical history from the patient, any witnesses or friends, and other staff.

- Review the patient's notes and charts:
  - study both absolute and trended values of vital signs
  - check that important routine medications are prescribed and being given
  - review the results of investigations including laboratory or radiological.

- Consider which level of care is required by the patient (e.g. ward, HDU, ICU).

- Make complete entries in the patient's records of your findings, assessment and treatment. Where necessary, hand over the patient to your colleagues.

- Record the patient's response to therapy.

- Consider definitive treatment of the patient's underlying condition.

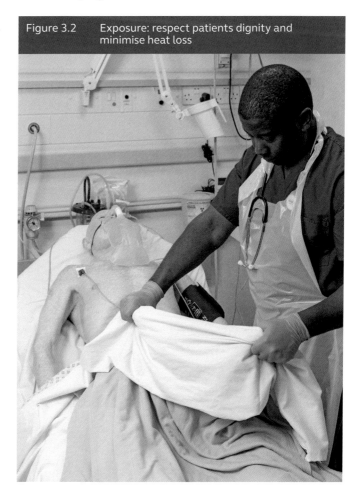

Figure 3.2   Exposure: respect patients dignity and minimise heat loss

03: Summary learning

Most patients who have an in-hospital cardiac arrest have warning signs and symptoms before the arrest.

Early recognition and treatment of the deteriorating patient will prevent some cardiac arrests.

Use strategies such as early warning scoring (EWS) systems to identify patients at risk of cardiac arrest.

Airway, breathing and circulation problems can cause cardiac arrest.

Use the ABCDE approach to assess and treat deteriorating patients.

My key take-home messages from this chapter are:

Further reading

National Confidential Enquiry into Patient Outcome and Death. An Acute Problem? London: National Confidential Enquiry into Patient Outcome and Death; 2005.

Healthcare Safety Investigation Branch. Recognising and responding to critically unwell patients. I2017/007 Independent report. 2019. https://www.hsib.org.uk/investigations-cases/recognising-and-responding-critically-unwell-patients/

National Early Warning Score (NEWS) 2: Standardising the assessment of acute-illness severity in the NHS. Updated report of a working party. Royal College of Physicians, London, 2017.

NICE Clinical Guideline 50 Acutely ill patients in hospital: recognition of and response to acute illness in adults in hospital. London: National Institute for Health and Clinical Excellence; 2007. https://www.nice.org.uk/guidance/cg50

NICE Clinical Guideline 174 Intravenous fluid therapy. Intravenous fluid therapy in adults in hospital. London: National Institute for Health and Clinical Excellence; 2017. https://www.nice.org.uk/guidance/cg174

Nolan JP, Soar J, Smith GB, et al. Incidence and outcome of in-hospital cardiac arrest in the United Kingdom National Cardiac Arrest Audit. Resuscitation 2014;85:987-92.

O'Driscoll BR, Howard LS, Earis J on behalf of the BTS Emergency Oxygen Guideline Development Group, et al. British Thoracic Society Guideline for oxygen use in adults in healthcare and emergency settings. BMJ Open Respiratory Research 2017;4:e000170.

Smith GB. In-hospital cardiac arrest: Is it time for an in-hospital 'chain of prevention'? Resuscitation 2010:81:1209-11.

Soar J, Berg KM, Andersen LW, Böttiger BW, Cacciola S, Callaway CW, et al; Adult Advanced Life Support Collaborators. Adult Advanced Life Support: 2020 International Consensus on Cardiopulmonary Resuscitation and Emergency Cardiovascular Care Science with Treatment Recommendations. Resuscitation. 2020;156:A80-A119.

Soar J, Böttiger BW, Carli P, Couper K, Deakin CD, Djärv T, Lott C, Olasveengen TM, Paal P, Pellis T, Perkins GD, Sandroni C, Nolan JP. European Resuscitation Council Guidelines 2021: Advanced Life Support. Resuscitation. 2021;161.

Stub D, Smith K, Bernard S, et al. Air Versus Oxygen in ST-Segment-Elevation Myocardial Infarction. Circulation 2015;131:2143-50.

The Hospital Management of Hypoglycaemia in Adults with Diabetes Mellitus. Joint British Diabetes Societies. Revised 2018.

Winters BD, Weaver SJ, Pfoh ER, Yang T, Pham JC, Dy SM. Rapid-response systems as a patient safety strategy: a systematic review. Annals of Internal Medicine 2013;158:417-25.

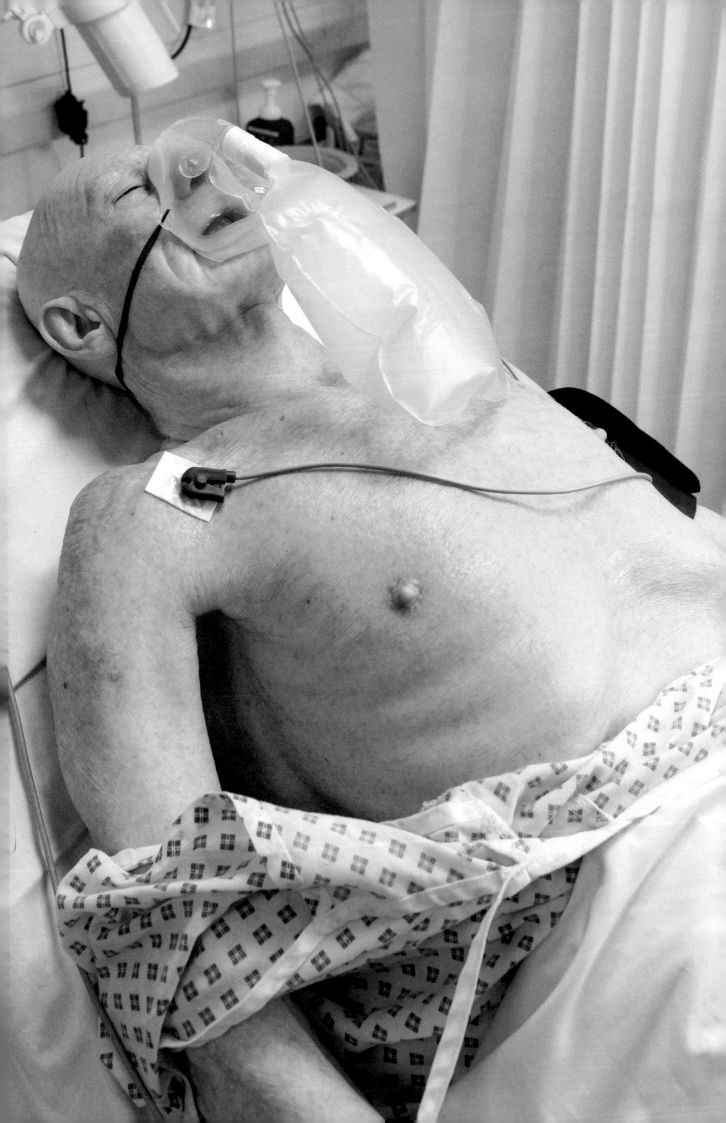

Cardiac causes of cardiac arrest

In this chapter

Recognition and treatment of acute coronary syndromes and the other conditions that may lead to cardiac arrest

Recognition of the features and events that may indicate high risk and interventions to prevent progression to cardiac arrest

The learning outcomes will enable you to:

Recognise and assess an acute coronary syndrome

Understand the disease process which causes acute coronary syndromes

Consider the immediate treatment of each type of acute coronary syndrome

Consider the treatment needed after recovery from an acute coronary syndrome

Recognise and respond to other cardiac conditions that may cause cardiac arrest

Introduction

Whilst rapid resuscitation offers the best chance of recovery from cardiac arrest, it is clearly better to prevent cardiac arrest whenever possible. Many cardiac arrests are caused by coronary artery disease (CAD) and occur most commonly in the context of an acute coronary syndrome (ACS).

It is therefore important that you:

- understand how to recognise an ACS
- understand how to assess a patient with an ACS
- know what treatments may reduce the risk of cardiac arrest and death
- know what actions are needed to achieve the best outcome when a person has a cardiac arrest as the presenting feature of a suspected ACS
- are aware of some of the other cardiac conditions that may cause cardiac arrest, and how to recognise and treat them to reduce the risk of cardiac arrest and death.

Acute coronary syndromes

Definitions and pathogenesis

The term acute coronary syndromes describes a group of clinical conditions, all of which usually present with chest pain or discomfort resulting from myocardial ischaemia. The distinct categories of ACS are distinguished initially by the presence or absence of ST-segment elevation on a 12-lead ECG and, in those without ST-segment elevation, by the presence or absence of a raised blood troponin concentration suggesting myocardial injury (Figure 4.1):

- ST-segment-elevation myocardial infarction (STEMI)
- Non-ST-segment-elevation acute coronary syndromes (NSTE ACS)
  - Non-ST-segment-elevation myocardial infarction (NSTEMI)
  - Unstable angina (UA).

These syndromes form part of a spectrum of the same disease process. In most cases this results from coronary artery disease and is initiated by the rupture or erosion of an atherosclerotic plaque within a coronary artery causing:

- acute thrombosis within the vessel lumen, often with haemorrhagic extension into the atherosclerotic plaque
- contraction of smooth muscle cells within the artery wall resulting in vasoconstriction that reduces the lumen of the artery
- associated partial or complete obstruction of the lumen, often with embolism of thrombus into the distal part of the vessel.

This process results in a sudden and critical reduction in blood flow to the myocardium. The degree and extent of this reduction in blood flow to the myocardium largely determines the clinical presentation and type of ACS.

Coronary artery disease

Coronary artery disease (CAD) is one of the leading causes of premature death in the world. It is characterised by accumulation of atherosclerotic plaques within the coronary arteries. CAD is a chronic process that can begin during adolescence and progress slowly throughout life. Risk factors for CAD include a family history of atherosclerosis, smoking, diabetes mellitus, hypertension, hyperlipidaemia, sedentary lifestyle and obesity. CAD is believed to be an abnormal response to vessel injury and these risk factors are thought to accelerate the inflammatory process that results in atherosclerosis. Over time atherosclerotic plaques can narrow the coronary artery lumen progressively. For many years such developing atherosclerosis may cause no symptoms.

However, if the plaque starts to impair the blood flow to the myocardium angina can occur. If a thrombus (blood clot) forms at the site of atherosclerosis myocardial infarction may result.

Angina (stable and unstable)

Typical stable angina is a constricting pain, tightness or discomfort in the front of the chest, and/or in the neck, shoulders, jaw, or arms that is provoked by physical exertion and relieved by stopping that exertion. It is usually caused by myocardial ischaemia, most commonly due to obstructive coronary artery disease.

Recognising stable angina is not always straightforward as some patients present with less typical symptoms. Patients may present with clear central chest pain or tightness but they may also report less typical discomfort, including symptoms that feel like indigestion. As with acute myocardial infarction (AMI), the pain/discomfort may radiate to the throat, into one or both arms, and into the back or upper abdomen. Some patients experience angina predominantly in one or more of these areas without chest pain. Some groups of people (including females, diabetics and the elderly) are more likely to present with atypical or less-specific symptoms such as breathlessness. Ischaemic chest pain (due to angina or AMI) may be misdiagnosed as indigestion or non-cardiac chest pain. Symptoms of this nature, which are provoked only by exercise, which settle promptly when exercise ceases, do not occur at rest and are not getting worse are referred to as stable angina. Although stable angina needs correct recognition and appropriate management it is not a medical emergency.

In contrast, unstable angina is defined by one or more of:

1. Angina on exertion, occurring with increasing frequency over a few days, provoked by progressively less exertion. This is sometimes referred to as 'crescendo angina'.

2. Episodes of angina-like pain occurring recurrently and unpredictably, without specific provocation by exercise. These episodes may be relatively short-lived (e.g. a few minutes) and may settle spontaneously or be relieved temporarily by sublingual glyceryl trinitrate, before recurring again.

3. An unprovoked and prolonged episode of chest pain, raising suspicion of AMI, but without definite ECG changes or laboratory evidence of AMI (see below).

In unstable angina (UA) the ECG may:

a) be normal

b) show evidence of acute myocardial ischaemia (usually ST-segment depression)

c) show non-specific abnormalities (e.g. T wave inversion).

In UA, by definition, biomarkers for myocardial necrosis (i.e. troponin release) are not present. The use of high-sensitivity troponin assays has resulted in a diagnosis of NSTEMI in many patients who would previously have been considered to have UA. Although the ECG may be normal or show non-specific features, ECG abnormalities (such as ST-segment depression) are a marker of increased risk. However, a normal ECG and an undetectable troponin level do not necessarily mean that an individual patient with UA is at low risk. Therefore all patients with UA should have their risk assessed using an established risk calculator, such as the Global Registry of Acute Coronary Events (GRACE) score (see below).

If the ECG and troponin concentration are normal and the estimated risk is low, patients can be considered for further risk assessment with non-invasive tests (e.g. exercise testing or non-invasive imaging) and other possible causes for their chest pain should be considered. In some patients who present with angina-like symptoms, coronary artery disease may later be excluded as the cause of those symptoms.

Acute coronary syndrome

History and clinical assessment suggest ACS

↓

12-lead ECG

ST-segment elevation or new* LBBB

Other ECG changes or normal ECG

STEMI
ST-segment-elevation myocardial infarction

Troponin concentration

Troponin release present

Troponin consistently negative

NSTEMI
Non-ST-segment-elevation myocardial infarction

Reconsider other causes of chest pain

Unstable angina

Higher risk NSTE ACS may be indicated by:
- ST-segment depression
- Dynamic ECG changes
- Unstable rhythm
- Unstable haemodynamics
- Diabetes mellitus
- High GRACE score

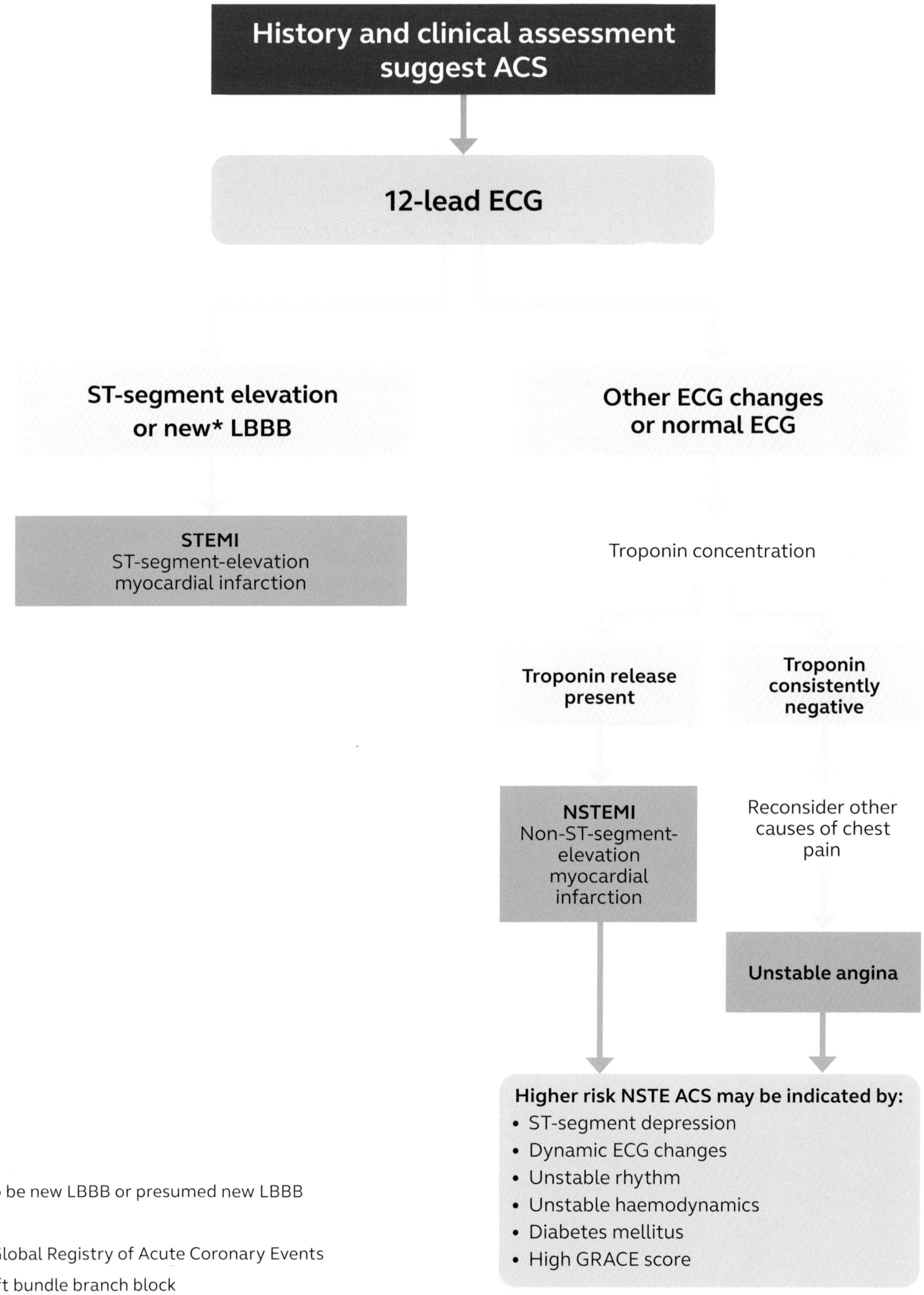

*Known to be new LBBB or presumed new LBBB

GRACE – Global Resigstry of Acute Coronary Events

LBBB – Left bundle branch block

NSTE ACS – Non-ST-segment-elevation acute coronary syndromes

NSTEMI – Non-ST-segment-elevation myocardial infarction

STEMI – ST-segment-elevation myocardial infarction

Figure 4.1   Algorithm for identifying the type of acute coronary syndrome

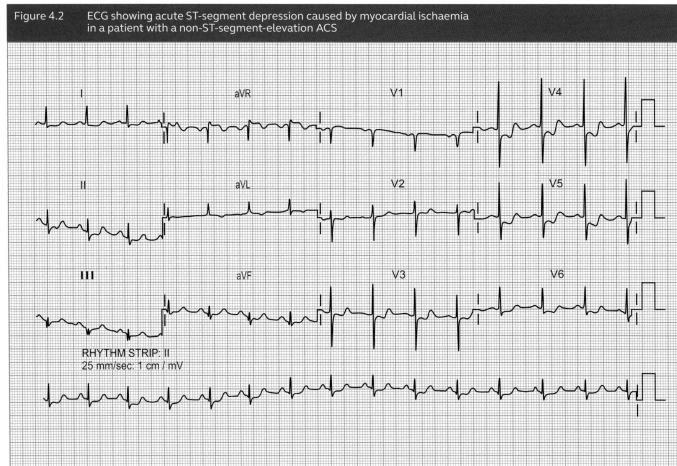

Figure 4.2 ECG showing acute ST-segment depression caused by myocardial ischaemia in a patient with a non-ST-segment-elevation ACS

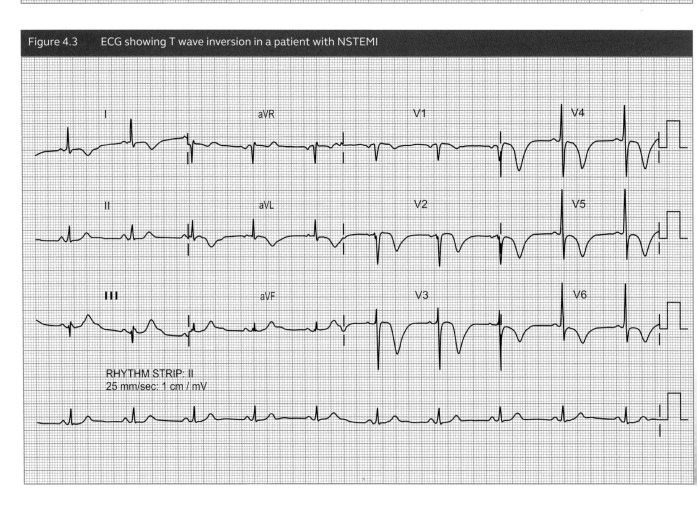

Figure 4.3 ECG showing T wave inversion in a patient with NSTEMI

Non-ST-segment-elevation myocardial infarction (NSTEMI)

Acute myocardial infarction presents typically with chest pain that is felt as a heaviness or tightness or indigestion-like discomfort in the chest or upper abdomen, usually sustained for at least 20 min. The chest pain/discomfort often radiates into the throat, into one or both arms, into the back or into the upper abdomen. Some patients experience the discomfort predominantly in one or more of these other areas rather than in the chest. The pain is usually accompanied by sweating; belching, nausea or vomiting may occur also. As with angina, some people with AMI experience less typical symptoms, such as acute breathlessness. A small proportion of people with AMI experience no symptoms.

When a patient presents with chest pain suggestive of AMI and has raised biomarkers (e.g. troponin) but has no ST-segment elevation on the ECG this is referred to as NSTEMI. The 12-lead ECG may be normal, show ST-segment depression or non-specific ECG abnormalities such as T wave inversion (Figures 4.2 and 4.3).

ECG changes are associated with increased risk. The confirmation of the release of cardiac-specific troponin indicates that myocardial damage has occurred

(in contrast to unstable angina which is not associated with troponin release). In this situation it is likely that there has been partial or intermittent occlusion of the 'culprit' coronary artery.

The amount of troponin released reflects the amount of myocardium damaged. Some patients with NSTEMI will be at high risk of progression to complete coronary occlusion, further myocardial infarction and sudden arrhythmic death. The risk of this is highest in the first few hours, days and months after the index event and diminishes progressively with time. The need for further treatment is largely determined by assessment of risk.

NSTEMI and unstable angina are classified together as 'non-ST-segment-elevation ACS (NSTE ACS)' because the treatment of the two is essentially the same. This is in contrast to the treatment of STEMI where immediate reperfusion is a major priority.

ST-segment-elevation myocardial infarction (STEMI)

A history of sustained acute chest pain typical of AMI, accompanied by acute ST-segment elevation (Figures 4.4, 4.5, 4.6) or new left bundle branch block (LBBB) on a 12-lead ECG, is the basis for the diagnosis of STEMI.

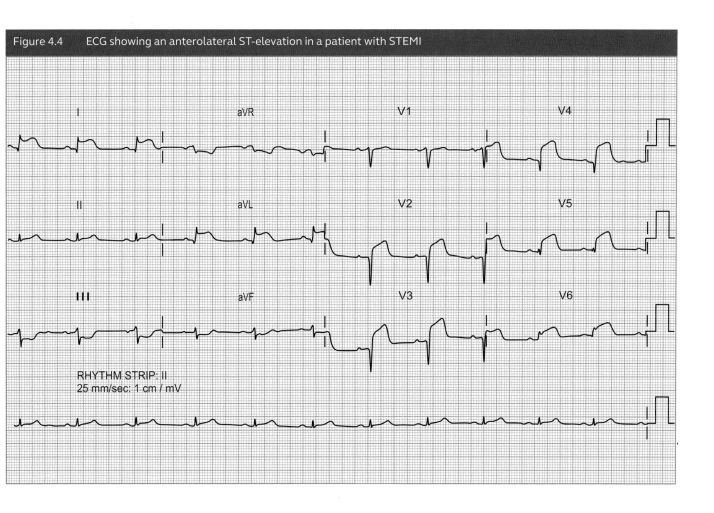

Figure 4.4   ECG showing an anterolateral ST-elevation in a patient with STEMI

RHYTHM STRIP: II
25 mm/sec: 1 cm / mV

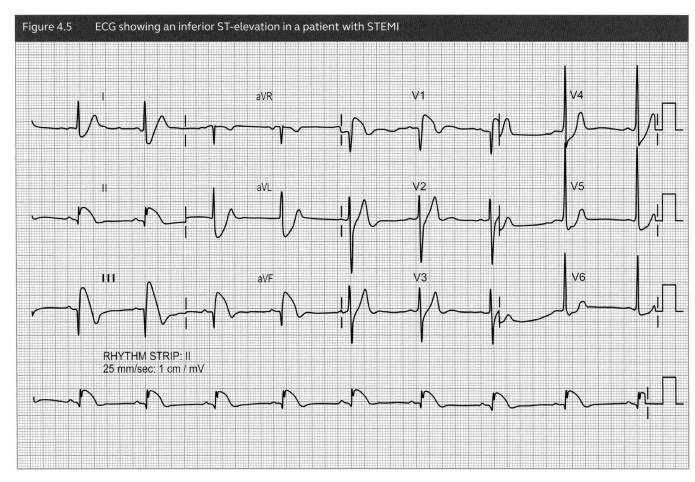

Figure 4.5   ECG showing an inferior ST-elevation in a patient with STEMI

RHYTHM STRIP: II
25 mm/sec: 1 cm / mV

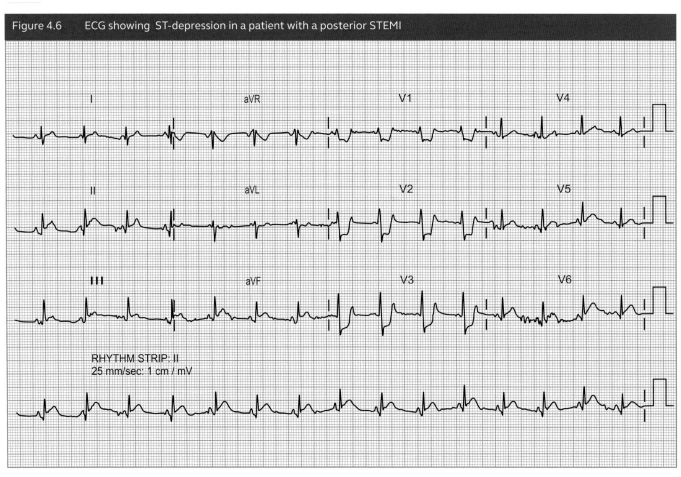

Figure 4.6   ECG showing ST-depression in a patient with a posterior STEMI

RHYTHM STRIP: II
25 mm/sec: 1 cm / mV

Figure 4.7 ECG showing onset of VF in a patient with acute anteroseptal STEMI

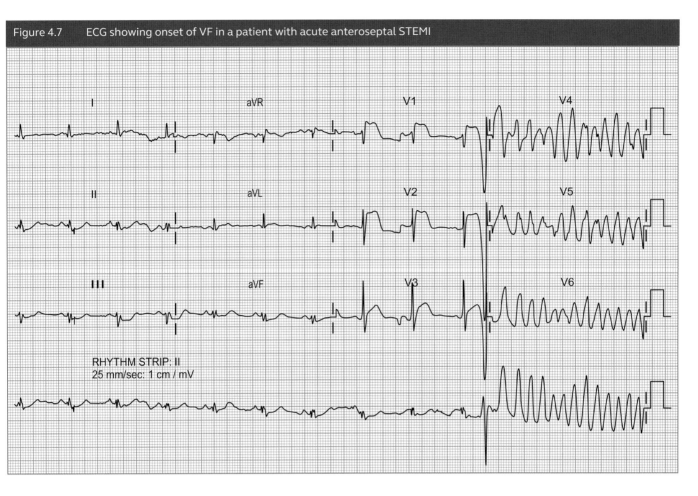

These findings indicate ongoing myocardial damage, typically caused by acute, complete, thrombotic occlusion of the 'culprit' coronary artery. Left untreated there will be further myocardial damage in the territory of the occluded artery. This may be shown by the development of Q waves on the ECG and by impairment of left ventricular function (seen on echocardiography).

During the acute phase of STEMI there is a substantial risk of ventricular tachycardia (VT), ventricular fibrillation (VF) (Figure 4.7) and sudden death. Confirmation of an elevated troponin is not required to make the initial diagnosis of STEMI or to ensure that the patient receives appropriate treatment without delay.

Diagnosis of acute coronary syndromes

History

An accurate history is the crucial first step in establishing a diagnosis, although it is important to realise that patients often present atypically. Some patient groups (e.g. elderly people, diabetics, females, people with renal disease and people during a peri-operative period) are more likely than others to develop an ACS with little or no chest discomfort. In such people, particularly diabetics, the dominant symptom may be breathlessness. The pain of angina or myocardial infarction may be mistaken for indigestion, both by patients and by healthcare professionals.

Symptoms such as belching, nausea or vomiting are not helpful in distinguishing cardiac pain from indigestion; they may accompany angina and myocardial infarction.

In addition to the history of chest pain, the presence of certain clinical findings and medical problems increases the probability of CAD and AMI. These include older age, males, a positive family history and known atherosclerosis (including in non-coronary territories, such as peripheral or carotid artery disease). The presence of risk factors such as hypertension, smoking, hypercholesterolemia and, in particular, diabetes mellitus and renal insufficiency all increase the likelihood of an ACS.

Clinical examination

Clinical examination is often of limited benefit in making a positive diagnosis of ACS. Severe pain of any source may provoke sweating, pallor and tachycardia, which commonly accompany ACS. However, a careful history and examination are essential in order to recognise other causes of chest pain and to aid the diagnosis of other life-threatening conditions.

Examination may identify other important abnormalities (e.g. a cardiac murmur or signs of heart failure) that will influence choices of investigation and treatment. In patients with acute chest pain remember to consider other important and potentially life-threatening differential diagnoses such as aortic dissection and pulmonary embolism. Major pulmonary embolism

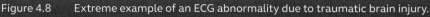

Figure 4.8   Extreme example of an ECG abnormality due to traumatic brain injury.
This shows marked ST-elevation in the anterolateral leads.

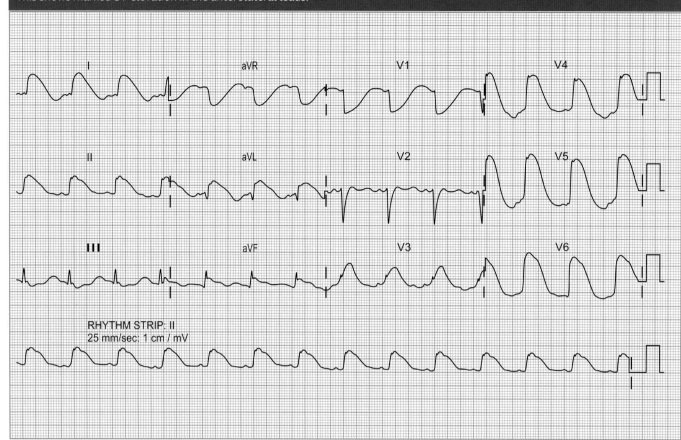

presents typically with unexplained breathlessness and hypoxia, sometimes with sudden collapse, and may cause ECG abnormalities (see below) and a raised troponin. The presence of aortic dissection may be suggested by acute, severe chest pain radiating to the back, which may be accompanied by other clinical signs. These include hypotension, loss of a peripheral pulse or asymmetry of pulses in the upper limbs, aortic regurgitation or signs of stroke from carotid artery involvement. Suspect aortic dissection in any patient who has acute chest pain and marked hypotension but no obvious ECG evidence of AMI. However, in a patient with a good history and typical ECG evidence of STEMI do not delay reperfusion therapy without strong clinical evidence to justify prior investigation for possible aortic dissection or pulmonary embolism.

Initial examination also serves as an important baseline to detect changes due to progression of the underlying condition or in response to treatment. Signs of shock and heart failure are especially important as they indicate a substantially increased risk of death.

The 12-lead ECG

Record a 12-lead ECG as soon as possible (within 10 min) during the initial assessment and repeat recordings subsequently to assess progression of the ACS and the response to treatment. For many patients an initial 12-lead ECG should form part of pre-hospital assessment by the ambulance service. Pre-hospital ECG recording in patients with STEMI expedites reperfusion therapy (see below), leading to a reduction in mortality.

The presence of ECG abnormalities on the initial recording may support the clinical suspicion of ACS and indicate the appropriate treatment. However, a single normal 12-lead ECG does not exclude an ACS and the ECG should be repeated at intervals to increase the chances of detecting an abnormality.

The ECG is the initial component of risk assessment and planning of treatment. Acute ST-segment elevation or new LBBB in a patient with a typical history of AMI establishes the diagnosis of STEMI. This diagnosis mandates immediate treatment to re-open the occluded coronary artery (reperfusion therapy), preferably by emergency primary percutaneous coronary intervention (PPCI). If this cannot be achieved within 120 min of the onset of chest pain, fibrinolytic therapy (given pre-hospital if appropriate) should be considered as an alternative. Reperfusion therapy should not be delayed whilst awaiting the result of troponin assays in patients with STEMI.

The ECG provides some information about the site and extent of myocardial damage in AMI, particularly in STEMI. This is important since the site and extent of myocardial ischaemia or damage influences prognosis and, in some cases, the appropriate choice of treatment:

*   Anterior or anteroseptal infarction is seen in leads V1–V4 and is typically caused by a lesion in the left anterior descending (LAD) coronary artery. Extension to involve leads V5–V6, I and aVL indicates an anterolateral infarct (Figure 4.4). An anterior infarct on average is more likely to cause substantial

Figure 4.9 ECG showing evidence of acute right ventricular pressure overload due to major pulmonary embolism.

An S wave in lead I and a deep Q wave and T wave inversion in lead III are accompanied by T wave inversion in the anterior chest leads (over the right ventricle). In this case the ECG changes were misinterpreted as evidence of an acute coronary syndrome, despite the history and clinical features suggesting pulmonary embolism.

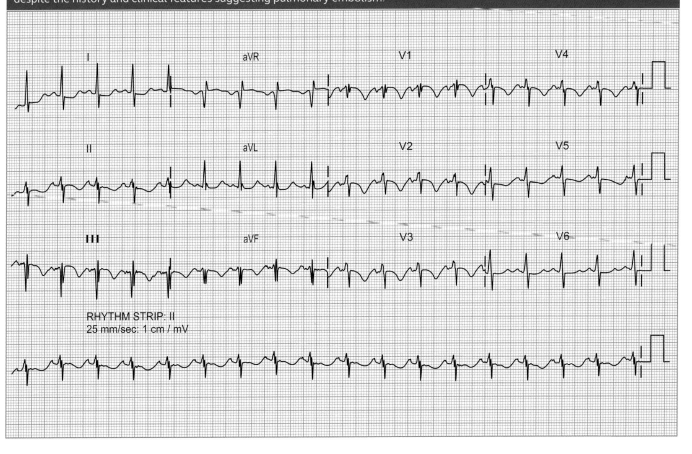

RHYTHM STRIP: II
25 mm/sec: 1 cm / mV

impairment of left ventricular function and has a worse prognosis than an inferior or lateral infarct.

- Inferior infarction is seen in leads II, III, and aVF (Figure 4.5), and is caused often by a lesion in the right coronary artery or, less commonly, the circumflex artery.

- Lateral infarction is seen in leads V5–V6 and/or leads I and aVL (sometimes aVL alone) and is caused usually by a lesion in the circumflex artery or diagonal branch of the LAD artery.

- Posterior myocardial infarction can be recognised when there is a reciprocal ST-segment depression in the anterior chest leads (Figure 4.6). ST-segment depression in these leads may reflect posterior ST-segment elevation, and development of a dominant R wave in V1 and V2 reflects posterior Q wave development. This is most commonly due to a right coronary artery occlusion but may be caused by a dominant circumflex artery lesion in individuals in whom this artery provides the main blood supply to the posterior part of the left ventricle and septum. Suspicion of posterior infarction can be confirmed by repeating the ECG using posterior leads. These leads (V8, V9 and V10) are placed in a horizontal line around the chest, continuing from V6 (mid-axillary line) and V7 (posterior axillary line). V9 is placed to the left of the spine, V8 half way between V7 and V9 and V10 to the right of the spine.

- Right ventricular (RV) infarction may be present in up to one third of patients with inferior and posterior STEMI. Extensive RV infarction may be seen on a conventional 12-lead ECG when ST-segment elevation in lead V1 accompanies an inferior (Figure 4.5) or posterior STEMI (Figure 4.6); use of right-sided precordial leads, especially V4R can also be useful in detecting RV infarction. In this case right-sided precordial leads, particularly V4R, may reveal RV infarction. Two-dimensional echocardiography is also very useful. A diagnosis of extensive RV infarction is suggested by fluid-responsive hypotension and signs of high systemic venous pressure (manifest as jugular venous distension) without pulmonary congestion.

- The ST-segment depression and T wave inversion that may occur in NSTEMI are less-clearly related to the site of myocardial damage than the changes in STEMI.

Acute ECG abnormalities may be caused by conditions other than an ACS. The ECGs of some people with subarachnoid haemorrhage or traumatic brain injury may show acute changes including ST-segment depression or elevation, or T wave inversion (Figure 4.8). The ECGs of some people with major pulmonary embolism may show acute changes that include T wave inversion in leads V1–V4, overlying an acutely dilated right ventricle. (Figure 4.9). Other conditions to consider include Brugada syndrome (ST-elevation in leads V1 and V2) and takotsubo (stress-induced) cardiomyopathy (chest pain and ST-elevation).

Laboratory tests

Laboratory tests are also an important component of diagnosis and risk assessment.

Cardiac-specific troponins (T and I) are two proteins that are components of the contractile structure of myocardial cells (the sarcomere). Because concentrations of troponin in the blood of healthy individuals are undetectably low, and cardiac-specific troponins measured by current assays do not detect troponin from other muscle types (e.g. skeletal muscle), troponin assays are very sensitive and specific markers of cardiac injury. In the context of a typical clinical presentation of an ACS, troponin release provides evidence of myocardial damage and therefore indicates that myocardial infarction has occurred (rather than unstable angina, which will be troponin negative).

Troponin values provide an important marker of risk. The greater the troponin concentration, the greater is the risk of a further event or death. A combination of ST-segment depression on the ECG and raised troponin identifies a particularly high-risk group for subsequent AMI and cardiac death.

The release of troponin does not in itself indicate a diagnosis of ACS. Troponin release aids diagnosis and is a marker of risk when the history indicates a high probability of AMI. Troponin may be released in other life-threatening conditions presenting with chest pain, such as pulmonary embolism, aortic dissection and myocarditis. Troponin values may also be elevated in acute or chronic heart failure, arrhythmias, chronic renal failure and acute sepsis. Troponin results must be interpreted in the context of the clinical history and presentation and the reference values of the local laboratory.

Echocardiography

Echocardiography is the most important non-invasive imaging modality in the acute setting because it is rapidly and widely available. Left ventricular (LV) systolic function is directly related to prognosis and, in a person with acute chest pain, regional wall motion abnormalities increase the likelihood of an ACS (but are not diagnostic).

Echocardiography may also allow prompt diagnosis of other conditions such as cardiomyopathies, valve disease, pericardial disease, aortic dissection and pulmonary embolism. Echocardiography can also confirm or exclude right ventricular (RV) dilatation and impairment when extensive RV infarction is suspected. In addition it can be used to diagnose complications of AMI such as a ventricular septal defect and severe mitral regurgitation, both of which may require urgent surgical correction.

Quantitative risk assessment scores: GRACE and CRUSADE

An ACS is a potentially unstable condition that is prone to further ischaemia, which may lead to death or AMI in the short or long term. The management of ACS includes anti-ischaemic and antithrombotic drug treatments in addition to coronary revascularisation. This is to prevent or reduce complications and improve outcomes but some of these treatments may also cause bleeding, which worsens prognosis. The timing and intensity of each of these interventions should be tailored to an individual patient's risk and be balanced between the risk of an adverse cardiac outcome and the risk of bleeding due to the treatment given.

Quantitative assessment of risk is useful for clinical decision-making as it is not uncommon for risk to be either over or under-estimated. The Global Registry of Acute Coronary Events (GRACE) risk score provides the most accurate stratification of risk, both on admission and over 6 months. The admission GRACE score is based on eight variables:

- age
- signs of heart failure
- heart rate at presentation
- blood pressure at presentation
- serum creatinine concentration
- ECG changes
- troponin concentration
- cardiac arrest at presentation.

The GRACE score has good discriminative power for predicting risk but because of its complexity is best calculated using an online calculator or app (www.outcomes-umassmed.org/grace/).

Bleeding is associated with an adverse prognosis in ACS, and all efforts should be made to avoid or reduce bleeding whenever possible. A few variables can help to classify patients into different levels of risk for major bleeding during hospital admission. These variables include:

- increased age
- known bleeding complications
- renal impairment
- low body weight.

Immediate treatment

General measures in all acute coronary syndromes

Patients presenting with a suspected ACS should have a rapid clinical assessment and a 12-lead ECG recorded. If the diagnosis of ACS is confirmed or likely, treat immediately to relieve symptoms, limit myocardial damage and reduce the risk of cardiac arrest. Connect the patient to a cardiac monitor. Immediate treatment for ACS comprises:

- aspirin 300 mg orally, crushed or chewed, as soon as possible
- sublingual glyceryl trinitrate (spray or tablet) unless the patient is hypotensive
- give oxygen only if the patient is hypoxic (saturation < 94% on air):
  - aim for saturation of 94–98%
  - in the presence of chronic obstructive pulmonary disease aim for 88–92%
- pain relief with IV opiate analgesia (morphine):
  - titrated to control symptoms whilst avoiding sedation and respiratory depression
  - given with an anti-emetic.

Treatment of STEMI (or AMI with new LBBB)

For patients presenting with STEMI within 12 h of symptom onset, mechanical or pharmacological reperfusion must be achieved without delay. The risk/benefit ratio for reperfusion therapy favours this treatment for those who are at highest risk of immediate major myocardial damage and death. In STEMI, coronary reperfusion may be achieved in one of two ways:

- Percutaneous coronary intervention (PCI) may be used to re-open the occluded artery. This is referred to as primary PCI (PPCI).
- Fibrinolytic therapy may be given in an attempt to dissolve the occluding thrombus that caused the AMI.

Primary percutaneous coronary intervention

Primary PCI is the preferred method of reperfusion. The aim is to restore the blood supply at the earliest possible time to myocardium that has not yet been damaged irreversibly. Clinical trials have confirmed the effectiveness of early reperfusion therapy in reducing infarct size, complications, and mortality from AMI. Reperfusion therapy is most effective when undertaken very soon after the onset of myocardial infarction and the benefit diminishes progressively with delay. Beyond 12 h from the onset of chest pain, there may be little or no benefit from reperfusion therapy in many patients, but emergency PCI should be considered in this situation if there is clinical or ECG evidence of ongoing ischaemia.

PPCI is the preferred treatment for STEMI provided it can be performed by an experienced team in a timely manner. Coronary angiography is used to identify the occluded coronary artery, following which a guidewire is passed through the occluding thrombus. Passage of the guidewire may restore blood flow but use of a balloon or aspiration devices may be required to restore flow within the vessel. In some settings glycoprotein IIb/IIIa inhibitors may be injected IV or directly into the coronary artery as adjunctive anti-thrombotic therapy. A stent is then inserted into the previously occluded segment of the artery, to reduce the risk of re-occlusion. PPCI is the most reliable method of re-opening and maintaining the patency of the culprit artery in the majority of patients.

There is a lower risk of major bleeding, particularly intracerebral, with PPCI than with fibrinolytic therapy.

For PPCI to provide reliable, timely reperfusion a fully-equipped catheter laboratory, staffed by an experienced team, must be available 24 h per day. A fail-safe pathway of communication and care must be in place to ensure that patients in whom STEMI is diagnosed can access the service, ideally by direct transfer to this facility (Figure 4.10). Services should aim to achieve a 'call-to-balloon' time (i.e. time from call for help to attempted re-opening of the culprit artery) of < 120 min whenever possible. Delays to treatment are associated with higher mortality. Where PPCI is not available immediately, the need to achieve reperfusion as early as possible remains a high priority and for those patients initial treatment with fibrinolytic therapy may offer the best chance of achieving early reperfusion.

Effective PPCI requires the use of appropriate anti-thrombotic therapy. In addition to aspirin, all patients should also be given one of the platelet ADP receptor blockers prior to PPCI, using one of the following loading doses:

- clopidogrel 600 mg
- prasugrel 60 mg (not if > 75 years, < 60 kg, history of bleeding or stroke)
- ticagrelor 180 mg.

Anticoagulation with unfractionated or low molecular weight heparin is given in the catheter laboratory and in high-risk cases a glycoprotein IIb/IIIa inhibitor may also be given. Bivalirudin, a direct thrombin inhibitor may be chosen as an alternative to heparin.

Fibrinolytic therapy

Fibrinolytic therapy substantially reduces mortality from AMI when given during the first few hours after the onset of chest pain, but is less effective than PPCI and therefore not commonly used. The advantage of fibrinolytic therapy is that it does not require a cardiac catheter laboratory or skilled angioplasty team. Early reperfusion may be achieved by pre-hospital fibrinolytic therapy with resulting clinical benefit, particularly when transport times to hospital are very long. Early treatment may also be achieved by minimising door-to-needle time (time from arrival at hospital to administration of fibrinolytic therapy).

Fibrinolytic therapy carries a risk of bleeding, including cerebral haemorrhage, and not all patients can be given this treatment safely. Table 4.1 lists typical indications for reperfusion therapy and the typical contraindications to fibrinolytic drugs are shown in Table 4.2.

The algorithm in Figure 4.10 provides a guide to choosing reperfusion therapy for STEMI.

Whilst fibrinolytic therapy may reopen an occluded artery, additional antithrombotic therapy must be given to minimise the risk of further thrombotic occlusion.

Give all patients receiving a fibrinolytic agent for STEMI:

- aspirin as a 300 mg and ticagrelor 180 mg loading doses, or in patients with a high bleeding risk, aspirin 300 mg and clopidogrel 300 mg loading doses, or aspirin alone.
- antithrombin therapy:
  - low molecular weight heparin (IV bolus then SC), or
  - unfractionated heparin (full dose), or
  - fondaparinux.

Table 4.1   Typical indications for immediate fibrinolytic therapy for acute myocardial infarction

Typical indications for immediate fibrinolytic therapy for AMI
Presentation within 12 hours of onset of chest pain suggestive of AMI and PCI not possible within 120 minutes AND:
ST-segment elevation > 0.2 mV in 2 adjacent chest leads, OR
> 0.1 mV in 2 or more 'adjacent' limb leads, OR
Dominant R waves and ST depression in V1-V3 (posterior infarction), OR
New-onset (or presumed new-onset) LBBB

Table 4.2   Typical contraindications to fibrinolytic therapy

Typical contraindications for fibrinolytic therapy	
Absolute	Previous haemorrhagic stroke
	Ischaemic stroke during the previous 6 months
	Central nervous system damage or neoplasm
	Recent (within 3 weeks) major surgery, head injury or other major trauma
	Active internal bleeding (menses excluded) or gastrointestinal bleeding within the past month
	Known or suspected aortic dissection
	Known bleeding disorder
Relative	Refractory hypertension (systolic blood pressure > 180 mm Hg)
	Transient ischaemic attack in preceding 6 months
	Oral anticoagulant treatment
	Pregnancy or less than 1 week post-partum
	Traumatic CPR
	Non-compressible vascular puncture
	Active peptic ulcer disease
	Advanced liver disease
	Infective endocarditis
	Previous allergic reaction to the fibrinolytic drug to be used

Rescue angioplasty

In 20–30% of patients receiving a fibrinolytic drug for STEMI, reperfusion is not achieved. Observe patients closely with cardiac monitoring during and after administration of a fibrinolytic. Record a 12-lead ECG at 60–90 min after giving fibrinolytic therapy. Failure of ST-segment elevation to resolve by more than 50% compared with the pre-treatment ECG suggests that fibrinolytic therapy has failed to re-open the culprit artery. In some people, the transient, often brief occurrence of an accelerated idioventricular rhythm occurs as a 'reperfusion arrhythmia' (Figure 4.11), indicating that the artery has reopened, but this does not occur in all cases and may not always be witnessed or its significance recognised.

Symptoms are not a reliable guide to reperfusion, partly because many patients will have received opiate analgesia. Even after initially successful thrombolysis there is a significant risk of re-occlusion and patients should be admitted to a cardiac care unit with continuous ECG monitoring.

In cases of failed reperfusion (or re-occlusion and further infarction with recurrence of ST-segment elevation) transfer the patient without delay to a cardiac catheter laboratory for PCI. This is referred to as 'rescue PCI' and has been shown to improve event-free survival and

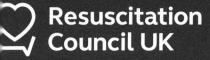
Adult reperfusion therapy (STEMI)

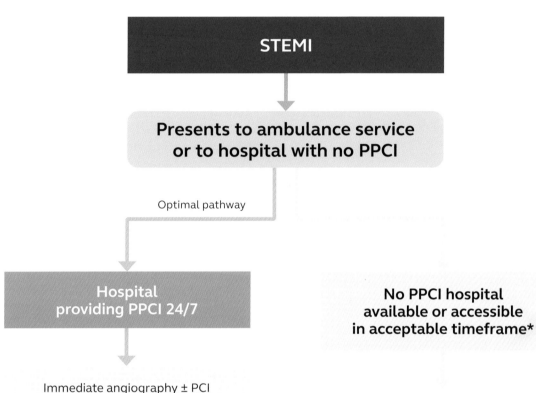

STEMI

Presents to ambulance service or to hospital with no PPCI

Optimal pathway

Hospital providing PPCI 24/7

Immediate angiography ± PCI

No PPCI hospital available or accessible in acceptable timeframe*

Pre-hospital or in-hospital fibrinolytic therapy

Failed thrombolysis

Successful thrombolysis

Immediate transfer to 24/7 PPCI hospital for rescue PCI

Angiography ± PCI during same admission

*see NICE CG 185 and ESC guidelines for STEMI

PCI – Percutaneous Coronary Intervention

PPCI – Primary PCI

Figure 4.10   Algorithm showing options for access to reperfusion therapy for STEMI

reduce heart failure when compared to more conservative therapy or repeat fibrinolytic therapy. Like PPCI, rescue PCI must be performed without any time delay in order to be effective.

Wherever possible, following initiation of fibrinolytic therapy, patients should be transferred to a PCI centre for early angiography (and PCI if indicated). Studies have shown that early routine angiography following thrombolysis, with PCI if required, reduced the rates of further infarction and recurrent ischaemia.

Treatment of NSTE ACS (unstable angina and NSTEMI)

In contrast to STEMI, there is no evidence of benefit from immediate reperfusion therapy in most patients with NSTE ACS (with ST-segment depression, T wave changes or normal ECGs), regardless of whether the ultimate diagnosis is UA or NSTEMI. There is no role for fibrinolytic therapy in these patients.

For patients with NSTE ACS, risk stratification to assess the likelihood of future events is required to guide further treatment. Patients with NSTEMI (positive biomarkers/ troponin) and patients with unstable angina (negative troponin) but other high-risk features have an increased risk of further coronary events and death. Patients who have been resuscitated from cardiac arrest due to suspected NSTE ACS are an especially high-risk group. All these higher-risk patients require immediate careful assessment (in most cases including coronary angiography to assess the need for revascularisation by PCI or coronary artery bypass surgery) and medical treatment (see below).

The immediate treatment objectives for all patients with these syndromes are:

- To prevent new thrombus formation, which may occlude an artery and lead to, or extend, myocardial damage.
- To reduce myocardial oxygen demand, providing myocardial cells with a better chance of survival in the presence of a limited supply of oxygen and glucose.

To prevent further thrombus formation:

- Give fondaparinux 2.5 mg once daily.
- Give aspirin 75 mg daily after the initial 300 mg loading dose.

In addition to aspirin, patients who have an elevated blood troponin (NSTEMI) or are planned for angiography +/- revascularisation should be given one of the platelet ADP receptor blockers in the following doses:

- Prasugrel 60 mg (contraindicated if > 75 years, < 60 kg, history of bleeding or stroke), then 10 mg daily maintenance dose.
- Ticagrelor 180 mg, then 90 mg twice daily maintenance dose.

Clopidogrel 300 mg, then 75 mg daily maintenance dose in patients who have another indication for anticoagulation.

In certain high-risk patients, if early PCI is planned, a glycoprotein IIb/IIIa inhibitor may be considered (tirofiban or eptifibatide). However it is not clear if they offer any additional benefit in patients on dual anti-platelet therapy and they are associated with increased bleeding.

To reduce myocardial oxygen demand:

- Start beta-adrenoceptor blockade (unless contraindicated).
- Consider diltiazem if beta blockade is contraindicated.
- Avoid dihydropyridine calcium channel blockers (e.g. nifedipine).
- Consider intravenous nitrate infusion if angina persists or recurs after sublingual nitrate.
- Consider early introduction of an angiotensin converting enzyme inhibitor (ACEI), especially if there is left ventricular systolic impairment or heart failure.
- Treat complications such as heart failure or tachyarrhythmia promptly and effectively.

Subsequent management of patients with acute coronary syndromes

Suspected unstable angina – low risk score

Patients with suspected unstable angina without high-risk features at presentation (ECG and troponin levels normal, low GRACE score) should undergo early further risk assessment by non-invasive imaging.

NSTEMI and high-risk unstable angina

Patients with unstable angina and high-risk features (e.g. resting ST-segment depression, high-risk features on non-invasive imaging or high GRACE score) should be considered for early investigation by percutaneous coronary angiography.

Patients with NSTEMI should be regarded as a high-risk group, requiring early assessment by coronary angiography within 72 h of presentation.

Many patients with high-risk NSTE ACS will benefit from revascularisation by PCI and some with complex coronary anatomy will require coronary artery bypass graft surgery. Use formal risk-scoring systems such as GRACE to guide clinical management. Those patients at the highest risk derive the greatest benefit from early intervention, in terms of reducing further major cardiac events.

STEMI

If fibrinolytic therapy has been used, many patients will be left with a severe stenosis or unstable plaque in the culprit coronary artery. PCI can stabilise this situation and reduce the risk of re-occlusion of the artery and resulting further myocardial infarction, cardiac arrest or sudden death.

Coronary angiography and, if indicated, PCI should be undertaken early during the same hospital admission. Patients who have had successful thrombolysis but are not in a PCI capable hospital should be transferred for angiography and possible PCI.

In patients with completed STEMI who have not been treated with reperfusion therapy (e.g. because of late presentation) it is usually recommended that coronary angiography is undertaken during the same hospital admission. Although the benefits of re-opening an occluded culprit artery late after STEMI are uncertain, there is often disease in other coronary vessels that can give rise to further major coronary events over subsequent months. Defining the severity and anatomy of such disease can help to identify those at highest risk, in whom early intervention may reduce that risk.

Cardiac rehabilitation

In all patients after an ACS, an effective programme of cardiac rehabilitation can speed the return to normal activity and encourage measures that will reduce future risk (see below). There is evidence that effective cardiac rehabilitation reduces readmission to hospital and improves overall prognosis and survival. Cardiac rehabilitation is a continuous process, beginning in the cardiac care unit and progressing through to a community-based approach to lifestyle modification and secondary prevention. Cardiac rehabilitation should include a supervised exercise programme.

Secondary prevention

In patients with established coronary disease, general measures to reduce cardiovascular risk ('secondary prevention') can reduce the likelihood of future coronary events (including sudden cardiac death) and stroke.

Anti-thrombotic therapy

Continued platelet inhibition is appropriate in all patients. They should receive low-dose aspirin (75 mg daily) for life, unless contraindicated. Give clopidogrel 75 mg daily/ or prasugrel 10 mg daily/ or ticagrelor 90 mg twice daily to patients with high-risk ACS and all those undergoing PCI; current guidelines recommend treatment for a minimum of one year. Clopidogrel alone may be used in patients who are intolerant of aspirin. In patients who develop atrial fibrillation as a complication of ischaemic heart disease, there is an additional risk of thromboembolism from the left atrium. Treatment with warfarin or a novel oral anticoagulant is more effective than aspirin or clopidogrel in preventing intra-cardiac thrombus formation, and should be considered in addition to, or instead of platelet inhibition.

Preservation of left ventricular function

Prognosis after AMI is partly determined by the severity of left ventricular impairment. Treatment after AMI with an ACEI can reduce the re-modelling that contributes to left ventricular dilatation and impairment, and where there is left ventricular systolic impairment, the use of ACEI therapy in adequate dose can reduce the risk and severity of subsequent heart failure, and the risk of future AMI and death. Echocardiographic examination of left ventricular function is appropriate during the first few days after an ACS to assess risk and identify those patients likely to benefit most from this treatment. The majority of patients should be considered for ACEI treatment during the first few days after AMI. Those with heart failure and reduced left ventricular ejection fraction should also be offered an aldosterone antagonist.

Beta-adrenoceptor blockade

Treatment with a beta-blocker, started early after AMI and continued, has been shown to reduce mortality. In the absence of a contraindication, a beta-blocker should be started in the acute phase of treatment and continued indefinitely. Careful dose adjustment is needed in each individual patient to achieve adequate beta blockade whilst avoiding adverse effects. There is evidence that prior treatment with beta blockade may reduce the size of subsequent myocardial infarction, so in patients with coronary disease this treatment may have a 'cardioprotective' effect, and it may help to protect against other complications such as arrhythmia. In patients with chronic heart failure and left ventricular systolic impairment there is evidence of symptomatic and prognostic benefit from some beta blocking drugs.

Reduction of cholesterol

Further reduction in risk can be achieved by effective suppression of cholesterol concentration in the blood, specifically suppression of LDL cholesterol. Statins reduce the risk of future coronary events by at least 30%. A low-fat, high-fibre diet and regular exercise will complement cholesterol suppression by drugs. High-dose statin treatment is usually advised after an ACS (e.g. atorvastatin 80 mg daily).

Stopping smoking

At least as important in reducing risk, is the removal of other avoidable risk factors such as smoking. Advise all people who smoke to stop and offer assistance from a smoking cessation service. Information, encouragement and support for patients to help them to stop smoking should begin at an early stage after presentation with an ACS.

Anti-hypertensive treatment

Effective control of raised blood pressure, using drugs as well as non-pharmacological methods, reduces the risk of stroke and of heart failure and contributes to some reduction in the risk of future coronary events.

Cardiac arrhythmia complicating acute coronary syndromes

Ventricular arrhythmia in ACS

In some people, cardiac arrest in VF or pulseless VT (pVT) may be the presenting feature of an ACS. If return of spontaneous circulation (ROSC) is achieved in a person whose cardiac arrest is a likely to be due to an ACS, record a 12-lead ECG as soon as possible. If this shows evidence of STEMI, emergency reperfusion therapy is needed, whenever possible by PPCI, together with all other treatment for STEMI. This also applies to those patients with STEMI who are unconscious and ventilated after ROSC (See Chapter 13). If NSTEMI is suspected as the cause of the arrest consider urgent coronary angiography with a view to PCI if necessary, together with all other treatment for a high-risk NSTE ACS. Where cardiac arrest is very likely to be due to an ACS but usual advanced life support measures fail to achieve ROSC, in some hospitals it is possible to consider the use of a mechanical chest compression device or extracorporeal CPR to enable coronary angiography and PCI to be performed as part of the ongoing resuscitation attempt.

When ventricular arrhythmia complicates an acute coronary syndrome (Figure 4.7), interpret its significance in the context of the clinical setting and the time of onset of the arrhythmia relative to the onset of the ACS. If an arrhythmia occurs within 24–48 h of a confirmed ACS an implantable cardioverter-defibrillator (ICD) is not indicated unless the patient has persistent severely impaired LV function at least 4 weeks post ACS. If a sustained ventricular arrhythmia occurs more than 24–48 h after an ACS an inpatient defibrillator is usually recommended unless the arrhythmia was associated with significant myocardial ischaemia which can be reversed by revascularisation. If the arrhythmia has occurred without evidence of severe ischaemia, the patient will be at risk of recurrent ventricular arrhythmia and should be referred to a heart rhythm specialist with a view to insertion of an ICD before discharge from hospital.

Patients who have a VF/pVT cardiac arrest as a late complication after myocardial infarction, or outside the context of an ACS, are at risk of recurrent cardiac arrest and should be seen by a heart rhythm specialist with a view to ICD implantation before discharge from hospital.

When an arrhythmia occurs in the setting of an ACS it is important to check for and treat other factors that may have predisposed to the arrythmia (e.g. hypokalaemia, heart failure).

It is important to recognise an accelerated idioventricular rhythm that is seen commonly and transiently after reperfusion of a previously occluded coronary artery, whether following PCI or after fibrinolysis. An example is shown in Figure 4.11.

After fibrinolytic therapy this may provide strong indication that thrombolysis has been achieved. These rhythms are usually transient and do not require treatment.

Other cardiac arrhythmia

The treatment of other cardiac arrhythmia will be covered in more detail in Chapter 11.

When atrial fibrillation occurs in the context of an ACS it may indicate left ventricular failure: treatment should address that as well as focusing on control of heart rate or rhythm.

When AV block occurs in the context of an inferior AMI there is often transient dysfunction of the conducting system and excessive vagal activity. QRS complexes are often narrow and the heart rate may not be especially slow. Treat symptomatic bradycardia in this setting with atropine; consider temporary cardiac pacing only if bradycardia and hypotension persist after atropine.

Complete AV block in this setting is usually transient and permanent cardiac pacing is rarely necessary. The heart block often resolves after PPCI, so do not delay arrangements for PPCI because of AV block in this setting.

When AV block occurs in the context of acute anterior myocardial infarction this usually implies extensive myocardial injury and a poor prognosis. The QRS complexes are usually broad and the heart rate is usually slow and resistant to atropine. Temporary cardiac pacing is usually needed and should not be delayed.

Cardiac arrest in the cardiac catheter laboratory

Data from the National Cardiac Arrest Audit show that around 4% of in-hospital cardiac arrests occur in the cardiac catheter laboratory. Patients who have a cardiac arrest in the catheter laboratory may have been stable prior to the procedure (e.g. having an elective procedure) or critically-ill (e.g. post-cardiac arrest patient with cardiogenic shock).

If the initial rhythm is shockable (VF/VT), up to three stacked shocks should be attempted. If there is no ROSC, then the standard ALS algorithm should be followed. Subsequent management will depend on whether the cardiologist wishes to proceed with angiography and intervention during cardiac arrest, or to delay until after ROSC. Return of spontaneous circulation may only be feasible after PCI. PCI is feasible during CPR either by use of a mechanical compression device, or in settings where it is available, extracorporeal-CPR (veno-arterial extra-corporeal membrane oxygenation (VA-ECMO)).

Other complications of ACS

Heart failure

Patients with heart failure complicating AMI or other ACS are at increased risk of deterioration, cardiac arrest and death: prompt, effective treatment of the heart failure is required to reduce risk. Give a loop diuretic (e.g. furosemide) and/or glyceryl trinitrate (sublingual and/or intravenous) for immediate symptomatic treatment. Give regular loop diuretic to maintain symptom control. Ensure that ACEI treatment has been started and increase the dose as tolerated, until the target dose is achieved. In patients intolerant of ACEI, consider an angiotensin receptor blocker. Maintain beta blockade and increase the dose as tolerated, unless contraindicated. For patients with heart failure or significant LV systolic impairment (ejection fraction 40% or less) start an aldosterone antagonist (e.g. eplerenone or spironolactone).

Cardiogenic shock

This consists of hypotension with poor peripheral perfusion, often accompanied by pulmonary oedema, drowsiness or mental confusion due to poor cerebral perfusion and oliguria caused by poor renal perfusion. The mortality is very high, but can be reduced by early revascularisation.

Some patients may improve with inotropic therapy, but this requires initiation and supervision by those experienced in its use. Other treatments such as intra-aortic balloon pumping, other forms of mechanical circulatory support and ventilatory support may be considered in selected patients. These require expert assessment and management in an ICU by a specialist multidisciplinary team.

When cardiogenic shock develops in a patient after STEMI, seek early expert help. Consider acute complications such as myocardial rupture, papillary muscle rupture, ventricular septal defect and interventions such as surgery, repeat angiography or mechanical circulatory support.

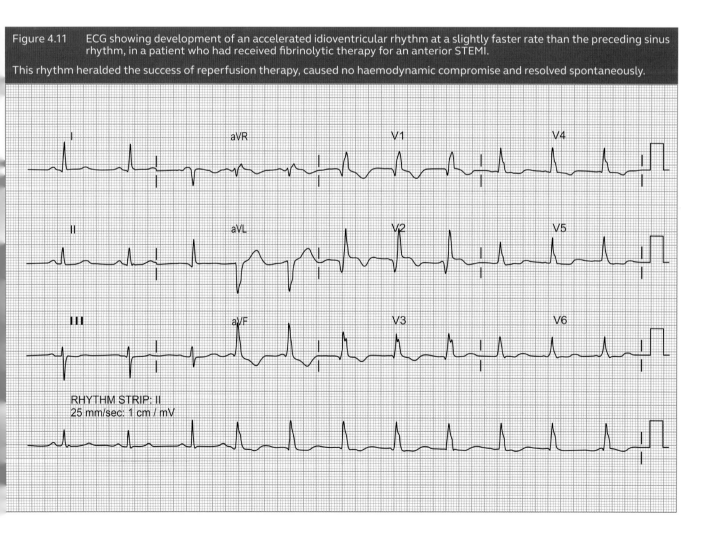

Figure 4.11   ECG showing development of an accelerated idioventricular rhythm at a slightly faster rate than the preceding sinus rhythm, in a patient who had received fibrinolytic therapy for an anterior STEMI.

This rhythm heralded the success of reperfusion therapy, caused no haemodynamic compromise and resolved spontaneously.

Table 4.3   Important causes of sudden cardiac death
Reproduced from: Pitcher D. Sudden Cardiac Death. In ABC of Resuscitation,
Sixth Edition 2012 Soar J, Perkins G, Nolan J eds. Wiley-Blackwell; Oxford.

Condition	Causes	Further detail
Long QT syndromes (LQTS)	Inherited (autosomal dominant) ion channel disorders Many different genotypes but types 1–3 are most common	Predispose to torsade de pointes VT and VF
Acquired QT interval prolongation	Drug therapy Ischaemic heart disease Myocarditis	Predisposes to torsade de pointes VT and VF
Brugada syndrome	Inherited (autosomal dominant) ion channel disorder	Occurs worldwide but more common in SE Asia Risk of SCD higher in young males
Short QT syndrome (SQTS)	Rare, inherited (autosomal dominant) ion channel disorder	Predisposes to torsade de pointes VT and VF
Catecholaminergic polymorphic ventricular tachycardia (CPVT)	Rare, inherited (autosomal dominant) ion channel disorder	Predisposes to torsade de pointes VT and VF, especially on exercise
Arrhythmogenic right ventricular cardiomyopathy (ARVC)	Inherited (autosomal dominant)	Predisposes to VT and VF
Hypertrophic cardiomyopathy (HCM)	Inherited (autosomal dominant) Several different genotypes	SCD risk is due to VT and VF. Risk varies with genotype and with individual factors
Wolff-Parkinson-White (WPW) syndrome	Mostly sporadic Infrequent familial incidence	Not all WPW patients are at risk of SCD. Risk is due to rapid transmission of AF to the ventricles, triggering VT or VF
High-grade atrioventricular block	Conducting system fibrosis Calcific aortic stenosis Myocardial diseases including ischaemic heart disease Cardiac surgery Drug therapy Occasionally congenital	Predisposes to ventricular standstill (asystole) Some people with extreme bradycardia develop torsade de pointes VT and VF
Severe aortic stenosis	Congenital bicuspid valve (becomes severe at age 50–70 or younger) Degenerative (becomes severe in elderly patients)	If untreated may progress to heart failure or SCD, probably mostly due to VT or VF
Dilated cardiomyopathy	Probably multiple causes Familial in a minority of cases	Many develop progressive heart failure but there is risk of SCD due to VT or VF
Ischaemic heart disease due to coronary atheroma	Partly genetic, partly acquired	SCD risk is mainly due to VT or VF, which may be in response to acute ischaemia or infarction or may be due to previous myocardial scarring SCD risk is mainly due to VT or VF, which may be in response to acute ischaemia or infarction or may be due to previous myocardial scarring
Other myocardial diseases	Hypertensive heart disease, sarcoid heart disease etc	May predispose to ventricular arrhythmia or AVB in some patients
Anomalous coronary artery anatomy	Congenital	Rare cause of SCD in young people, often on exercise. Risk varies with the anomalous anatomical pattern
Adult congenital heart disease	Congenital	Patients with adult congenital heart disease often remain at risk of cardiac arrest due to tachycardia and bradycardia even when they have had corrective surgery as a child

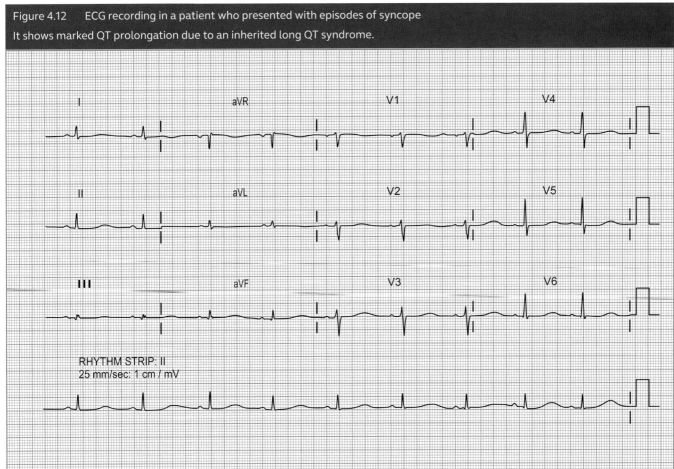

Figure 4.12 ECG recording in a patient who presented with episodes of syncope
It shows marked QT prolongation due to an inherited long QT syndrome.

Other cardiac causes of cardiac arrest and sudden cardiac death

Whilst coronary artery disease is the commonest cause of cardiac arrest and sudden cardiac death (SCD) in adults over the age of 35 years, other (mostly acquired) conditions can cause SCD in this age group. Inherited conditions are a less common cause in older adults but predominate as the causes of SCD in people under the age of 35. Table 4.3 lists some of the important causes.

Identifying the cause of a cardiac arrest or sudden death

When someone has a cardiac arrest or dies suddenly, it is important to obtain as much detail as possible of the circumstances of the event in order to assist in identifying the cause. Following SCD, the autopsy is crucial as it may identify some inherited conditions (e.g. hypertrophic cardiomyopathy, arrhythmogenic right ventricular cardiomyopathy) and enable screening of family members to identify others at risk in whom treatment may prevent SCD. Detailed examination of hearts of SCD patients by an expert cardiac pathologist is recommended as these conditions may not always be easy to confirm or exclude at a routine autopsy. In addition tissue samples for a 'molecular autopsy' may identify inherited conditions (e.g. channelopathies). If no abnormality is found at autopsy to explain SCD, this is termed sudden arrhythmic death syndrome (SADS). This should always raise suspicion of an 'electrical' inherited cardiac condition that may affect other family members and place them at similar risk.

When a person has a cardiac arrest it is important that those attempting resuscitation consider from the outset the likely cause of the arrest. This may identify a reversible cause, but may also lead to early recognition of a cause that will guide management of the resuscitation effort and/or post-resuscitation care. This is equally important in out-of-hospital and in-hospital cardiac arrest. A detailed history of the event, clinical examination following ROSC, a 12-lead ECG recorded as soon as possible after ROSC and echocardiography as soon as practicable may each provide evidence that allows early recognition of one of the conditions listed in Table 4.3.

Identifying people at risk

Whilst is important to consider the cause in every instance of cardiac arrest and sudden death, you should be alert also for warning symptoms that may allow recognition and treatment of a life-threatening condition, so preventing cardiac arrest or SCD. For example, in people with severe aortic stenosis those symptoms might be angina, breathlessness or syncope. People at risk of sudden death from cardiac arrhythmia may experience syncope (Figure 4.12). Assess people who experience one or more episodes of syncope to identify features of common problems that do not carry a significant risk of death (such as uncomplicated faints) and to identify the small minority of people in whom syncope may be the only warning of a preventable risk of SCD. Syncope that occurs during exertion should raise particular concern and lead to urgent, expert assessment.

Increasingly, screening of asymptomatic people may lead to identification of clinical signs, or of ECG or echocardiographic abnormalities that lead to diagnosis of a condition predisposing to cardiac arrest and SCD. There is international debate about the cost-effectiveness of screening low-risk groups and the screening techniques that are appropriate. Various groups of people may undergo screening including sportspeople, pilots and family members of people with inherited cardiac conditions (ICCs) or suspected ICCs. In the latter group screening is best coordinated through a dedicated cardiology-genetics clinic dealing specifically with ICCs.

Avoidance of cardiac arrest in people at risk

The treatment needed to minimise the risk of cardiac arrest and SCD depends largely on the underlying condition, but also varies according to individual circumstances in people with the same condition. In some people, reducing risk of SCD requires avoidance of specific activities or circumstances that predispose to SCD in their specific situation. In many people with a long QT syndrome, beta blockade may be the only treatment needed to reduce risk to a minimum, but in others beta blockade may provide insufficient protection and an ICD may be needed. In severe aortic stenosis, aortic valve replacement is likely to offer an opportunity for risk reduction. In complete AV block pacemaker implantation restores average life expectancy to normal for the person's age. These examples are not exhaustive and are mentioned to illustrate the range of conditions and treatments that must be considered. Urgent, detailed specialist assessment is needed. Refer anyone thought to be at risk to the most appropriate specialist without delay.

04: Summary learning

The acute coronary syndromes comprise unstable angina, NSTEMI and STEMI.

Rapid initial assessment by history, examination and 12-lead ECG will help to determine the diagnosis and immediate risk.

Give aspirin to patients presenting with ACS.

Give nitroglycerine and, if required, morphine (with an anti-emetic) to relieve pain.

Do not routinely give oxygen unless the patient is hypoxaemic. Aim to achieve SpO_2 94–98% (88–92% in hypercapnic respiratory failure).

Consider immediate reperfusion therapy (preferably by PPCI) in people with STEMI or AMI with new LBBB.

Consider early coronary angiography (+/- revascularisation) in people with NSTEMI or high-risk unstable angina.

Effective assessment and immediate treatment of patients with ACS will reduce the risk of cardiac arrest and death.

A range of other cardiac conditions can cause cardiac arrest and sudden death.

When a person has a cardiac arrest or SCD obtain detailed information about the event and consider the most likely cause.

Assess people with syncope to identify those in whom it may be a warning symptom of a risk of SCD that may be prevented.

Refer people who may be at risk (and/or their families where appropriate) for appropriate expert assessment.

My key take-home messages from this chapter are:

Further reading

Collet JP, Thiele H, Barbato E, et al. 2020 ESC Guidelines for the management of acute coronary syndromes in patients presenting without persistent ST-segment elevation. Eur Heart J. 2020: ehaa575.

Lott C, Truhlár A, Alfonzo A, Barelli A, González-Salvado V, Hinkelbein J, Nolan JP, Paal P, Perkins GD, Thies K-C, Yeung J, Zideman DA, Soar J. European Resuscitation Council Guidelines 2021: Cardiac arrest in special circumstances. Resuscitation. 2021;161.

National Institute for Health and Care Excellence. Clinical Guideline 185. Acute coronary syndromes. NICE 2020 - https://www.nice.org.uk/guidance/ng185

Nolan JP, Böttiger BW, Cariou A, Cronberg T, Friberg H, Gengrugge C, Haywood K, Lilja G, Moulaert VRM, Nikolaou N, Olasveengen TM, Skrifvars MB, Taccone FS, Soar J. European Resuscitation Council and European Society of Intensive Care Medicine Guidelines 2021: Post-resuscitation Care. Resuscitation. 2021;161.

Soar J, Böttiger BW, Carli P, Couper K, Deakin CD, Djärv T, Lott C, Olasveengen TM, Paal P, Pellis T, Perkins GD, Sandroni C, Nolan JP. European Resuscitation Council Guidelines 2021: Advanced Life Support. Resuscitation. 2021;161.

Thygesen K, Alpert JS, Jaffe AS, et al. Executive Group on behalf of the Joint European Society of Cardiology (ESC)/American College of Cardiology (ACC)/American Heart Association (AHA)/World Heart Federation (WHF) Task Force for the Universal Definition of Myocardial Infarction. Fourth Universal Definition of Myocardial Infarction (2018). Circulation. 2018 Nov 13;138(20):e618-e651.

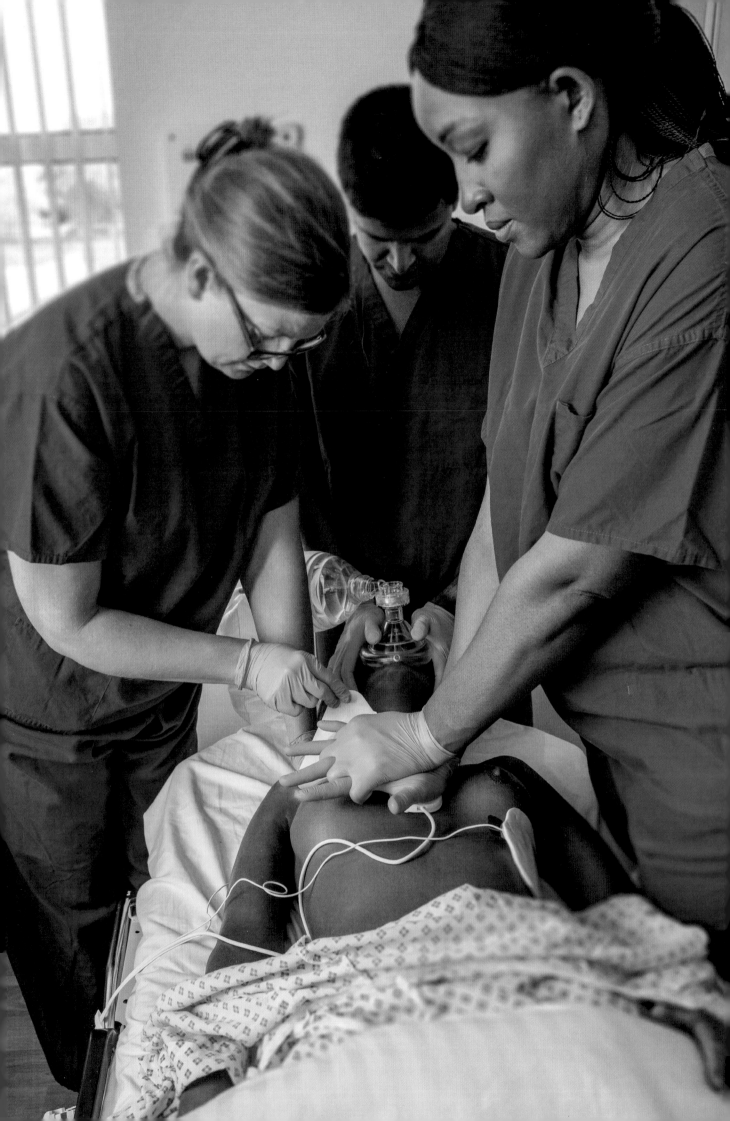

In-hospital resuscitation

In this chapter

Features specific to in-hospital resuscitation

Sequence for the collapsed patient in hospital

The learning outcomes will enable you to:

Start resuscitation in hospital

Maintain high-quality cardiopulmonary resuscitation (CPR) with minimal interruption

Prioritise your actions according to the in-hospital algorithm

Introduction

After in-hospital cardiac arrest, the division between basic life support (BLS) and advanced life support (ALS) is arbitrary; in practice, the resuscitation process is a continuum. The public expect that all clinical staff can undertake CPR.

For every in-hospital cardiac arrest, ensure that:

- cardiorespiratory arrest is recognised immediately
- help is summoned using a standard telephone number (2222 in the UK)
- CPR is started immediately and, if indicated, defibrillation is attempted as soon as possible (within 3 min).

This chapter is primarily for healthcare professionals who are first to respond to an in-hospital cardiac arrest, but may also be relevant to healthcare professionals working in other clinical settings.

Features specific to in-hospital resuscitation

The exact sequence of actions after in-hospital cardiac arrest depends on several factors including:

- location (clinical/non-clinical area; monitored/unmonitored area)
- skills of the first responders
- number of responders
- equipment available
- hospital response system to cardiac arrest and medical emergencies (e.g. medical emergency team (MET), resuscitation team).

Location

In patients who are being monitored closely, clinical deterioration and cardiorespiratory arrest is usually identified rapidly. Patients in areas without facilities for close monitoring can have unobserved deterioration and an unwitnessed cardiorespiratory arrest. All patients who are at high risk of cardiac arrest should be cared for in a monitored area where facilities for immediate resuscitation are available. Patients, visitors or staff may also have a cardiac arrest in non-clinical areas (e.g. car parks, corridors).

Cardiac arrest patients may have to be moved to enable effective resuscitation. Resuscitation Council UK has published guidance for safer handling during resuscitation in healthcare settings:

https://www.resus.org.uk/library/publications/publication-guidance-safer-handling

Training of first responders

All healthcare professionals should be able to recognise cardiac arrest, call for help and start resuscitation. Staff should do what they have been trained to do; for example, staff in critical care and emergency medicine may have more advanced resuscitation skills and greater experience in resuscitation than those who are not involved regularly in resuscitation in their normal clinical role. Hospital staff responding to a cardiac arrest may have different levels of skill to manage the airway, breathing and circulation. Rescuers must undertake tasks and procedures in which they are trained and proficient or with appropriate clinical supervision.

Number of responders

The single responder must first ensure help is coming. Usually, other staff are nearby and the resuscitation team called whilst other staff start CPR simultaneously. Hospital staff numbers tend to be fewer at night and weekends. This may influence patient monitoring, recognition, treatment and outcomes; studies show that survival rates from in-hospital cardiac arrest are lower during nights and weekends.

Equipment available

Staff in all clinical areas should have immediate access to resuscitation equipment and drugs to facilitate rapid resuscitation of the patient in cardiorespiratory arrest. The equipment used for CPR (including defibrillators) and the layout of equipment and drugs should be standardised throughout the hospital. You should be familiar with the resuscitation equipment used in your clinical area.

A review by Resuscitation Council UK of serious patient safety incidents associated with CPR and patient deterioration showed that equipment problems during resuscitation (e.g. equipment missing or not working) are common. All resuscitation equipment needs to be checked on a regular basis to ensure it is ready for use. Specially designed trolleys or sealed tray systems can improve speed of access to equipment and reduce adverse incidents.

Defibrillators with automated rhythm recognition should be considered for use in clinical and non-clinical areas where staff do not have rhythm recognition skills or rarely need to use a defibrillator. However, manual defibrillators used by trained staff who are able to recognise a shockable rhythm and deliver a shock rapidly are associated with increased survival after in-hospital cardiac arrest compared with when automated external defibrillators (AEDs) are used. Use an AED when someone trained to use a manual defibrillator is not immediately available, or when only an AED is available.

Waveform capnography must be used to confirm correct tracheal tube placement during resuscitation and can also help guide resuscitation interventions (Chapter 6). Waveform capnography monitoring is available on newer defibrillators, as part of portable monitors or as a hand held device. After successful resuscitation, patients often need transferring to other clinical areas (e.g. intensive care unit) or other hospitals. Transfer equipment and drugs should be available to enable this.

Resuscitation team

Hospitals should have a system to recognise patients at risk of cardiac arrest and allow staff to call a resuscitation team before cardiac arrest occurs. For example, the medical emergency team (MET) deals with patients who are deteriorating and at risk of cardiac arrest. In-hospital cardiac arrests are rarely sudden or unexpected. A strategy of recognising patients at risk of cardiac arrest may enable some of these arrests to be prevented or prevent futile resuscitation attempts in those who are unlikely to benefit from CPR (Chapter 3).

Resuscitation teams should have formal briefings for introductions and to plan their roles and responsibilities during actual resuscitation events. Team members should also participate in a debriefing after each event to allow performance and concerns to be discussed openly. This has most benefit when discussions are based on data collected during the event.

Sequence for a collapsed patient in hospital

An algorithm for the initial management of in-hospital cardiac arrest is shown in Figure 5.1.

1. Ensure personal safety

- There are very few reports of harm to rescuers during resuscitation.
- Your personal safety and that of resuscitation team members is the first priority during any resuscitation attempt.
- Check that the patient's surroundings are safe.
- Put on gloves as soon as possible. Other personal protective equipment (PPE) (eye protection, face masks, aprons, gowns) may be necessary especially when the patient has a serious infection. The risk of transmitting severe acute respiratory distress syndrome coronavirus 2 (SARS-CoV-2) through mouth-to-mouth is extremely high and confirmed or suspected coronavirus disease 2019 (COVID-19) is a contraindication to mouth-to-mouth ventilation in clinical settings. Check the Resuscitation Council UK website for the latest guidance regarding PPE for CPR: https://www.resus.org.uk/
- Be careful with sharps; a sharps box must be available.
- Use safe handling techniques for moving patients during resuscitation.
- Take care with patients exposed to poisons. For example, avoid mouth-to-mouth ventilation and exhaled air in hydrogen cyanide or hydrogen sulphide poisoning. Avoid contact with corrosive chemicals (e.g. strong acids, alkalis, paraquat) or substances such as organophosphates that are easily absorbed through the skin or respiratory tract.

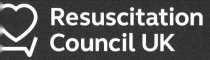
Adult in-hospital resuscitation

Maintain
personal
safety

**Collapsed/sick
patient**

**Shout for HELP
and assess patient**

Signs of life?
- Check for consciousness and normal breathing
- Experienced ALS providers should simultaneously check for carotid pulse

**NO
(or any doubt)**

YES

CARDIAC ARREST

Call and collect*
CALL resuscitation team
COLLECT resuscitation equipment

High-quality CPR*
Give high-quality CPR with oxygen
and airway adjuncts*
Switch compressor at every
rhythm assessment

Defibrillation*
Apply pads/turn on defibrillator/AED
Attempt defibrillation if indicated**

Advanced life support
When sufficient skilled personnel
are present

Handover
Handover to
resuscitation team

MEDICAL EMERGENCY

Call and collect*
CALL resuscitation / medical
emergency team if needed
COLLECT resuscitation equipment

Assess*
ABCDE assessment –
recognise and treat
Give high-flow oxygen
(titrate to SpO_2 when able)
Attach monitoring
Vascular access
Consider call for resuscitation/
medical emergency team
(if not already called)

Handover
Handover to resuscitation/
medical emergency team

* Undertake actions concurrently
if sufficient staff available

** Use a manual defibrillator if trained
and device available

Figure 5.1   Adult in-hospital resuscitation algorithm   63

2. Check the patient for a response

- If you see a patient collapse, or find a patient apparently unconscious, assess if they are responsive (shake and shout). Gently shake their shoulders and ask loudly: "Are you all right?" (Figure 5.2).
- If other members of staff are nearby it will be possible to undertake actions simultaneously.

3A. If they respond

- Urgent medical assessment is required. Call for help according to local protocols. This may include calling a resuscitation team (e.g. MET).
- While waiting for the team, assess the patient using the ABCDE (Airway, Breathing, Circulation, Disability, Exposure) approach.

  A B C D E

- Give the patient oxygen. Use a pulse oximeter to guide oxygen therapy.
- Attach monitoring: a minimum of pulse oximetry, ECG and blood pressure. Record vital signs observations and calculate the early warning score.
- Obtain venous access, and take blood samples for investigation.
- Prepare for handover using SBARD (Situation, Background, Assessment, Recommendation, Decision) or RSVP (Reason, Story, Vital signs, Plan).

3B. If no response

- The exact sequence will depend on your training and experience in assessment of breathing and circulation in sick patients.
- Shout for help (if not already).
- Turn the patient on to their back.
- Open the airway using head tilt and chin lift (Figure 5.3).
- If there is a risk of cervical spine injury, establish a clear upper airway by using jaw thrust or chin lift in combination with manual in-line stabilisation (MILS) of the head and neck by an assistant (if enough people are available). If life-threatening airway obstruction persists despite effective application of jaw thrust or chin lift, add head tilt a small amount at a time until the airway is open; establishing a patent airway, oxygenation and ventilation takes priority over concerns about a potential cervical spine injury.
- Keeping the airway open, look, listen, and feel to determine if the patient is breathing normally. This is a rapid check and should take less than 10 s:
  - Look for chest movement (breathing or coughing)
  - Look for any other movement or signs of life
  - Listen at the patient's mouth for breath sounds
  - Feel for air on your cheek.

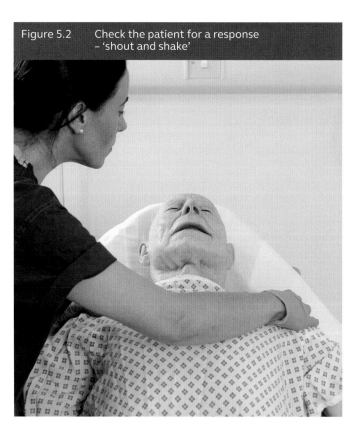

Figure 5.2   Check the patient for a response – 'shout and shake'

- If trained and experienced in the assessment of sick patients, check for breathing and assess the carotid pulse at the same time (Figure 5.4).
- Agonal breathing (occasional, irregular gasps) is common in the early stages of cardiac arrest and is a sign of cardiac arrest and should not be confused as a sign of life/circulation. Agonal breathing and limb movement can also occur during chest compressions as cerebral perfusion improves, but is not indicative of a return of spontaneous circulation.
- A very short period of seizure-like movements can occur at the start of cardiac arrest.
- Starting CPR on a very sick patient with a low cardiac output rarely causes significant damage and can be beneficial. However, a delay in diagnosis of cardiac arrest and starting CPR will affect survival adversely and must be avoided.
- If there is any doubt about the presence or absence of signs of life or a pulse, start CPR immediately (step 4B). Delays in diagnosis of cardiac arrest and starting CPR will affect survival adversely and must be avoided. Several studies show that even trained healthcare staff cannot assess the breathing and pulse sufficiently reliably to confirm cardiac arrest. If the patient is already attached to monitoring in a critical care area this will add to, rather than replace, the assessment for signs of life.

Figure 5.3	Head tilt and chin lift

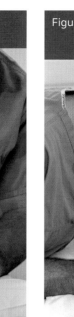

Top view

Side view

Figure 5.4	Simultaneous check for breathing, pulse and signs of life

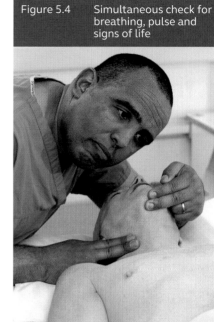

4A. If there are signs of life or a pulse

- Urgent medical assessment is required. Depending on the local protocols, this may take the form of a resuscitation team. While awaiting the team, assess and treat the patient using the ABCDE approach, give oxygen, attach monitoring and insert an intravenous cannula.

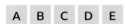

A B C D E

- Follow the steps in 3A whilst waiting for the team.

- The patient is at high risk of further deterioration and cardiac arrest and needs continued observation until the team arrives.

4B. If there are no signs of life and no pulse

- Start CPR and get a colleague to call the resuscitation team and collect the resuscitation equipment and a defibrillator.

- If alone, leave the patient to get help and equipment.

- Give 30 chest compressions followed by 2 ventilations.

- The correct hand position for chest compression is the middle of the lower half of the sternum.

- This hand position can be found quickly if you have been taught to 'place the heel of one hand in the centre of the chest with the other hand on top' and your teaching included a demonstration of placing hands in the middle of the lower half of the sternum (Figure 5.5).

- Ensure high-quality chest compressions:
  - depth of 5–6 cm
  - rate of 100–120 compressions min^{-1}
  - allow the chest to recoil completely after each compression
  - take approximately the same amount of time for compression and relaxation
  - minimise any interruptions to chest compression (hands-off time).

- If available, use a prompt and/or feedback device to help ensure high-quality chest compressions. Do not rely on a palpable carotid or femoral pulse to assess effective arterial flow.

- Each time compressions are resumed, place your hands without delay in the centre of the chest.

- The quality of chest compressions delivered by a single rescuer can decay over time, often even before they feel tired. If there are enough team members, this person should change about every 2 min or

Figure 5.5	Hand position for chest compressions

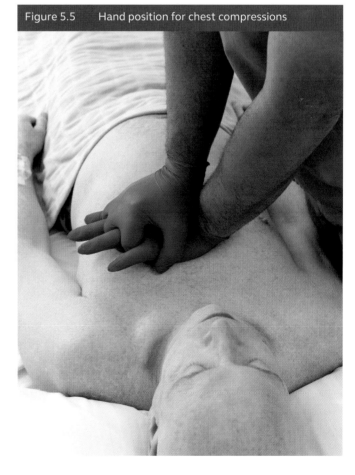

sooner if they are unable to maintain high-quality chest compressions. This change should be done with minimal interruption to compressions and this should be done during planned pauses in chest compressions such as during rhythm assessment.

- Use whatever equipment is available immediately for airway and ventilation; for example, a self-inflating bag-mask (Figure 5.6), or a supraglottic airway (e.g. i-gel) and bag. In practice patients can have several airway techniques used during a cardiac arrest as equipment arrives and according to the skills of the rescuer.

- Although previously advocated, mouth-to-mask was not a popular technique because of the requirement for the rescuer to be close to the patient's face. The COVID-19 pandemic has raised awareness of infection risk particularly when undertaking airway manoeuvres; consequently the use of a pocket mask technique is no longer recommended in clinical settings.

- Use an inspiratory time of about 1 s and give enough volume to produce a visible rise of the chest wall. Add supplemental oxygen as soon as possible.

- Avoid rapid or forceful breaths.

- Tracheal intubation should be attempted only by those who are trained, competent and experienced in this skill, and can insert the tracheal tube with minimal interruption (less than 5 s) to chest compressions. Waveform capnography must be routinely used for confirming that a tracheal tube is in the patient's airway and subsequent monitoring during CPR. Waveform capnography can also be used to monitor the quality of CPR, as an indicator of a return of spontaneous circulation (ROSC) and as a prognostic indicator. Once the patient's trachea

has been intubated, continue chest compressions uninterrupted (except for defibrillation or pulse checks when indicated), at a rate of 100–120 min^{-1}, and ventilate the lungs at approximately 10 breaths min^{-1} (i.e. do not stop chest compressions for ventilation). If a supraglottic airway (e.g. i-gel) has been inserted it may also be possible to ventilate the patient without stopping chest compressions.

- Early defibrillation is the priority if the rhythm is shockable. As soon as the defibrillator arrives, apply the self-adhesive defibrillation electrodes to the patient and analyse the rhythm. These should be applied whilst chest compressions are ongoing (Figure 5.7) The use of adhesive electrode pads will enable rapid assessment of heart rhythm compared with the use of ECG electrodes.

- For manual defibrillation, minimise the interruption to CPR to deliver a shock (Chapter 9). Using a manual defibrillator, it is possible to reduce the pause between stopping and restarting of chest compressions to less than 5 s.

- Once the pads are applied, pause briefly for a rapid rhythm check – aim for a pause in chest compressions of less than 5 s for the rhythm check. If the rhythm is ventricular fibrillation/pulseless ventricular tachycardia (VF/pVT), restart chest compressions. All other team members must now be informed to stand clear of the patient whilst the defibrillator is charged and a safety check performed (Figure 5.8). Once the defibrillator is charged and the safety check completed, stop chest compressions, deliver the shock and restart chest compressions immediately.

- The length of the pre-shock pause, the interval between stopping chest compressions and delivering a shock, is inversely proportional to the chance of

| Figure 5.6 | Two-person bag-mask ventilation during CPR |
| Figure 5.7 | Maintain chest compressions while self-adhesive pads are applied |

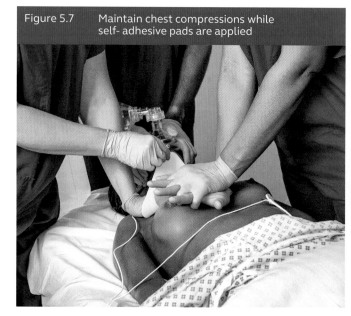

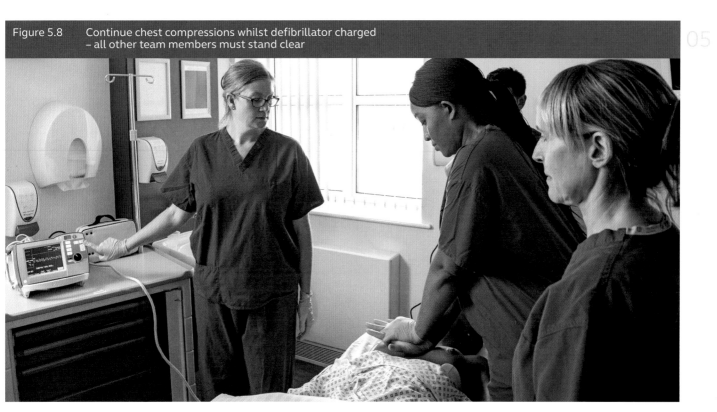

Figure 5.8   Continue chest compressions whilst defibrillator charged – all other team members must stand clear

successful defibrillation. Every 5 s increase in the duration of the pre-shock pause almost halves the chance of successful defibrillation; therefore it is critical to minimise this interval.

- If using an automated external defibrillator (AED), switch on the machine and follow the AED's audio-visual prompts.

- Rescuers must not compromise on safety. All actions should be planned by the team before pausing chest compressions. If there are delays caused by difficulties in rhythm analysis or if individuals are still in contact with the patient, chest compressions should be restarted whilst a decision is made what to do when compressions are next paused.

- Continue resuscitation until the resuscitation team arrives or the patient shows signs of life. Follow the Advanced Life Support algorithm (Chapter 6).

- Once resuscitation is underway, and if there are sufficient staff present, prepare intravenous cannulae and drugs likely to be used by the resuscitation team (e.g. adrenaline).

- Use a watch or clock for timing between rhythm checks. Any interruption to CPR should be planned. Assess the cardiac rhythm about every two minutes.

- The importance of uninterrupted chest compressions cannot be over-emphasised. Even short interruptions to chest compressions are disastrous for outcome and every effort must be made to ensure that continuous, effective chest compression is maintained throughout the resuscitation attempt.

- Identify one person to be responsible for handover to the resuscitation team leader. Use a structured communication tool for handover (e.g. SBARD, RSVP).

- Locate the patient's records.

4C. If the patient is not breathing and has a pulse (respiratory arrest)

- Ventilate the patient's lungs (as described above) and check for a pulse every minute.

- This diagnosis can be made only if you are confident in assessing breathing and pulse or the patient has other signs of life (e.g. warm and well-perfused, normal capillary refill).

- If there are any doubts about the presence of a pulse, start chest compressions and continue ventilations until more experienced help arrives.

- All patients in respiratory arrest will develop cardiac arrest if the respiratory arrest is not treated rapidly and effectively.

5. If the patient has a monitored and witnessed cardiac arrest

- If a patient has a monitored and witnessed cardiac arrest in the catheter laboratory, coronary care unit, a critical care area, or whilst monitored after cardiac surgery, and a manual defibrillator is rapidly available:

- Confirm cardiac arrest and shout for help.

- If the initial rhythm is VF/pVT, give up to three quick successive (stacked) shocks.

- Rapidly check for a rhythm change and, if appropriate check for a pulse and other signs of ROSC after each defibrillation attempt.

- Start chest compressions and continue CPR for 2 min if the third shock is unsuccessful. These initial three stacked shocks are considered as giving the first shock in the ALS algorithm.

- This three-shock strategy may also be considered for an initial, witnessed VF/pVT cardiac arrest if the patient is already connected to a manual defibrillator – these circumstances are rare.

- A precordial thump rarely works. Delivery of a precordial thump must not delay calling for help or accessing a defibrillator. Consider a precordial thump only when it can be used without delay whilst awaiting the arrival of a defibrillator in a monitored VF/pVT arrest. Using the ulnar edge of a tightly clenched fist, deliver a sharp impact to the lower half of the sternum from a height of about 20 cm, then retract the fist immediately to create an impulse-like stimulus.

05: Summary learning

The exact sequence of actions after in-hospital cardiac arrest depends on the location, skills of the first responders, number of responders, equipment available, and the hospital response system to cardiac arrest and medical emergencies.

Check for responsiveness, normal breathing, signs of life and if trained a carotid pulse to confirm cardiac arrest. This should take less than 10 s. Call for help and start CPR with chest compressions.

Deliver high-quality chest compressions with a depth of 5–6 cm, rate of 100–120 min^{-1}, and allow complete recoil between compressions.

Minimise interruptions to chest compressions for other interventions – this means all interruptions must be planned before stopping compressions.

Check the latest local and national guidance on requirements for personal protective equipment during CPR.

My key take-home messages from this chapter are:

Further reading

Couper K, Kimani PK, Abella BS, et al. The System-Wide Effect of Real-Time Audiovisual Feedback and Postevent Debriefing for In-Hospital Cardiac Arrest: The Cardiopulmonary Resuscitation Quality Improvement Initiative. Crit Care Med. 2015 Jul 16. doi: 10.1097/CCM.0000000000001202.

Davies M, Couper, K., Bradley, J al. A simple solution for improving reliability of cardiac arrest equipment provision in hospital. Resuscitation 2014;85:1523-6.

Edelson DP, Abella BS, Kramer-Johansen J, et al. Effects of compression depth and pre-shock pauses predict defibrillation failure during cardiac arrest. Resuscitation 2006;71:137-45.

Nolan JP, Soar J, Smith GB, et al. Incidence and outcome of in-hospital cardiac arrest in the United Kingdom National Cardiac Arrest Audit. Resuscitation 2014;85:987-92.

Perkins GD, Handley AJ, Koster RM et al. Part 2: Adult basic life support and automated external defibrillation. Resuscitation 2015;95:81-98.

Resuscitation Council (UK). Guidance for safer handling during resuscitation in healthcare settings. July 2015. https://www.resus.org.uk/library/publications/publication-guidance-safer-handling

Resuscitation Council (UK). Quality standards for cardiopulmonary resuscitation and training. https://www.resus.org.uk/library/quality-standards-CPR

Soar J, Berg KM, Andersen LW, Böttiger BW, Cacciola S, Callaway CW, et al; Adult Advanced Life Support Collaborators. Adult Advanced Life Support: 2020 International Consensus on Cardiopulmonary Resuscitation and Emergency Cardiovascular Care Science with Treatment Recommendations. Resuscitation. 2020;156:A80-A119.

Soar J, Böttiger BW, Carli P, Couper K, Deakin CD, Djärv T, Lott C, Olasveengen TM, Paal P, Pellis T, Perkins GD, Sandroni C, Nolan JP. European Resuscitation Council Guidelines 2021: Advanced Life Support. Resuscitation. 2021;161.

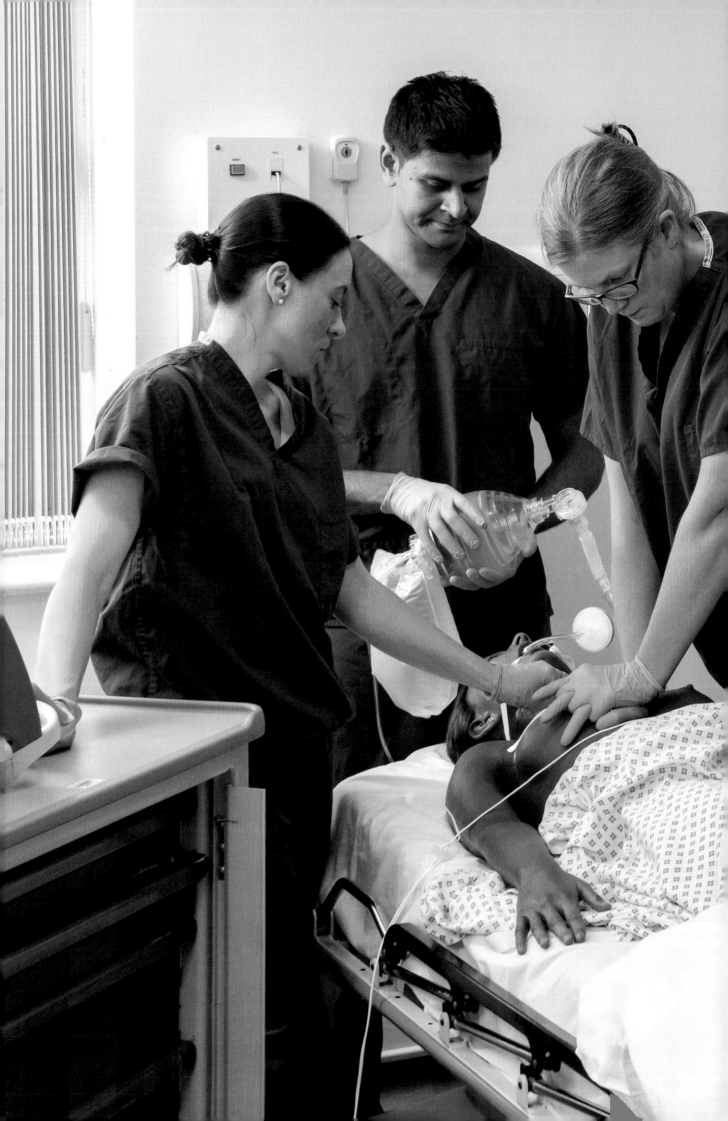

In this chapter

The Advanced Life Support (ALS) algorithm

Treatment of shockable and non-shockable rhythms

Monitoring during CPR including waveform capnography

Identification and treatment of reversible causes of cardiac arrest

The learning outcomes will enable you to:

Manage a cardiac arrest using the ALS algorithm

Understand the importance of minimising interruptions to chest compressions during CPR

Appropriately and promptly treat shockable and non-shockable rhythms

Know when and how to give drugs during cardiac arrest

Identify and treat the relevant reversible causes of cardiac arrest

Understand the role of waveform capnography during CPR

Introduction

Heart rhythms associated with cardiac arrest are divided into two groups:

- **shockable rhythms (ventricular fibrillation/pulseless ventricular tachycardia (VF/pVT))**

- **non-shockable rhythms (asystole and pulseless electrical activity (PEA)).**

The principle difference in the management of these two groups of arrhythmias is the need for attempted defibrillation in patients with VF/pVT. Subsequent actions, including chest compressions, airway management and ventilation, venous access, injection of adrenaline and the identification and correction of reversible factors, are common to both groups.

The ALS algorithm (Figure 6.1) is a standardised approach to cardiac arrest management. This has the advantage of enabling treatment to be delivered expediently and without protracted discussion. It enables each member of the resuscitation team to predict and prepare for the next stage in the patient's treatment, further enhancing efficiency of the team. Although the ALS algorithm is applicable to most cardiac arrests, additional interventions may be indicated for cardiac arrest in special circumstances (Chapter 12).

The interventions that unquestionably contribute to improved survival after cardiac arrest are prompt and effective bystander cardiopulmonary resuscitation (CPR), uninterrupted, high-quality chest compressions, and early defibrillation for VF/pVT. Although drugs and advanced airways are still included among ALS interventions, they are of secondary importance to high-quality, uninterrupted chest compressions and when appropriate early defibrillation. During ALS there is an increase in emphasis on monitoring during CPR to help guide interventions. This includes the use of waveform capnography and the use of focused cardiac and lung ultrasound assessment to help identify reversible causes of cardiac arrest.

The ALS algorithm has the advantage of enabling treatment to be delivered expediently and without protracted discussion

Drugs and advanced airways are of secondary importance to high-quality, uninterrupted chest compressions and, when appropriate, early defibrillation

Shockable rhythms (VF/pVT)

The first monitored rhythm is VF/pVT in approximately 20% of cardiac arrests, both in- or out-of-hospital. VF/pVT will also occur at some stage during resuscitation in about 25% of cardiac arrests with an initial documented rhythm of asystole or PEA.

Treatment of shockable rhythms (VF/pVT)

A manual defibrillator is used in the sequence described below. Further information about defibrillation can be found in Chapter 9.

1. Confirm cardiac arrest – check for signs of life or if trained to do so, normal breathing and pulse simultaneously.

2. Call the resuscitation team.

3. Perform uninterrupted chest compressions while applying self-adhesive defibrillation/monitoring pads – one below the right clavicle and the other in the V6 position in the midaxillary line.

4. Plan actions before pausing CPR for rhythm analysis and communicate these to the team.

5. Stop chest compressions; confirm VF/pVT from the ECG. This pause in chest compressions should be brief – aim for less than 5 s.

6. Resume chest compressions immediately; warn all rescuers other than the individual performing the chest compressions to "stand clear" and remove any oxygen delivery device as appropriate.

7. The designated person selects the appropriate energy on the defibrillator and presses the charge button (Figure 6.2). Choose an energy setting of at 120 to 150 J for the first shock, the same or a higher energy for subsequent shocks, or follow the manufacturer's guidance for the particular defibrillator.

8. Ensure that the rescuer giving the compressions is the only person touching the patient.

9. Once the defibrillator is charged and the safety check is complete, tell the rescuer doing the chest compressions to "stand clear"; when clear, give the shock (Figure 6.3).

10. After shock delivery immediately restart CPR using a ratio of 30:2, starting with chest compressions. Do not pause to reassess the rhythm or feel for a pulse. This pause in chest compressions should be very brief and no longer than 5 s.

11. Continue CPR for 2 min; the team leader prepares the team for the next pause in CPR.

12. Pause briefly to check the monitor.

13. If VF/pVT, repeat steps 6–12 above and deliver a second shock.

14. If VF/pVT persists, repeat steps 6–8 above and deliver a third shock. Resume chest compressions immediately. Give adrenaline 1 mg IV (intravenous) and amiodarone 300 mg IV while performing a further 2 min CPR. Withhold adrenaline if there are signs of return of spontaneous circulation (ROSC) during CPR.

15. Repeat this 2 min CPR – rhythm/pulse check – defibrillation sequence if VF/pVT persists.

16. Give further adrenaline 1 mg IV after alternate shocks (i.e. approximately every 3–5 min).

17. If organised electrical activity compatible with a cardiac output is seen during a rhythm check, seek evidence of ROSC (check for signs of life, a central pulse and end-tidal CO_2 if available).

a) If there is ROSC, start post-resuscitation care.

b) If there are no signs of ROSC, despite an organised rhythm (PEA), continue CPR and switch to the non-shockable algorithm.

18. If asystole is seen, continue CPR and switch to the non-shockable algorithm.

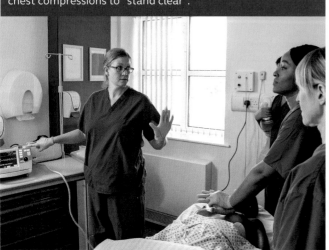

Figure 6.2   Continuous chest compressions during charging with a manual defibrillator.

Warn all rescuers other than the individual performing the chest compressions to "stand clear".

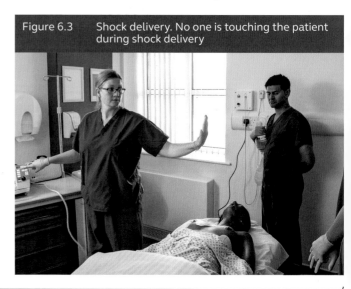

Figure 6.3   Shock delivery. No one is touching the patient during shock delivery

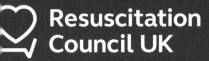
Adult advanced life support

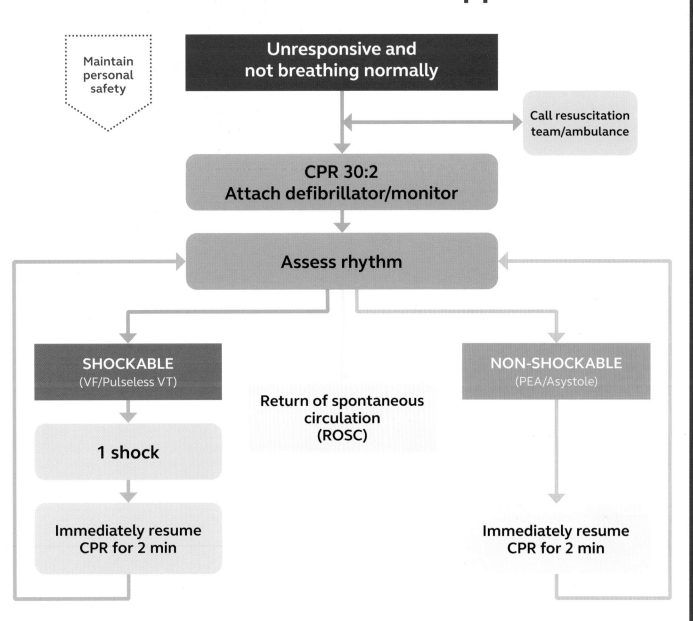

Maintain personal safety

Unresponsive and not breathing normally

Call resuscitation team/ambulance

CPR 30:2
Attach defibrillator/monitor

Assess rhythm

SHOCKABLE
(VF/Pulseless VT)

NON-SHOCKABLE
(PEA/Asystole)

Return of spontaneous circulation (ROSC)

1 shock

Immediately resume CPR for 2 min

Immediately resume CPR for 2 min

Give high-quality chest compressions, and:
- Give oxygen
- Use waveform capnography
- Continuous compressions if advanced airway
- Minimise interruptions to compressions
- Intravenous or intraosseous access
- Give adrenaline every 3–5 min
- Give amiodarone after 3 shocks
- Identify and treat reversible causes

Identify and treat reversible causes
- Hypoxia
- Hypovolaemia
- Hypo-/hyperkalaemia/metabolic
- Hypo/hyperthermia
- Thrombosis – coronary or pulmonary
- Tension pneumothorax
- Tamponade – cardiac
- Toxins
Consider ultrasound imaging to identify reversible causes

Consider
- Coronary angiography/percutaneous coronary intervention
- Mechanical chest compressions to facilitate transfer/treatment
- Extracorporeal CPR

After ROSC
- Use an ABCDE approach
- Aim for SpO_2 of 94–98% and normal $PaCO_2$
- 12-lead ECG
- Identify and treat cause
- Targeted temperature management

Figure 6.1   Adult Advanced Life Support algorithm

73

The interval between stopping compressions and delivering a shock must be minimised. Longer interruptions to chest compressions reduce the chance of a shock restoring a spontaneous circulation. Chest compressions are resumed immediately after delivering a shock (without checking the rhythm or a pulse) because:

- Even if the defibrillation attempt is successful in restoring a perfusing rhythm, it is very rare for a pulse to be palpable immediately after defibrillation. The time taken from ROSC and return of a palpable pulse may be longer than 2 min in as many as 25% of successful shocks.

- The delay in trying to palpate a pulse will further compromise the myocardium if a perfusing rhythm has not been restored.

- If a perfusing rhythm has been restored, giving chest compressions does not increase the chance of VF recurring.

- In the presence of post-shock asystole chest compressions may usefully induce VF.

Current evidence is insufficient to support or refute the routine use of any particular drug or sequence of drugs during CPR. The use of both adrenaline and amiodarone is currently recommended, based largely on an increased short-term survival in humans.

The first dose of adrenaline is given during the 2 min cycle of CPR after delivery of the third shock.

Give amiodarone 300 mg after three defibrillation attempts. Do not stop CPR to check the rhythm before giving drugs unless there are clear signs of ROSC.

Subsequent doses of adrenaline are given after alternate 2 min cycles of CPR (which equates to every 3–5 min) for as long as cardiac arrest persists. If VF/pVT persists, or recurs, a further dose of 150 mg amiodarone may be given after a total of five defibrillation attempts. Lidocaine, 1 mg kg^{-1}, may be used as an alternative if amiodarone is not available, but do not give lidocaine if amiodarone has been given already.

It is important in shock-refractory VF/pVT to check the position and contact of the defibrillation pads. The duration of any individual resuscitation attempt is a matter of clinical judgement, and should take into account the perceived prospect of a successful outcome. If it was considered appropriate to start resuscitation, it is usually considered worthwhile continuing as long as the patient remains in identifiable VF/pVT. Consider changing the pad position in refractory VF/pVT (e.g. to anterior-posterior).

When the rhythm is checked 2 min after giving a shock, if a non-shockable rhythm is present, and the rhythm is one that could be compatible with a pulse, try to palpate a central pulse and look for other evidence of ROSC (e.g. sudden increase in end-tidal CO_2 or evidence of cardiac output on any invasive monitoring equipment). Rhythm checks must be brief, and pulse checks undertaken only if a rhythm that could be compatible with a pulse is observed. If a rhythm compatible with a pulse is seen during a 2 min period of CPR, do not interrupt chest compressions to palpate a pulse unless the patient shows signs of life suggesting ROSC. If there is any doubt about the presence of a palpable pulse, resume CPR. If the patient has ROSC, begin post-resuscitation care. If the patient's rhythm changes to asystole or PEA, see non-shockable rhythms, below.

Do not spend time attempting to distinguish fine VF from coarse VF, or extremely fine VF from asystole during the 5 s rhythm check. If the rhythm appears to be VF give a shock, and if it appears to be asystole continue chest compressions. Avoid excessive interruptions in chest compression for rhythm analysis.

Precordial thump

A precordial thump has a very low success rate for cardioversion of a shockable rhythm. Its routine use is therefore not recommended. Consider a precordial thump only when it can be used without delay whilst awaiting the arrival of a defibrillator in a monitored VF/pVT arrest. Using the ulnar edge of a tightly clenched fist, deliver a sharp impact to the lower half of the sternum from a height of about 20 cm, then retract the fist immediately to create an impulse-like stimulus.

Witnessed and monitored VF/pVT cardiac arrest

If a patient has a monitored and witnessed cardiac arrest in the catheter laboratory, coronary care unit, a critical care area, or whilst monitored after cardiac surgery, and a manual defibrillator is rapidly available:

- Confirm cardiac arrest and shout for help.

- If the initial rhythm is VF/pVT, give up to three quick successive (stacked) shocks.

- Rapidly check for a rhythm change and, if appropriate check for a pulse and other signs of ROSC after each defibrillation attempt.

- Start chest compressions and continue CPR for 2 min if the third shock is unsuccessful.

This three-shock strategy may also be considered for an initial, witnessed VF/pVT cardiac arrest if the patient is already connected to a manual defibrillator – these circumstances are rare. Although there are no data supporting a three-shock strategy in any of these circumstances, it is unlikely that chest compressions will improve the already very high chance of ROSC when defibrillation occurs immediately after onset of VF/pVT.

If this initial three-shock strategy is unsuccessful for a monitored VF/pVT cardiac arrest, follow the ALS algorithm and treat these three-shocks as if only the first single shock has been given. These initial three stacked shocks are considered as giving the first shock in the ALS algorithm (i.e. the first dose of adrenaline should be given after another two shock attempts if VF/pVT persists).

Amiodarone is given after three shock attempts irrespective of when they are given during the cardiac arrest (i.e. give amiodarone during the 2 min of CPR after the three stacked-shock attempts).

Non-shockable rhythms (PEA and asystole)

Pulseless electrical activity (PEA) is defined as cardiac arrest in the presence of electrical activity (other than ventricular tachyarrhythmia) that would normally be associated with a palpable pulse. These patients often have some mechanical myocardial contractions but they are too weak to produce a detectable pulse or blood pressure. PEA may be caused by reversible conditions that can be treated (see below). Survival following cardiac arrest with asystole or PEA is unlikely unless a reversible cause can be found and treated quickly and effectively.

Asystole is the absence of electrical activity on the ECG trace. During CPR, ensure the ECG pads are attached to the chest and the correct monitoring mode is selected. Ensure the gain setting is appropriate. Whenever a diagnosis of asystole is made, check the ECG carefully for the presence of P waves because in this situation ventricular standstill may be treated effectively by cardiac pacing. Attempts to pace true asystole are unlikely to be successful.

Treatment for PEA and asystole

- Start CPR 30:2.
- Give adrenaline 1 mg IV as soon as intravascular access is achieved.
- Continue CPR 30:2 until the airway is secured, then continue chest compressions without pausing during ventilation.
- Recheck the rhythm after 2 min:
- If electrical activity compatible with a pulse is seen, check for a pulse and/or signs of life:
  - if a pulse and/or signs of life are present, start post-resuscitation care
  - if no pulse and/or no signs of life are present (PEA OR asystole):
    - continue CPR
    - recheck the rhythm after 2 min and proceed accordingly
    - give further adrenaline 1 mg IV every 3–5 min (during alternate 2 minute cycles of CPR).
- If VF/pVT at rhythm check, change to shockable side of algorithm.

During CPR

During the treatment of persistent VF/pVT or PEA/asystole, emphasis is placed on high-quality chest compression between defibrillation attempts, recognising and treating reversible causes (4 Hs and 4 Ts), obtaining a secure airway and vascular access.

During CPR with a 30:2 ratio, the underlying rhythm may be seen clearly on the monitor as compressions are paused to enable ventilation. If VF is seen during this brief pause (whether on the shockable or non-shockable side of the algorithm) do not attempt defibrillation at this stage; instead, continue with high-quality CPR until the 2 minute period is completed. Knowing that the rhythm is VF, the team should be fully prepared to deliver a shock with minimal delay at the end of the 2 minute period of CPR.

Maintain high-quality, uninterrupted chest compressions

The quality of chest compressions and ventilations are important determinants of outcome, yet are frequently performed poorly by healthcare professionals. Avoid interruptions in chest compressions because pauses cause coronary perfusion pressure to decrease substantially. Ensure compressions are of adequate depth (5–6 cm) and rate (100–120 min⁻¹), and ensure there is full recoil of the chest at the end of each compression.

As soon as the airway is secured, continue chest compressions without pausing during ventilation.

To reduce fatigue, change the individual undertaking compressions every 2 min or earlier if necessary.

Airway and ventilation

A bag-mask, or preferably, a supraglottic airway (SGA) (e.g. i-gel) should be used in the absence of personnel skilled in tracheal intubation (Chapter 7). Once a SGA has been inserted, attempt to deliver continuous chest compressions, uninterrupted during ventilation. Ventilate the lungs at 10 breaths min⁻¹; do not hyperventilate the lungs. If excessive gas leakage causes inadequate ventilation of the patient's lungs, interrupt chest compressions to enable ventilation (using a compression-ventilation ratio of 30:2).

No studies have shown that tracheal intubation increases survival after cardiac arrest compared with bag-mask ventilation or use of an SGA. Long pauses in chest compression or incorrect placement of the tracheal tube are common in cardiac arrest if intubation is attempted by unskilled personnel. Tracheal intubation should be attempted only if the healthcare provider is properly trained and has regular, ongoing experience with the technique. Avoid stopping chest compressions during laryngoscopy and intubation; if necessary, a brief pause in chest compressions may be required as the tube is passed between the vocal cords, but this pause should not exceed 5 s.

Alternatively, to avoid any interruptions in chest compressions, the intubation attempt may be deferred until after ROSC. After intubation, confirm correct tube position with waveform capnography, and secure the tube adequately. Once the patient's trachea has been intubated, continue chest compressions at a rate of 100–120 min^{-1} without pausing during ventilation.

Monitoring during CPR

Several methods can be used to monitor the patient during CPR and potentially help guide ALS interventions. These include:

- **Clinical signs** such as breathing efforts, movements and eye opening can occur during CPR. These can indicate ROSC and require verification by a rhythm and pulse check, but can also occur because high-quality CPR can generate a sufficient circulation to restore signs of life including consciousness.

- **Pulse checks** can be used to identify ROSC when there is an ECG rhythm compatible with a pulse, but may not detect pulses in those with low cardiac output states and a low blood pressure. The value of attempting to feel arterial pulses during chest compressions to assess the effectiveness of chest compressions is unclear. A pulse that is felt in the femoral triangle can indicate venous rather than arterial blood flow. Carotid pulsation during CPR does not necessarily indicate adequate myocardial or cerebral perfusion.

- **Monitoring the heart rhythm** through pads, paddles or ECG electrodes is a standard part of ALS. Motion artefacts can prevent reliable heart rhythm assessment during chest compressions.

- **End-tidal carbon dioxide measured with waveform capnography.** The use of waveform capnography during CPR is addressed in more detail below.

- **Feedback or prompt devices** can monitor CPR quality data such as compression rate and depth during CPR, and provide real-time feedback to rescuers.

  Be aware that some devices fail to compensate for compression of the underlying mattress during CPR on a bed when providing feedback. The use of these devices should be as part of a broader system of care that includes CPR quality improvement initiatives such as debriefing based on the data collected.

- **Blood sampling and analysis** during CPR can be used to identify potentially reversible causes of cardiac arrest. Avoid finger prick samples because they may not be reliable; instead, use samples from veins or arteries. Blood gas values are difficult to interpret during CPR. During cardiac arrest, arterial gas values may be misleading and bear little relationship to the tissue acid-base state. Analysis of central venous blood may provide a better estimation of tissue pH.

- **Invasive cardiovascular monitoring** in critical care settings (e.g. continuous arterial blood pressure and central venous pressure monitoring). Invasive arterial pressure monitoring will enable the detection of even very low blood pressure values when ROSC is achieved.

- The use of **focused echocardiography/ultrasound** to identify and treat reversible causes of cardiac arrest, and identify low cardiac output states ('pseudo-PEA') is discussed below.

Waveform capnography during advanced life support

Carbon dioxide (CO_2) is a waste product of metabolism; approximately 400 L are produced each day. It is carried in the blood to the lungs where it is exhaled. The concentration in the blood is measured as the partial pressure of CO_2 (PCO_2) and in arterial blood ($PaCO_2$) is normally 5.3 kPa (range 4.7–6.0 kPa). The concentration of CO_2 can also be measured in expired air and is expressed as either a percentage by volume or as a partial pressure, both of which are very similar numerically. The concentration varies throughout expiration, being maximal at the end and it is this value, the end-tidal CO_2 that is most useful.

End-tidal CO_2 is the partial pressure of CO_2 at the end of an exhaled breath. It reflects cardiac output and pulmonary blood flow (CO_2 is transported by the venous system to the right side of the heart and then pumped to the lungs by the right ventricle), as well as the ventilation minute volume. During CPR, end-tidal CO_2 values are low, reflecting the low cardiac output generated by chest compression. Waveform capnography enables continuous real time end-tidal CO_2 to be monitored during CPR. It works most reliably in patients who have a tracheal tube, but can also be used with a supraglottic airway device or bag mask.

The role of waveform capnography during CPR

- **Ensuring tracheal tube placement in the trachea.** Correct tube placement also relies on observation and auscultation to ensure both lungs are ventilated.

- **Monitoring ventilation rate during CPR** and avoiding hyperventilation.

- **Monitoring the quality of chest compressions** during CPR. End-tidal CO_2 values are associated with compression depth and ventilation rate and a greater depth of chest compression will increase the value.

- **Identifying ROSC during CPR.** An increase in end-tidal CO_2 during CPR may indicate ROSC, and prevent unnecessary and potentially harmful administration of adrenaline in a patient with ROSC. If ROSC is suspected during CPR, withhold adrenaline. Give adrenaline if cardiac arrest is confirmed at the next rhythm check.

- **Prognostication during CPR.** Precise values of end-tidal CO_2 depend on several factors including the cause of cardiac arrest, bystander CPR, chest compression quality, ventilation rate and volume, time from cardiac arrest and the use of adrenaline. Values are higher after an initial asphyxial arrest and with bystander CPR, and decline over time after cardiac arrest. Low end-tidal CO_2 values during CPR have been associated with lower ROSC rates and increased mortality, and high values with better ROSC and survival. End-tidal CO_2 values should be considered only as part of a multi-modal approach to decision-making for prognostication during CPR.

Practical aspects of waveform capnography

A capnograph is a device that displays a waveform of the concentration of CO_2 as it varies during expiration and a numerical value. This is usually referred to as waveform capnography and is the most useful display for clinical use.

Equipment

- Portable monitors that measure the end-tidal CO_2 and display the waveform are now readily available (Figure 6.4).
- Most capnographs use side-stream sampling. A connector (T-piece) is placed in the breathing system, usually on the end of the tracheal tube or supraglottic airway device. This has a small port on the side to which is attached a fine bore sampling tube. A continuous sample of gas is aspirated (about 50 mL min^{-1}) and analysed by using the property of absorption of infrared light.

Figure 6.4 Example of a monitor screen showing end-tidal CO_2 waveform (waveform capnography)

This patient had a return of spontaneous circulation, and chest compressions have stopped. The ECG shows sinus rhythm with a rate of 70 min^{-1}. The end-tidal CO_2 waveform shows an end-tidal CO_2 value of 4.4 kPa, and a ventilation rate (RR) of 12 min^{-1}. On clinical assessment the patient had a palpable carotid pulse.

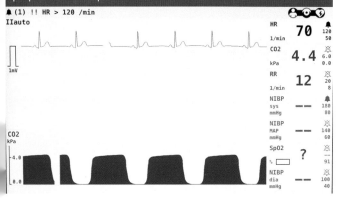

- An alternative system is mainstream sampling in which the infrared source and detector are contained within a cell or cuvette which is placed directly in the breathing system, usually between the tracheal tube or supraglottic airway device and circuit. Gas is analysed as it passes through the sensor and none is removed from the system.

The capnography waveform

The shape of the waveform that is displayed will depend upon the time scale and the patient's condition. (Figure 6.5).

A-B: This is the baseline and indicates the end of inspiration. In effect the concentration of CO_2 is being measured in air (or whatever gas is being delivered) which is virtually zero.

B-C: This represents the start of expiration, with a rapid rise in the concentration of expired CO_2. The expired gas initially contains no CO_2 as it has come from the anatomical dead space (i.e. the volume of the respiratory tract that does not take part in gas exchange (larynx, trachea, main bronchi)). As gas from alveoli that contains CO_2 starts to be expired, it mixes with this gas and the concentration rises.

C-D: Eventually the alveolar plateau is reached. This represents gas from alveoli taking part in gas exchange. The slight gradual increase during this phase is due to the fact that not all alveoli empty at the same rate.

D: At the end of expiration the concentration of CO_2 is maximal, this is the end-tidal CO_2. In healthy patients, this is normally 4.8 kPa (4.3–5.5 kPa), slightly lower than would be obtained if the arterial $PaCO_2$ was measured at the same point in time.

D-E: As inspiration starts, air containing no CO_2 is mixed with a small amount of residual expired gas in the breathing circuit. This is rapidly diluted until gas containing no CO_2 is being inspired.

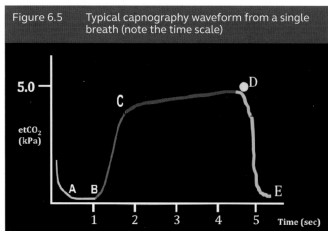

Figure 6.5 Typical capnography waveform from a single breath (note the time scale)

End-tidal CO$_2$ during CPR

Reliable end-tidal CO$_2$ monitoring during CPR will usually require a tracheal tube or, when there is a good seal, a supraglottic airway device. Figure 6.6 shows how end-tidal CO$_2$ values can change during CPR.

- The presence of an end-tidal CO$_2$ waveform indicates the tracheal tube is positioned in the airway. Check that both lungs are being ventilated by looking and by listening with a stethoscope as the tube may have passed down into a bronchus and only be ventilating one lung.

- The rate of ventilation is 10 min^{-1} (Figure 6.6).

- Soon after the second defibrillation attempt there is a significant increase in the end-tidal CO$_2$ value during CPR. This is often the first indicator of ROSC and often precedes other indicators such as the presence of a palpable pulse. It is a result of the improved circulation transporting accumulated CO$_2$ from the tissues to the lungs. If ROSC is suspected during CPR, withhold adrenaline. Give adrenaline if cardiac arrest is confirmed at the next rhythm check.

- Failure to achieve an end-tidal CO$_2$ value > 1.33 kPa (10 mmHg) after 20 min of CPR is associated with a poor outcome in observational studies. A specific end-tidal CO$_2$ value at any time during CPR should not be used alone to stop CPR efforts. End-tidal CO$_2$ values should be considered only as part of a multi-modal approach to decision-making for prognostication during CPR.

Signs of life during CPR

If there is a combination of clinical and physiological signs of return of spontaneous circulation (ROSC) such as waking, purposeful movement, arterial blood pressure waveform or a sharp rise in end-tidal CO$_2$, consider briefly stopping chest compressions for rhythm analysis, and if appropriate a pulse check. If a pulse is palpable, continue post-resuscitation care and/or treatment of peri-arrest arrhythmias if appropriate. If no pulse is present, continue CPR.

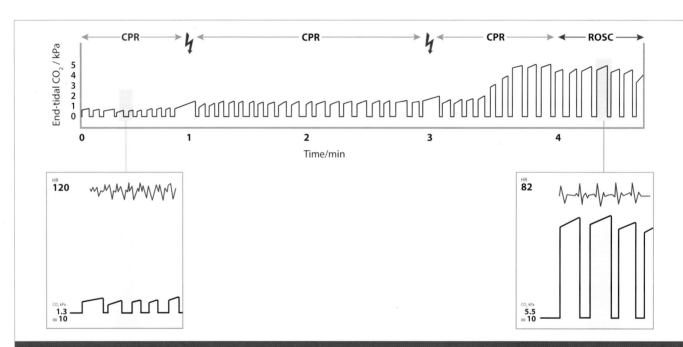

Figure 6.6   Waveform capnography showing changes in the end-tidal CO$_2$ during CPR and after ROSC.

The boxes show the monitor displays at the times indicated. In this example the patient's trachea is intubated at zero minutes. The patient is ventilated at 10 min^{-1} and given chest compressions (indicated by CPR) at about two per second. A minute after tracheal intubation, there is a pause in chest compressions and ventilation followed by a defibrillation attempt, and chest compressions and ventilation then continue. Higher-quality chest compressions lead to an increased end-tidal CO$_2$ value. There is a further defibrillation attempt after 2 min of chest compressions. There are then further chest compressions and ventilation. There is a

significant increase in the end-tidal CO$_2$ value during chest compressions and the patient starts moving and eye opening. Chest compressions are stopped briefly the monitor shows sinus rhythm and there is a pulse indicating ROSC. Ventilation continues at 10 min^{-1}.

CPR – cardiopulmonary resuscitation

ROSC – return of spontaneous circulation

HR – heart rate

RR – respiratory rate

Vascular access

Some patients will already have IV access before they have a cardiac arrest. If this is not the case ensure CPR had started and defibrillation, if appropriate, attempted before considering vascular access. Although peak drug concentrations are higher and circulation times shorter when drugs are injected into a central venous catheter compared with a peripheral cannula, insertion of a central venous catheter requires interruption of CPR and is associated with several potential complications. Peripheral venous cannulation is quicker, easier, and safer. Drugs injected peripherally must be followed by a flush of at least 20 mL of fluid and elevation of the extremity for 10–20 s to facilitate drug delivery to the central circulation.

If rapid IV access is difficult or impossible, consider the intraosseous (IO) route (Figure 6.7). Intraosseous injection of drugs achieves adequate plasma concentrations in a time comparable with injection through a vein.

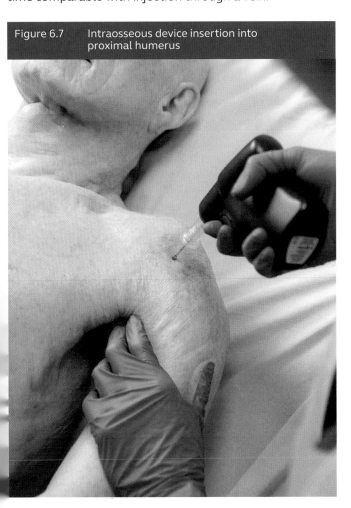

Figure 6.7   Intraosseous device insertion into proximal humerus

Use of intraosseous access during resuscitation

- The three main insertion sites for IO access recommended for use in adults are the proximal humerus, proximal tibia and distal tibia.

- Contraindications to IO access include trauma, infection or a prosthesis (e.g. joint replacement) at the target site, recent IO access (previous 48 h) in the same limb including a failed attempt, or a failure to identify the anatomical landmarks.

- Training in the specific device to be used in clinical practice is essential. Site of insertion, identification of landmarks and technique for insertion will differ depending on the device being used.

- Once inserted, confirm correct placement before delivery of drugs or infusion of fluids. Attempt to aspirate from the needle; presence of IO blood indicates correct placement, absence of aspirate does not necessarily imply a failed attempt.

- Flush the needle to ensure patency and observe for leakage or extravasation. This is best achieved using an extension set flushed with 0.9% saline attached to the hub of the needle before use.

- Once IO access has been confirmed, resuscitation drugs including adrenaline and amiodarone can be infused. Fluids and blood products can also be delivered but pressure will be needed to achieve reasonable flow rates using either a pressure bag or a syringe.

- Follow the manufacturer's guidance both for securing the needle and the maximum length of time it can be left in place.

- Complications associated with IO access include extravasation into the soft tissues surrounding the insertion site, dislodgement of the needle, compartment syndrome due to extravasation, fracture or chipping of the bone during insertion, pain related to the infusion of drugs/fluid, fat emboli and infection/osteomyelitis.

Identification and treatment of reversible causes

Potential causes or aggravating factors for which specific treatment exists must be considered during any cardiac arrest. For ease of memory, these are divided into two groups of four based upon their initial letter – either H or T (Figure 6.8). More details on many of these conditions are covered in Chapter 12.

- Hypoxia
- Hypovolaemia
- Hyperkalaemia, hypokalaemia, hypoglycaemia, hypocalcaemia, and other metabolic disorders
- Hypothermia/hyperthermia
- Thrombosis (coronary or pulmonary)
- Tension pneumothorax
- Tamponade – cardiac
- Toxins.

The four Hs

Minimise the risk of hypoxia by ensuring that the patient's lungs are ventilated adequately with 100% oxygen during CPR. Make sure there is adequate chest rise and bilateral breath sounds. Using the techniques described in Chapter 7, check carefully that the tracheal tube is not misplaced in a bronchus or the oesophagus. If ROSC is achieved adjust the inspired oxygen to target an oxygen saturation of 94–98% (Chapter 13).

PEA caused by hypovolaemia is usually due to severe haemorrhage. Evidence of haemorrhage may be obvious, (e.g. trauma (Chapter 12)), or occult (e.g. gastrointestinal bleeding, or rupture of an aortic aneurysm). Intravascular volume should be restored rapidly with fluid and blood, coupled with urgent interventions to stop the haemorrhage – effective chest compressions require an adequate circulating volume.

Hyperkalaemia, hypokalaemia, hypoglycaemia, hypocalcaemia, and other metabolic disorders are detected by biochemical tests or suggested by the patient's medical history (e.g. renal failure (Chapter 12)). Intravenous calcium chloride is indicated in the presence of hyperkalaemia, hypocalcaemia, and calcium channel-blocker overdose. Hypoglycaemia as a sole reversible cause of cardiac arrest is controversial. A very low blood glucose can however cause irreversible brain damage and should be corrected during CPR.

Suspect hypothermia in any drowning incident (Chapter 12); use a low reading thermometer.

The four Ts

Coronary thrombosis is a common cause of cardiac arrest. If an acute coronary syndrome is expected as the cause of a refractory cardiac arrest, it may be feasible to perform percutaneous coronary angiography and percutaneous coronary intervention during ongoing CPR. This would require an automated mechanical chest compression device and/or extracorporeal CPR to maintain a circulation during the procedure. A decision to transport a patient with ongoing CPR should take into consideration a realistic chance of survival (e.g. witnessed cardiac arrest with initial shockable rhythm (VF/pVT) and bystander CPR). Intermittent ROSC also strongly favours a decision to transport.

The commonest cause of thromboembolic or mechanical circulatory obstruction is massive pulmonary embolism. If pulmonary embolism is thought to be the cause of cardiac arrest, consider giving a fibrinolytic drug immediately. Following fibrinolysis during CPR for acute pulmonary embolism, survival and good neurological outcome have been reported, even in cases requiring in excess of 60 min of CPR. If a fibrinolytic drug is given in these circumstances, consider performing CPR for at least 60–90 min before termination of resuscitation attempts.

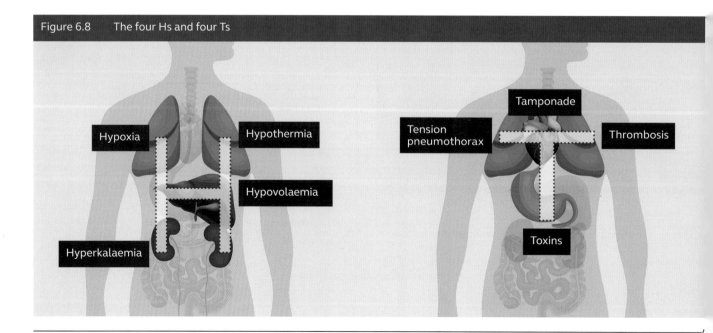

Figure 6.8   The four Hs and four Ts

In settings where it is available, extracorporeal CPR, and/or surgical or mechanical thrombectomy should also be considered in select patients to treat pulmonary embolism.

A tension pneumothorax may be the primary cause of PEA. The diagnosis is made clinically or by focused ultrasound of the chest. Decompress rapidly by thoracostomy or needle thoracocentesis and then insert a chest drain.

Cardiac tamponade is difficult to diagnose because the typical signs of distended neck veins and hypotension cannot be assessed during cardiac arrest. Focused cardiac ultrasound performed during CPR can be used to diagnose a pericardial effusion during CPR (see below). Cardiac arrest after penetrating chest trauma or after cardiac surgery should raise strong suspicion of tamponade and the need for resuscitative thoracotomy should be considered in this setting (Chapter 12).

In the absence of a specific history of accidental or deliberate ingestion, poisoning by therapeutic or toxic substances may be difficult to detect but in some cases may be revealed later by laboratory investigations (Chapter 12). Where available, the appropriate antidotes should be used but most often treatment is supportive. Again, in settings where it is available, extracorporeal CPR, should also be considered in select patients to treat cardiac arrest caused by a toxin.

Ultrasound during advanced life support

In skilled hands, focused echocardiography/ultrasound can be useful for the detection of potentially reversible causes of cardiac arrest (e.g. cardiac tamponade, pulmonary embolism, ischaemia (regional wall motion abnormality), aortic dissection, hypovolaemia, pneumothorax). The integration of ultrasound into advanced life support requires training if interruptions to chest compressions are to be minimised. A sub-xiphoid probe position is recommended (Figure 6.9).

Placement of the probe just before chest compressions are paused for a planned rhythm assessment enables a well-trained operator to obtain views within 10 s. The Focused Echocardiography in Emergency Life Support (FEEL) course provides a valuable introduction to focused echocardiography/ultrasound in this setting.

The use of automated mechanical chest compression devices

Automated mechanical chest compression devices should not be used routinely to replace manual chest compressions. Automated mechanical chest compression devices may enable the delivery of high-quality compressions in circumstances where this is not possible with manual compressions – CPR in a moving ambulance where safety is at risk, prolonged CPR (e.g. hypothermic

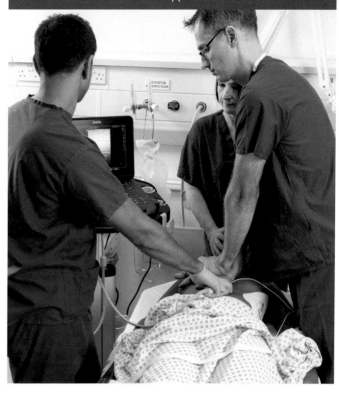

arrest), and CPR during certain procedures (e.g. coronary angiography or preparation for extracorporeal CPR (ECPR)).

More recently, mechanical devices have been used to minimise close proximity to patients with COVID-19. Avoid interruptions to compressions during device deployment. Healthcare personnel who use mechanical chest compression devices should do so only within a structured, monitored programme, which should include comprehensive competency-based training and regular opportunities to refresh skills.

Extracorporeal CPR

Extracorporeal resuscitation techniques require vascular access and a circuit with a pump and oxygenator and can provide a circulation of oxygenated blood to restore tissue perfusion. This has the potential to buy time for restoration of an adequate spontaneous circulation, and treatment of reversible underlying conditions. This is commonly called extracorporeal life support (ECLS), and more specifically ECPR when started during cardiac arrest. These techniques are becoming more commonplace and have been used for both in-hospital and out-of-hospital.

Evidence suggests ECPR can improve the chances of survival in select patients in whom there is a reversible cause for cardiac arrest (e.g. myocardial infarction, pulmonary embolism, severe hypothermia, poisoning), there is little comorbidity, the cardiac arrest is witnessed, the individual receives immediate high-quality CPR, and ECPR is implemented early and certainly within 1 h of collapse. The implementation of ECPR requires considerable resource and training, and availability is therefore limited.

The duration of a resuscitation attempt

If attempts at obtaining ROSC are unsuccessful the resuscitation team leader should discuss stopping CPR with the team. The decision to stop CPR requires clinical judgement and a careful assessment of the likelihood of achieving ROSC and longer term survival.

The duration of any resuscitation attempt should be based on the individual circumstances of the case and is a matter of clinical judgement, taking into consideration the circumstances and the perceived prospect of a successful outcome. If it was considered appropriate to start resuscitation, it is usually considered worthwhile continuing, as long as the patient remains in VF/pVT, or there is a potentially reversible cause that can be treated. The use of mechanical compression devices and ECPR techniques make prolonged attempts at resuscitation feasible in selected patients. It is generally accepted that asystole for more than 20 min in the absence of a reversible cause and with ongoing ALS constitutes reasonable grounds for stopping further resuscitation attempts, although a shorter or longer time could be appropriate based on the circumstances of cardiac arrest.

Diagnosing death after unsuccessful resuscitation

If CPR is unsuccessful at achieving ROSC and a decision is made to discontinue CPR efforts, after stopping CPR observe the patient for a minimum of 5 min before confirming death. The absence of mechanical cardiac function is normally confirmed using a combination of the following:
- absence of a central pulse on palpation
- absence of heart sounds on auscultation.

One or more of the following can supplement these criteria:
- asystole on a continuous ECG display
- absence of pulsatile flow using direct intra-arterial pressure monitoring
- absence of contractile activity using echocardiography.

Any return of cardiac or respiratory activity during this period of observation should prompt a further 5 min observation from the next cardiorespiratory arrest. After 5 min of continued cardiorespiratory arrest, the absence of pupillary responses to light, corneal reflexes, and motor response to supra-orbital pressure should be confirmed. The time of death is recorded as the time at which these criteria are fulfilled.

Post-event tasks

At the end of the resuscitation further tasks include:
- Ongoing care of the patient, and allocation of further team roles and responsibilities including handover to other teams.
- Documentation of the resuscitation attempt. Use information from defibrillators and monitors to help document events and times.
- Communication with relatives (Chapter 17).
- An immediate post-event debriefing ('Hot' debriefing). This is normally led by the resuscitation team leader, focuses on immediate issues and concerns, and is usually of short duration. This can be difficult if the patient has a ROSC, as focus then inevitably shifts to post-resuscitation care. A delayed facilitated debriefing ('Cold' debriefing) is also useful (Chapter 2).
- Ensuring equipment and drug trolleys are replenished.
- Ensuring audit forms are completed.

06: Summary learning

The ALS algorithm provides a framework for the standardised resuscitation of all adult patients in cardiac arrest.

The delivery of high-quality chest compressions with minimal interruptions is an important determinant of outcome.

Treatment depends on the underlying rhythm.

Look for reversible causes and treat early.

Secure the airway early to enable continuous chest compressions.

Use waveform capnography to help assess and guide resuscitation interventions.

My key take-home messages from this chapter are:

Further reading

Academy of Medical Royal Colleges. A code of practice for the diagnosis and confirmation of death. 2008. http://www.aomrc.org.uk

Cook TM, Woodall N, Harper J, Benger J; Fourth National Audit Project. Major complications of airway management in the UK: results of the Fourth National Audit Project of the Royal College of Anaesthetists and the Difficult Airway Society. Part 2: intensive care and emergency departments. Br J Anaesth. 2011 May;106(5):632-42.

Couper K, Kimani PK, Abella BS, et al. The System-Wide Effect of Real-Time Audiovisual Feedback and Postevent Debriefing for In-Hospital Cardiac Arrest: The Cardiopulmonary Resuscitation Quality Improvement Initiative. Crit Care Med. 2015 Jul 16. doi: 10.1097/CCM.0000000000001202.

Diagnosis of death after cessation of cardiopulmonary resuscitation. Signal 1329. National Reporting and Learning System (NRLS) and National Patient Safety Agency (NPSA). February 2012.

FEEL - Focused Echocardiography in Emergency Life Support. https://www.resus.org.uk/information-on-courses/focused-echocardiography-in-emergency-life-support/

Gates S, Quinn T, Deakin CD, Blair L, Couper K, Perkins GD. Mechanical chest compression for out-of-hospital cardiac arrest: Systematic review and meta- analysis. Resuscitation 2015;94:91-7.

Nolan JP, Soar J, Smith GB, et al. Incidence and outcome of in-hospital cardiac arrest in the United Kingdom National Cardiac Arrest Audit. Resuscitation 2014;85:987-92.

Soar J, Berg KM, Andersen LW, Böttiger BW, Cacciola S, Callaway CW, et al; Adult Advanced Life Support Collaborators. Adult Advanced Life Support: 2020 International Consensus on Cardiopulmonary Resuscitation and Emergency Cardiovascular Care Science with Treatment Recommendations. Resuscitation. 2020;156:A80-A119.

Soar J, Böttiger BW, Carli P, Couper K, Deakin CD, Djärv T, Lott C, Olasveengen TM, Paal P, Pellis T, Perkins GD, Sandroni C, Nolan JP. European Resuscitation Council Guidelines 2021: Advanced Life Support. Resuscitation. 2021;161.

Lott C, Truhlár A, Alfonzo A, Barelli A, González-Salvado V, Hinkelbein J, Nolan JP, Paal P, Perkins GD, Thies K-C, Yeung J, Zideman DA, Soar J. European Resuscitation Council Guidelines 2021: Cardiac arrest in special circumstances. Resuscitation. 2021;161.

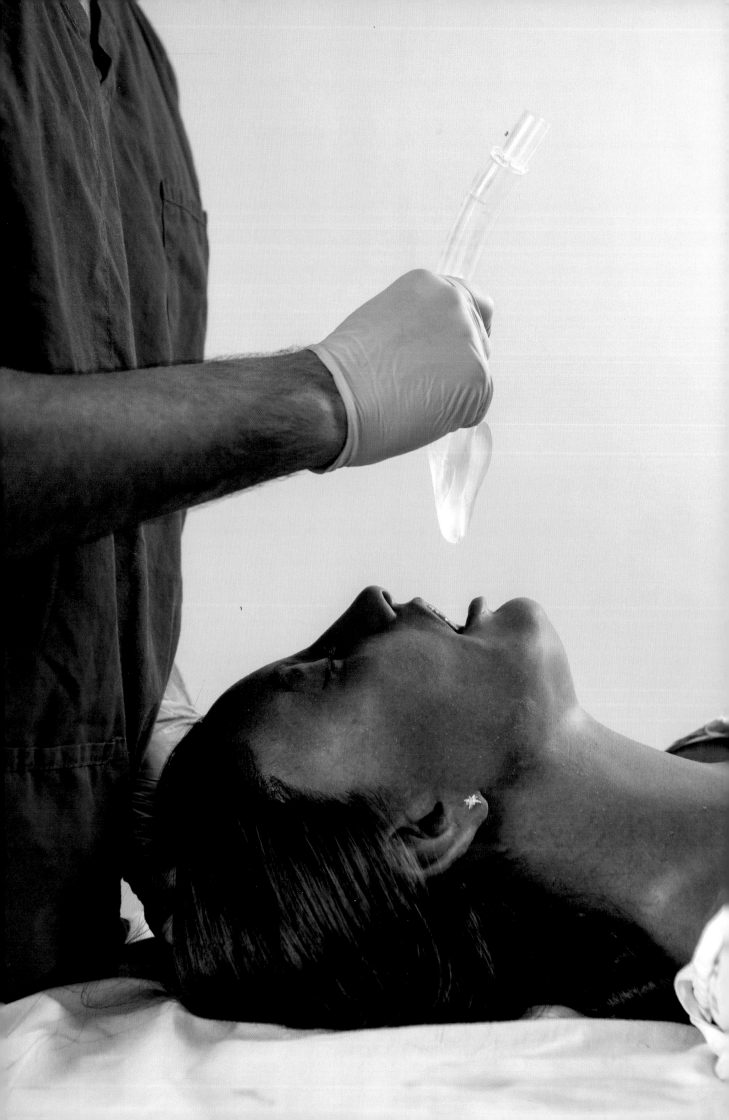

Airway management and ventilation

07

In this chapter

Causes and recognition of airway obstruction

Techniques for airway management when starting resuscitation

The use of simple adjuncts to maintain airway patency

Techniques for ventilating the lungs

Supraglottic airway devices

Tracheal intubation and cricothyroidotomy

The learning outcomes will enable you to:

Recognise the causes of airway obstruction

Manage the airway effectively during resuscitation

Understand the role of simple techniques and devices for maintaining the airway and ventilating the lungs

Understand the role of supraglottic airways during CPR

Consider the role of tracheal intubation during CPR

Understand the role of surgical cricothyroidotomy

Introduction

Patients requiring resuscitation often have an obstructed airway, usually caused by loss of consciousness, but occasionally it may be the primary cause of cardiorespiratory arrest.

Prompt assessment, with control of airway patency and provision of ventilation if required are essential. This will help to prevent secondary hypoxic damage to the brain and other vital organs. Without adequate oxygenation it may be impossible to restore an organised, perfusing cardiac rhythm. These principles may not apply to the witnessed primary cardiac arrest in the vicinity of a defibrillator; in this case, the priority is immediate defibrillation followed by attention to the airway.

Causes of airway obstruction

Obstruction of the airway may be partial or complete. It may occur at any level from the nose and mouth down to the level of the carina and bronchi. In the unconscious patient, the commonest site of airway obstruction is the pharynx – more often at the soft palate and epiglottis rather than the tongue. Obstruction may also be caused by vomit or blood, following regurgitation of gastric contents or trauma, or by foreign bodies. Laryngeal obstruction may be caused by oedema from burns, inflammation or anaphylaxis. Upper airway stimulation or inhalation of foreign material may cause laryngeal spasm.

Obstruction of the airway below the larynx is less common, but may be caused by excessive bronchial secretions, mucosal oedema, bronchospasm, pulmonary oedema, or aspiration of gastric contents. Extrinsic compression of the airway may also occur above or below the larynx (e.g. trauma, haematoma or tumour).

Recognition of airway obstruction

Airway obstruction can be subtle and is often not recognised by healthcare professionals. Recognition is best achieved by the look, listen and feel approach.

LOOK for chest and abdominal movements.

LISTEN and FEEL for airflow at the mouth and nose.

In partial airway obstruction, air entry is diminished and usually noisy:

- **Inspiratory stridor** – caused by obstruction at the laryngeal level or above.
- **Expiratory wheeze** – suggests obstruction of the lower airways, which tend to collapse and obstruct during expiration.
- **Gurgling** – suggests the presence of liquid or semisolid foreign material in the upper airways.
- **Snoring** – arises when the pharynx is partially occluded by the tongue or palate.

Complete airway obstruction in a patient who is making respiratory efforts causes paradoxical chest and abdominal movement, described as 'see-saw breathing'. As the patient attempts to breathe in, the chest is drawn in and the abdomen expands; the opposite occurs in expiration. This contrasts with the normal breathing pattern of synchronous movement of the abdomen upwards and outwards (pushed down by the diaphragm) with lifting of the chest wall. During airway obstruction, accessory muscles of respiration are used – the neck and the shoulder muscles contract to assist movement of the thoracic cage. There may also be intercostal and subcostal recession and a tracheal tug. Full examination of the neck, chest and abdomen should enable differentiation of the movements associated with complete airway obstruction from those of normal breathing. Listen for airflow: normal breathing should be quiet, completely obstructed breathing will be silent, and noisy breathing indicates partial airway obstruction.

During apnoea, when spontaneous breathing movements are absent, complete airway obstruction is recognised by failure to inflate the lungs during attempted positive pressure ventilation. Unless airway obstruction can be relieved to enable adequate lung ventilation within a few minutes it will cause injury to the brain and other vital organs, and cardiac arrest if this has not already occurred.

Whenever possible, give high-concentration oxygen during the attempt to relieve airway obstruction. Arterial blood oxygen saturation (SaO_2) measurements (normally using pulse oximetry (SpO_2)) will guide further use of oxygen as airway patency improves. If airway patency remains poor and SpO_2 remains low, continue to give high inspired oxygen concentration. As airway patency improves, blood oxygen saturation levels will be restored more rapidly if the inspired oxygen concentration is initially high. Inspired oxygen concentrations can then be adjusted to maintain SpO_2 at 94%–98%. Lower oxygen saturations (82–92%) may be appropriate in some patients with chronic obstructive pulmonary disease (COPD) after airway patency is improved.

Patients with tracheostomies or permanent tracheal stomas

A patient with a tracheostomy tube, or a permanent tracheal stoma (usually following a laryngectomy) may develop airway obstruction from blockage of the tracheostomy tube or stoma – the source of airway obstruction in these patients will not be at the level of the pharynx or larynx. Remove any obvious foreign material from the stoma or tracheostomy tube. Remove the tracheostomy liner (inner tube) if one is present. If it is still not possible to ventilate the lungs, try to pass a suction catheter. If this is successful, perform tracheal suctioning and attempt to ventilate. If a suction catheter will not pass remove the tracheostomy tube and exchange it if possible.

If a blocked tracheostomy tube is removed it may be possible to ventilate the patient's lungs by sealing the stoma and using a bag-mask applied to the face, or by intubating the trachea orally with a standard tracheal tube. This might not be possible if the tracheostomy was created because of significant upper airway obstruction (e.g. tumour).

In a patient with a laryngectomy and permanent tracheal stoma, give oxygen and, if required, assist ventilation via the stoma, and not the mouth.

The National Tracheostomy and Safety Project in collaboration with Resuscitation Council UK has produced emergency guidelines and resources that are available at: http://www.tracheostomy.org.uk

Choking

Recognition

Foreign bodies may cause either mild or severe airway obstruction. The signs and symptoms enabling differentiation between mild and severe airway obstruction are summarised in Table 7.1.

Table 7.1 Signs of choking

General signs of choking	
Attack occurs while eating	
Patient may clutch their neck	
Signs of severe airway obstruction	
Response to question 'Are you choking?'	Patient unable to speak
	Patient may respond by nodding
Other signs	Patient unable to breathe
	Breathing sounds wheezy
	Attempts at coughing are silent
	Patient may be unconscious
Signs of mild airway obstruction	
Response to question 'Are you choking?'	Patient speaks and answers yes
Other signs	Patient is able to speak, cough and breathe

Sequence for the treatment of adult choking

1. If the patient shows signs of mild airway obstruction (Table 7.1):
   - Encourage them to continue coughing, but do nothing else (Figure 7.1).

2. If the patient shows signs of severe airway obstruction and is conscious:
   - Give up to 5 back blows.
     - Stand to the side and slightly behind the patient.
     - Support the chest with one hand and lean the patient well forwards.
     - Give up to 5 sharp blows between the scapulae with the heel of the other hand.

Adult choking

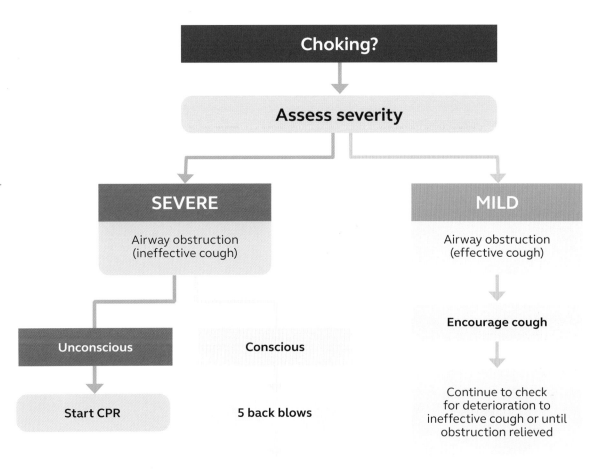

Choking?

Assess severity

SEVERE

Airway obstruction (ineffective cough)

Unconscious

Conscious

Start CPR

5 back blows

5 abdominal thrusts

MILD

Airway obstruction (effective cough)

Encourage cough

Continue to check for deterioration to ineffective cough or until obstruction relieved

- Check to see if each back blow has relieved the airway obstruction.
- If 5 back blows fail to relieve the airway obstruction give up to 5 abdominal thrusts.
  - Stand behind the patient and put both arms round the upper part of their abdomen.
  - Place a clenched fist just under the xiphisternum;
  - Grasp this hand with your other hand and pull sharply inwards and upwards.
  - Repeat up to 5 times.
- If the obstruction is still not relieved, continue alternating 5 back blows with abdominal thrusts.

3. If the patient becomes unconscious, call the resuscitation team and start CPR – chest compressions may aid in dislodging any foreign body.

4. As soon as an individual with appropriate skills is present, undertake laryngoscopy and attempt to remove any foreign body with Magill's forceps.

Basic techniques for opening the airway

Once airway obstruction is recognised, take immediate action to relieve the obstruction and maintain a clear airway. Three manoeuvres that can be used to relieve upper airway obstruction are:

- head tilt
- chin lift
- jaw thrust.

Head tilt and chin lift

Place one hand on the patient's forehead and tilt the head back gently; place the fingertips of the other hand under the point of the patient's chin, and gently lift to stretch the anterior neck structures (Figure 7.2).

Jaw thrust

Jaw thrust is an alternative manoeuvre for bringing the mandible forward and relieving obstruction by the tongue, soft palate and epiglottis (Figure 7.3). It is most successful when applied with a head tilt.

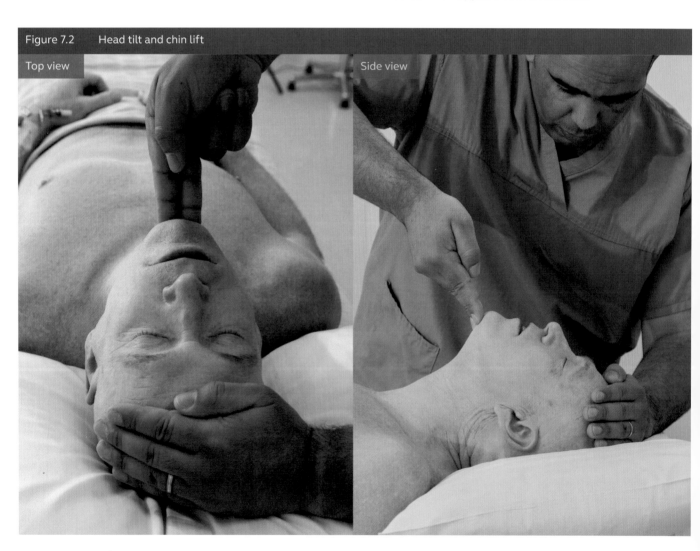

Figure 7.2   Head tilt and chin lift

Top view

Side view

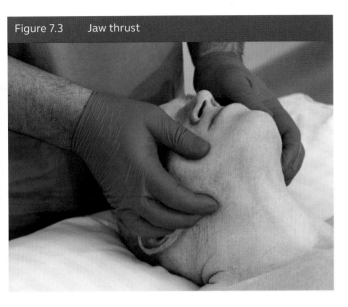

Figure 7.3 Jaw thrust

Procedure for jaw thrust

- Identify the angle of the mandible.
- With the index and other fingers placed behind the angle of the mandible, apply steady upwards and forward pressure to lift the mandible.
- Using the thumbs, slightly open the mouth by downward displacement of the chin.

These simple positional methods are successful in most cases where airway obstruction is caused by loss of muscle tone in the pharynx. After each manoeuvre, check for success using the look, listen and feel sequence. If a clear airway cannot be achieved, look for other causes of airway obstruction. Carefully remove any visible foreign body with forceps or suction. Remove broken or displaced dentures but leave well-fitting dentures in place as they help to maintain the contours of the mouth, facilitating a good seal for ventilation by mouth-to-mask or bag-mask techniques.

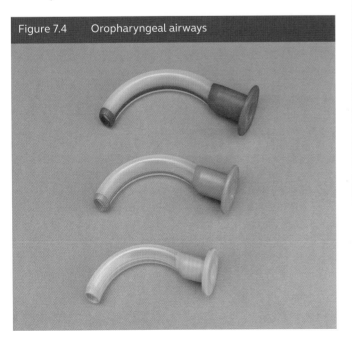

Figure 7.4 Oropharyngeal airways

Adjuncts to basic airway techniques

Simple airway adjuncts are often helpful, and sometimes essential to maintain an open airway, particularly when resuscitation is prolonged. The position of the head and neck must be maintained to keep the airway aligned. Oropharyngeal and nasopharyngeal airways are designed to overcome soft palate obstruction and backward tongue displacement in an unconscious patient, but head tilt and jaw thrust may also be required.

Oropharyngeal airway

The oropharyngeal or Guedel airway is a curved plastic tube, flanged and reinforced at the oral end with a flattened shape to ensure that it fits neatly between the tongue and hard palate (Figure 7.4). It is available in sizes suitable for small and large adults. An estimate of the size required may be obtained by selecting an airway with a length corresponding to the vertical distance between the patient's incisors and the angle of the jaw (Figure 7.5). The most common sizes are 2, 3 and 4 for small, medium and large adults respectively. An oropharyngeal airway that is slightly too big will be more beneficial than one that is slightly too small.

During insertion of an oropharyngeal airway, the tongue can occasionally be pushed backwards, exacerbating obstruction instead of relieving it. The oropharyngeal airway may lodge in the vallecula, or the epiglottis may obstruct the lumen. Ensuring a correct insertion technique should avoid this problem. Attempt insertion only in unconscious patients: vomiting or laryngospasm may occur if glossopharyngeal or laryngeal reflexes are present.

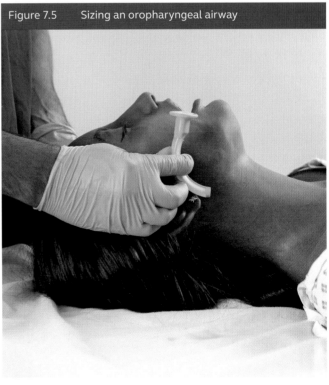

Figure 7.5 Sizing an oropharyngeal airway

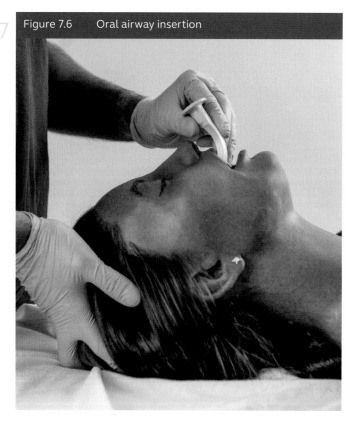

Figure 7.6   Oral airway insertion

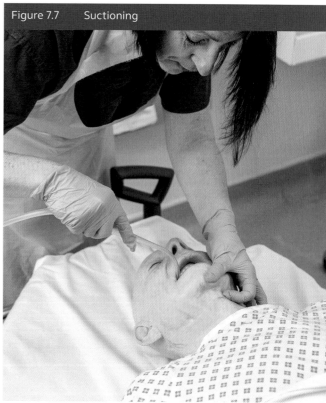

Figure 7.7   Suctioning

Technique for insertion of an oropharyngeal airway

Open the patient's mouth and ensure that there is no foreign material that may be pushed into the larynx (if there is any, then use suction to remove it).

Insert the airway into the oral cavity in the 'upside-down' position as far as the junction between the hard and soft palate and then rotate it through 180° (Figure 7.6). Advance the airway until it lies within the pharynx. This rotation technique minimises the chance of pushing the tongue backwards and downwards. Remove the airway if the patient gags or strains. Correct placement is indicated by an improvement in airway patency and by the seating of the flattened reinforced section between the patient's teeth or gums (if edentulous). A jaw thrust may further aid final placement of the airway as it is finally pushed into the correct position.

After insertion, maintain head-tilt/chin-lift or jaw thrust, and check the patency of the airway and ventilation using the look, listen and feel technique. Where there is suspicion of an injury to the cervical spine, maintain alignment and immobilisation of the head and neck. Suction is usually possible through an oropharyngeal airway using a fine-bore flexible suction catheter.

Nasopharyngeal airway

This is made from soft malleable plastic, bevelled at one end and with a flange at the other. In patients who are not deeply unconscious, it is better tolerated than an oropharyngeal airway. It may be life-saving in patients with clenched jaws, trismus or maxillofacial injuries.

Inadvertent insertion of a nasopharyngeal airway through a fracture of the skull base and into the cranial vault is possible, but extremely rare. In the presence of a known or suspected basal skull fracture an oral airway is preferred, but if this is not possible, and the airway is obstructed, gentle insertion of a nasopharyngeal airway may be life-saving (i.e. the benefits may far outweigh the risks).

The tubes are sized in millimetres according to their internal diameter, and the length increases with diameter. The traditional methods of sizing a nasopharyngeal airway (measurement against the patient's little finger or anterior nares) do not correlate with the airway anatomy and are unreliable. Sizes 6–7 mm are suitable for adults. Insertion can cause damage to the mucosal lining of the nasal airway, resulting in bleeding in up to 30% of cases. If the tube is too long it may stimulate the laryngeal or glossopharyngeal reflexes to produce laryngospasm or vomiting.

Oxygen

In the absence of data indicating the optimal SaO_2 during CPR, ventilate the lungs with the highest feasible oxygen inspired concentration until return of spontaneous circulation (ROSC) is achieved.

After ROSC is achieved and in any acutely ill, or unconscious patient, give high-flow oxygen until the SaO_2 can be measured reliably. A standard oxygen face mask will deliver up to 50%, providing the flow of oxygen is high enough. Initially, give the highest possible oxygen concentration – a face mask with reservoir bag (non-rebreathing mask) can deliver an inspired oxygen concentration of 85% at flows of 10 L min^{-1}. Monitor the SpO_2 or arterial blood gases to enable titration of the inspired oxygen concentration. When blood oxygen saturation can be measured reliably, try to maintain the SpO_2 at 94–98%; or 88–92% if the patient has chronic obstructive pulmonary disease (COPD).

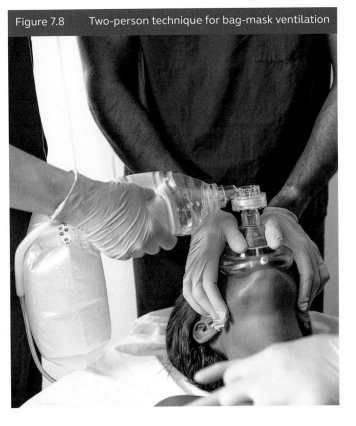

Figure 7.8   Two-person technique for bag-mask ventilation

Suction

Use a wide-bore rigid sucker (Yankauer) to remove liquid (blood, saliva and gastric contents) from the upper airway (Figure 7.7). Use the sucker cautiously if the patient has an intact gag reflex – it can provoke vomiting. Fine-bore flexible suction catheters may be required in patients with limited mouth opening. These suction catheters can also be passed through oropharyngeal or nasopharyngeal airways.

Ventilation

Artificial ventilation is started as soon as possible in any patient in whom spontaneous ventilation is inadequate or absent. Expired air ventilation (rescue breathing) is effective but the rescuer's expired oxygen concentration is only 16–17%; so it must be replaced as soon as possible by ventilation with oxygen-enriched air. Although mouth-to-mouth ventilation has the benefit of not requiring any equipment, the technique is aesthetically unpleasant, particularly when vomit or blood is present, and the rescuer may be reluctant to place themselves in intimate contact with the patient who may be unknown to them.

There are some reports of individuals acquiring infections after providing CPR (e.g. tuberculosis and severe acute respiratory distress syndrome (SARS)). The risk of transmitting severe acute respiratory distress syndrome coronavirus 2 (SARS-CoV-2) through mouth-to-mouth is extremely high and confirmed or suspected coronavirus disease 2019 (COVID-19) is a contraindication to mouth-to-mouth ventilation. Check the Resuscitation Council UK website for the latest guidance regarding COVID-19: https://www.resus.org.uk/

The pocket resuscitation mask is similar to an anaesthetic face mask and enables mouth-to-mask ventilation. Although previously advocated, mouth-to-mask was not a popular technique because of the requirement for the rescuer to be close to the patient's face. The COVID-19 pandemic has raised awareness of infection risk particularly when undertaking airway manoeuvres, consequently this technique is no longer recommended for clinical settings.

Self-inflating bag

The self-inflating bag can be connected to a face mask, tracheal tube, or supraglottic airway (SGA). As the bag is squeezed, the contents are delivered to the patient's lungs. On release, the expired gas is diverted to the atmosphere via a one-way valve; the bag then refills automatically via an inlet at the opposite end. When used without supplemental oxygen, the self-inflating bag ventilates the patient's lungs with ambient air (oxygen concentration 21%) only. This is increased to around 45% by attaching high-flow oxygen directly to the bag adjacent to the air intake. An inspired oxygen concentration of approximately 85% is achieved if a reservoir system is attached and the oxygen flow is maximally increased. As the bag re-expands it fills with oxygen from both the reservoir and the continuous flow from the attached oxygen tubing.

Although the bag-mask enables ventilation with high concentrations of oxygen, its use by a single person requires considerable skill. When used with a face mask, it is often difficult to achieve a gas-tight seal between the mask and the patient's face, and maintain a patent airway with one hand whilst squeezing the bag with the other.

Any significant leak will cause hypoventilation and if the airway is not patent, gas may also be directed into the stomach. This will reduce ventilation further and greatly increase the risk of regurgitation and aspiration. There is a natural tendency to try to compensate for a leak by excessive compression of the bag, which causes high peak airway pressures and forces more gas into the stomach. Some self-inflating bags have flow restrictors that limit peak airway pressure with the aim of reducing gastric inflation.

The two-person technique for bag-mask ventilation is preferable (Figure 7.8). One person holds the face mask in place using a jaw thrust with both hands and an assistant squeezes the bag. In this way, a better seal can be achieved and the patient's lungs can be ventilated more effectively and safely. This assistant can also be the person delivering chest compressions. An oropharyngeal airway should always be considered when using bag-mask ventilation.

Automatic resuscitators

Various small portable automatic ventilators may be used during resuscitation; they are more likely to be used pre-hospital rather than in-hospital. Most automatic resuscitators provide a constant flow of gas to the patient during inspiration; the volume delivered is dependent on the inspiratory time (a longer time provides a greater tidal volume). Because pressure in the airway rises during inspiration, these devices are often pressure-limited to protect the lungs against barotrauma.

Automatic resuscitators have some advantages over alternative methods of ventilation:

- In unintubated patients, the rescuer has both hands free for mask and airway alignment.
- In intubated patients they free the rescuer for other tasks.
- Once set, they provide a constant tidal volume, respiratory rate and minute ventilation; thus, they may help to avoid excessive ventilation.

Passive oxygen delivery

In the presence of a patent airway, chest compressions alone may result in some ventilation of the lungs. Oxygen can be delivered passively, either via an adapted tracheal tube or with the combination of an oropharyngeal airway and standard oxygen mask with non-rebreathe reservoir. There is insufficient evidence to support or refute the use of passive oxygen delivery during CPR to improve outcome when compared with oxygen delivery by positive pressure ventilation and until further data are available, passive oxygen delivery without ventilation is not currently recommended for routine use during CPR.

Supraglottic airways

Effective bag-mask ventilation requires a reasonable level of skill and experience; the inexperienced are likely to achieve ineffective tidal volumes and cause gastric inflation with risk of regurgitation and pulmonary aspiration. In comparison with bag-mask ventilation, use of SGAs may enable more effective ventilation and reduce the risk of gastric inflation. Furthermore, SGAs are easier to insert than a tracheal tube and, unlike tracheal intubation, they can generally be positioned without interrupting chest compressions.

Without adequate training and experience, the incidence of complications associated with attempted tracheal intubation is unacceptably high. Unrecognised oesophageal intubation is disastrous and prolonged attempts at tracheal intubation are harmful; the pause in chest compressions during this time will severely compromise coronary and cerebral perfusion. Alternative airway devices should be used by all personnel not skilled in regular intubation of the trachea and if attempted tracheal intubation by those highly skilled to perform the technique has failed.

There are no data supporting the routine use of any specific approach to airway management during cardiac arrest. The best technique is dependent on the precise circumstances of the cardiac arrest and the competence of the rescuer.

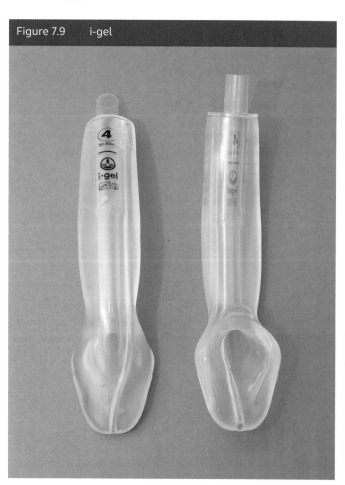

Figure 7.9   i-gel

i-gel airway

The i-gel incorporates a cuff made of thermoplastic elastomer gel and does not require inflation; the stem of the i-gel incorporates a bite block and a narrow oesophageal drain tube (Figure 7.9). It is easy to insert, requiring only minimal training, and a laryngeal seal pressure of 20–24 cmH$_2$O can be achieved. Insertion of the i-gel is faster than most other airway devices. Ventilation using the i-gel is more efficient and easier than with a bag-mask apparatus; provided high inflation pressures (> 24 cmH$_2$O) are avoided, gastric inflation is minimised. When an i-gel can be inserted without delay it is preferable to avoid bag-mask ventilation altogether: the risk of gastric inflation and regurgitation is reduced.

Supraglottic airway devices like the i-gel are particularly valuable if attempted tracheal intubation by skilled personnel has failed and bag-mask ventilation is proving difficult or impossible (the cannot ventilate, cannot intubate scenario).

The ease of insertion of the i-gel and its favourable leak pressure make it very attractive as a resuscitation airway device for those inexperienced in tracheal intubation. The i-gel is in widespread use in the UK for both in-hospital and out-of-hospital cardiac arrest.

Technique for insertion of an i-gel

- Try to maintain chest compressions throughout the insertion attempt; if it is necessary to stop chest compressions during the insertion attempt, limit this pause in chest compressions to a maximum of 5 s.

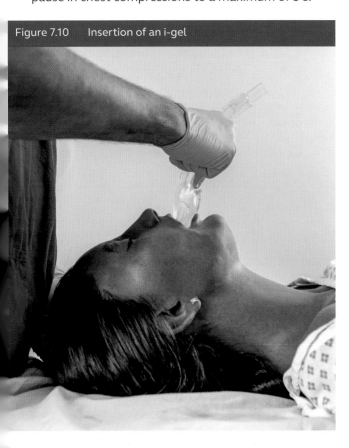

Figure 7.10   Insertion of an i-gel

- Select an appropriately sized i-gel: a size 4 will function well in most adults although small adults may require a size 3 and tall adults a size 5.
- Lubricate the back, sides and front of the i-gel cuff with a thin layer of lubricant.
- Grasp the lubricated i-gel firmly along the integral bite block. Position the device so that the i-gel cuff outlet is facing towards the chin of the patient.
- Ensure the patient is in the 'sniffing the morning air' position with head extended and neck flexed. Gently press the chin down to open the mouth before inserting the i-gel.
- Introduce the leading soft tip into the mouth of the patient in a direction towards the hard palate (Figure 7.10).
- Do not apply excessive force to the device during insertion. It is not normally necessary to insert fingers or thumbs into the patient's mouth during the process of inserting the device. If there is early resistance during insertion, get an assistant to apply a jaw thrust or slightly rotate the device.
- Glide the device downwards and backwards along the hard palate with a continuous but gentle push until a definitive resistance is felt.
- At this point the tip of the airway should be located at the upper oesophageal opening and the cuff should be located against the larynx. The incisors should be resting on the integral bite-block.
- A horizontal line at the middle of the integral bite-block represents the approximate position of the teeth when the i-gel is positioned correctly. However, this line is only a guide – there is considerable variation in its location relative to the incisors. In short patients, this line may be higher than the teeth, even when correctly positioned. In tall patients, the line may not be visible above the teeth.

Limitations of the i-gel

- In the presence of high airway resistance or poor lung compliance (pulmonary oedema, bronchospasm, chronic obstructive pulmonary disease) there is a risk of a significant leak around the cuff causing hypoventilation. Most of the gas leaking around the cuff normally escapes through the patient's mouth but some gastric inflation may occur.
- Uninterrupted chest compressions are likely to cause at least some gas leak from the i-gel cuff when ventilation is attempted. Attempt continuous compressions initially but if gas leakage results in inadequate ventilation, pause compressions for ventilation using a compression-ventilation ratio of 30:2.
- There is a theoretical risk of aspiration of stomach contents because the i-gel does not sit within the larynx like a tracheal tube; however, this complication is rarely documented in clinical practice.

- If the patient is not deeply unconscious, insertion of the i-gel may cause coughing, straining or laryngeal spasm. This will not occur in patients in cardiorespiratory arrest.

- If an adequate airway is not achieved, withdraw the i-gel and attempt reinsertion ensuring a good alignment of the head and neck.

Laryngeal mask airway

The laryngeal mask airway (LMA) consists of a wide-bore tube with an elliptical inflated cuff designed to seal around the laryngeal opening (Figures 7.11, 7.12). It was introduced into anaesthetic practice in the middle of the 1980s and is a reliable and safe device, which can be introduced easily, with a high success rate after a short period of training.

Ventilation using the LMA is more efficient and easier than with a bag-mask apparatus; provided high inflation pressures (> 20 cmH$_2$O) are avoided, gastric inflation is minimised. When an LMA can be inserted without delay it is preferable to avoid bag-mask ventilation altogether: the risk of gastric inflation and regurgitation is reduced.

Though not guaranteeing protection of the airway from gastric contents, pulmonary aspiration during use of the LMA is uncommon. The LMA does protect against sources of aspiration from above the larynx. Use of the LMA by nursing, paramedical and medical staff during resuscitation has been studied and reported to be effective. The LMA, like the i-gel is particularly valuable if attempted tracheal intubation by skilled personnel has failed and bag-mask ventilation is impossible (the cannot ventilate, cannot intubate scenario). The original LMA (classic LMA (cLMA)), which is reusable, has been studied during CPR, but none of these studies has compared it directly with the tracheal tube. The cLMA has been superseded by several second generation SGAs that have more favourable characteristics, particularly when used for emergency airway management. Most of these SGAs are single-use devices and achieve higher oropharyngeal seal pressures than the cLMA, and some incorporate gastric drain tubes e.g. i-gel.

Tracheal intubation

Randomised controlled trials undertaken in out-of-hospital cardiac arrest have failed to show a survival advantage with any particular airway management strategy. No randomised trials of airway management have been undertaken for in-hospital cardiac arrest. In practice, airway management is most commonly undertaken using a stepwise approach, starting with basic techniques and moving on to more advanced techniques, depending on available skills, until effective ventilation and satisfactory airway protection is achieved. Tracheal intubation should be attempted only when trained personnel are available to carry out the procedure with a high level of skill and competence. Expert consensus has defined this skill threshold as a 95%

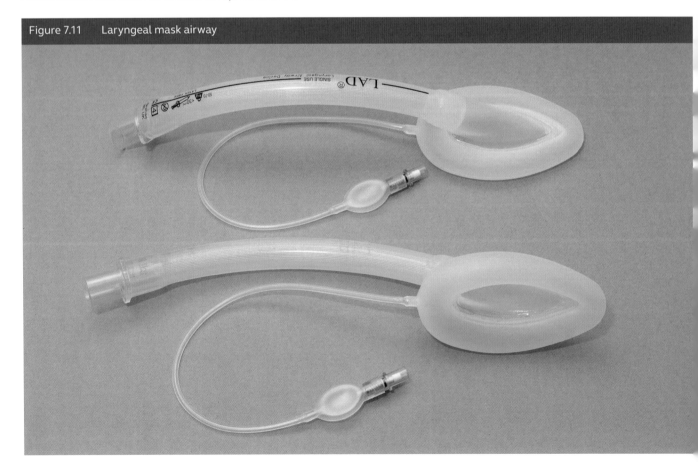

Figure 7.11   Laryngeal mask airway

success rate with up to two intubation attempts. The perceived advantages of tracheal intubation over bag-mask ventilation include maintenance of a patent airway which is protected from aspiration of gastric contents or blood from the oropharynx, the ability to provide an adequate tidal volume reliably even when chest compressions are uninterrupted, the potential to free the rescuer's hands for other tasks, and the ability to suck-out airway secretions. Use of a bag-mask is more likely to cause gastric distension, which, theoretically, is more likely to cause regurgitation and the risk of aspiration. This theoretical risk has not been realised in the randomised clinical trials undertaken to date.

The perceived disadvantages of tracheal intubation over bag-mask ventilation include the risk of an unrecognised misplaced tracheal tube (which is as high as 17% in some older studies of out-of-hospital cardiac arrest), a prolonged time without chest compressions while tracheal intubation is attempted (tracheal intubation attempts accounted for almost 25% of all CPR interruptions in one pre-hospital study) and a comparatively high failure rate (50% in a recent pre-hospital study). Tracheal intubation success rates depend on the intubation experience attained by the rescuer. Healthcare personnel who undertake pre-hospital intubation should do so only within a structured, monitored program, which should include comprehensive competency-based training and regular opportunities to refresh skills.

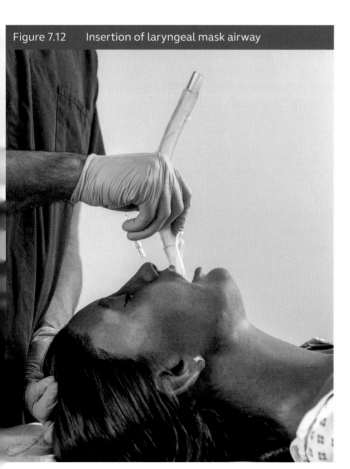

Figure 7.12   Insertion of laryngeal mask airway

Rescuers must weigh the risks and benefits of tracheal intubation against the need to provide effective chest compressions. To avoid any interruptions in chest compressions, unless alternative airway management techniques are ineffective, it is reasonable to defer tracheal intubation until after ROSC. In settings with personnel skilled in advanced airway management laryngoscopy should be undertaken without stopping chest compressions; a brief pause in chest compressions will be required only as the tube is passed through the vocal cords. The tracheal intubation attempt should interrupt chest compressions for less than 5 s; if intubation is not achievable within these constraints, recommence bag-mask ventilation. After tracheal intubation, tube placement must be confirmed immediately (see below) and the tube must be secured adequately.

In some cases, laryngoscopy and attempted intubation may prove impossible or cause life-threatening deterioration in the patient's condition. Such circumstances include acute epiglottitis, pharyngeal and laryngeal disease, head injury (where coughing or straining may cause further increase in intracranial pressure), or in patients with cervical spine injury. In these circumstances, specialist skills such as the use of anaesthetic drugs, videolaryngoscopy or flexible fibreoptic laryngoscopy may be required. Such techniques require a high level of skill and training.

Post-intubation procedures

- After successful intubation, connect the tracheal tube (via a catheter mount if necessary) to a ventilating device (e.g. self-inflating bag), and ventilate with the highest oxygen concentration available.

- Inflate the cuff of the tracheal tube just sufficiently to stop an air leak during inspiration.

- Confirm correct placement of the tracheal tube using clinical assessment AND waveform capnography. Unrecognised oesophageal intubation is the most serious complication of attempted tracheal intubation. Routine use of waveform capnography to confirm correct placement of the tracheal tube will reduce this risk and is mandatory regardless of location.

- Continue ventilation with a high-concentration of oxygen until ROSC and oxygen saturations are recordable.

- Secure the tube with a bandage or tie. Adhesive tape is not reliable if the face is moist.

- An oropharyngeal airway may be inserted alongside the tracheal tube to maintain the position of the tube, and prevent damage from biting if consciousness returns.

Clinical assessment

Primary assessment includes observation of chest expansion bilaterally, auscultation over the lungs bilaterally in the axillae (breath sounds should be equal and adequate) and over the epigastrium (breath sounds should not be heard). Clinical signs of correct tube placement (condensation in the tube, chest rise, breath sounds on auscultation of lungs, and inability to hear gas entering the stomach) are all unreliable.

Secondary confirmation of tracheal tube placement by waveform capnography (see below) will reduce the risk of unrecognised oesophageal intubation; however, this will not differentiate between a tube placed in a main bronchus and one placed correctly in the trachea.

Carbon dioxide detectors

Carbon dioxide (CO_2) detector devices measure the concentration of exhaled carbon dioxide from the lungs. The persistence of exhaled CO_2 after six ventilations indicates placement of the tracheal tube in the trachea or a main bronchus. Confirmation of correct placement above the carina will require auscultation of the chest bilaterally in the mid-axillary lines. Broadly, there are two types of CO_2 detector devices that can be used during CPR:

1. End-tidal CO_2 detectors that include a waveform graphical display (capnograph) are the most reliable for verification of tracheal tube position during cardiac arrest. Studies of waveform capnography to verify tracheal tube position in patients of cardiac arrest demonstrate 100% sensitivity and 100% specificity in identifying correct tracheal tube placement.

2. Non-waveform electronic digital end-tidal CO_2 devices generally measure end-tidal CO_2 using an infrared spectrometer and display the results with a number; they do not provide a waveform graphical display of the respiratory cycle on a capnograph and are not sufficiently reliable to confirm tracheal intubation in cardiac arrest.

Waveform capnography is the most sensitive and specific way to confirm and continuously monitor the position of a tracheal tube in patients of cardiac arrest and must supplement clinical assessment (auscultation and visualisation of tube through cords). Waveform capnography will not discriminate between tracheal and bronchial placement of the tube – careful auscultation is essential. Existing portable monitors make capnographic initial confirmation and continuous monitoring of tracheal tube position feasible in all settings, including out-of-hospital, emergency department, and in-hospital locations where tracheal intubation is performed. Waveform capnography is also a sensitive indicator of ROSC and a monitor for the delivery of effective CPR (see Chapter 6).

The 'No Trace = Wrong Place' campaign emphasises that exhaled CO_2 will be detectable by waveform capnography even during cardiac arrest; failure to detect any CO_2 indicates that the tube is in the oesophagus. The use of waveform capnography to confirm tracheal tube placement is now a standard of care. Do not attempt tracheal intubation if waveform capnography is not immediately available and use a supraglottic airway device if advanced airway management is required.

Aids to intubation

Videolaryngoscopes

Videolaryngoscopes are being used increasingly in anaesthetic and critical care practice. In comparison with direct laryngoscopy, they enable a better view of the larynx and improve the success rate of intubation. They also enable the intubator to be further from the patient's airway, which is an advantage if the risk of infection transmission is a concern. Studies indicate that use of videolaryngoscopes improves laryngeal view and intubation success rates during CPR. The use of a videolaryngoscope requires device specific training as a number of different types of videolaryngoscope are available. Use direct (standard) or video laryngoscopy for tracheal intubation according to local protocols.

Suction

Use a wide-bore rigid suction end (Yankauer) to remove liquid (blood, saliva and gastric contents) from the upper airway. This is done best under direct vision during intubation but must not delay achieving a definitive airway. Apply suction to the trachea as briefly as possible and ventilate the lungs with 100% oxygen before and after the procedure. Use fine-bore suction catheters for tracheal suction and pass them directly down the tracheal tube.

Cricothyroidotomy

Occasionally it will be impossible to ventilate an apnoeic patient with a bag-mask, SGA, or to pass a tracheal tube. This may occur in patients with extensive facial trauma or laryngeal obstruction caused by oedema (e.g. anaphylaxis, or foreign material). In these circumstances, it will be necessary to create a surgical airway below the level of the obstruction. A tracheostomy is contraindicated in an emergency because it is time consuming, hazardous and requires considerable surgical skill and equipment. Substantial bleeding can occur. Surgical cricothyroidotomy provides a definitive airway that can be used to ventilate the patient's lungs until semi-elective intubation or tracheostomy is performed. Needle cricothyroidotomy is no longer recommended. Surgical cricothyroidotomy should only be performed by those trained in the technique.

07: **Summary learning**

During CPR, start with basic airway techniques and progress stepwise according to the skills of the rescuer until effective ventilation is achieved.

Use of simple airway manoeuvres, with or without basic adjuncts, will often achieve a patent airway.

Give all patients high-concentration oxygen until the arterial oxygen saturation can be measured.

Supraglottic airways are excellent alternatives to a bag-mask and are used instead of a bag-mask technique wherever possible.

Supraglottic airways are used instead of tracheal intubation unless individuals highly skilled in intubation are immediately available. They are also used if attempted intubation is unsuccessful.

In skilled hands, tracheal intubation is an effective airway management technique during cardiopulmonary resuscitation; however, to avoid any interruptions in chest compressions, it is reasonable to defer intubation until after ROSC.

In unskilled hands, prolonged interruptions of chest compressions, a high risk of failure and other complications (e.g. unrecognised oesophageal intubation) make attempted tracheal intubation potentially extremely harmful and it should not be attempted.

My key take-home messages from this chapter are:

Further reading

Granfeldt A, Avis SR, Nicholson TC, et al. Advanced airway management during adult cardiac arrest: a systematic review. Resuscitation 2019;139:133–143.

Higgs A, McGrath BA, Goddard C, Rangasami J, Suntharalingam G, Gale R, Cook TM; Difficult Airway Society. DAS guidelines on the airway management of critically ill patients. Anaesthesia. 2018;73:1035-1036.

Soar J, Berg KM, Andersen LW, et al. Advanced life support: 2020 International Consensus on Cardiopulmonary Resuscitation and Emergency Cardiovascular Care Science With Treatment Recommendations. Resuscitation 2020;156:A80–A119.

Soar J, Böttiger BW, Carli P, Couper K, Deakin CD, Djärv T, Lott C, Olasveengen TM, Paal P, Pellis T, Perkins GD, Sandroni C, Nolan JP. European Resuscitation Council Guidelines 2021: Advanced Life Support. Resuscitation. 2021;161.

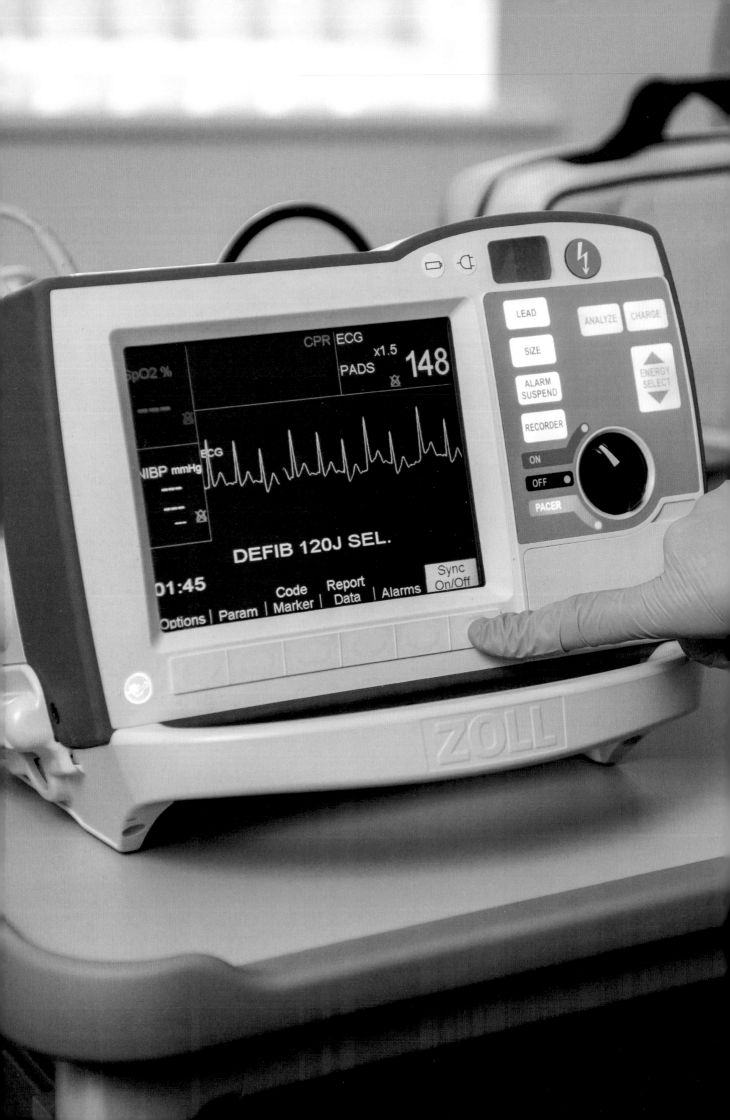

Rhythm recognition

In this chapter

Indications and techniques
for ECG monitoring

The basis of the ECG signal

Reading an ECG rhythm strip

Common arrhythmias

**The learning outcomes
will enable you to:**

Understand the reasons
for ECG monitoring

Know how to monitor the ECG

Consider the origin of the ECG

Understand the importance of
recording the ECG

Identify the cardiac rhythms
associated with cardiac arrest

Systematically interpret rhythms
on an ECG

Introduction

During cardiac arrest, assessment of the cardiac rhythm is crucial to enable you to make the correct choice of treatment (Chapter 6). Establish ECG monitoring as soon as possible. In many patients who have been resuscitated from cardiac arrest there is a substantial risk of further arrhythmia and cardiac arrest. Maintain ECG monitoring in people who have been resuscitated from cardiac arrest until you are confident that the risk of recurrence is very low.

Some patients present with an arrhythmia that may lead to cardiac arrest or other serious deterioration in their condition. Early detection and treatment of the arrhythmia may prevent cardiac arrest in some patients and prevent life-threatening deterioration in others. Patients at risk include those with persistent arrhythmia associated with structural heart disease, chest pain, heart failure, reduced conscious level or shock. In all patients who have persistent arrhythmia and are at risk of deterioration, establish ECG monitoring and as soon as possible record a good-quality 12-lead ECG. Monitoring alone will not always enable accurate rhythm recognition and it is important to document the arrhythmia in 12-leads for future reference if required.

Some people experience symptoms (usually syncope) caused by an intermittent cardiac arrhythmia that, if not documented and treated, could lead to cardiac arrest or sudden death. However, the arrhythmia may not be present at the time of initial assessment. In people who present with syncope undertake careful clinical assessment and record a 12-lead ECG. People who have experienced uncomplicated faints, situational syncope (such as cough syncope or micturition syncope) or syncope due to orthostatic hypotension do not require continuous ECG monitoring and do not usually require hospital admission. In those who have had unexplained syncope, especially during exercise, those who have had syncope and have evidence of structural heart disease, and those who have had syncope and have an abnormal ECG (especially a prolonged QT interval) start ECG monitoring and arrange further expert cardiovascular assessment.

Monitoring the ECG by looking at only one of the 12-leads is not a reliable technique for detecting evidence of myocardial ischaemia (e.g. ST-segment depression). Record serial 12-lead ECGs in people experiencing chest pain suggestive of an acute coronary syndrome.

During cardiac arrest, prompt recognition of ventricular fibrillation/pulseless ventricular tachycardia (VF/pVT) as shockable rhythms will allow you to deliver effective treatment with minimum delay. Automated external defibrillators (AEDs) and shock-advisory defibrillators can identify these rhythms reliably by electronic analysis. If a shockable rhythm is present, the defibrillator will charge to the appropriate energy level and instruct the operator that a shock should be given. AEDs enable resuscitation from VF/pVT to be achieved by people who do not have skill in rhythm recognition and little or no training in AED use, both in hospitals and in the wider community.

Accurate analysis of some rhythm abnormalities requires experience and expertise; however, the non-expert can interpret most rhythms sufficiently to identify what immediate treatment is needed. The main priority is to recognise that the rhythm is abnormal and that the heart rate is inappropriately slow or fast. Use the structured approach to rhythm interpretation described in this chapter to help you to avoid errors. Any need for immediate treatment will be determined largely by the effect of the arrhythmia on the patient rather than by the nature of the arrhythmia. When an arrhythmia is present, first assess the patient (use the ABCDE approach), and then interpret the rhythm as accurately as possible. Always treat the patient and not their ECG.

Techniques for ECG monitoring

ECG monitors

ECG monitors display the ECG on a screen in real time. The signal is obtained from adhesive electrodes on the patient's skin and transmitted to the monitor either by wires or by telemetry. Many monitor systems have other features, such as the ability to print samples of the ECG rhythm display or to store samples of the ECG. Most monitors include a display of heart rate, and some have alarms that can be programmed to provide an alert when the heart rate goes below or exceeds preset limits.

Many systems enable monitoring of other variables such as blood pressure and oxygen saturation, which are important in the assessment of patients at risk. Digital processing of the ECG offers the potential for electronic analysis of the cardiac rhythm. If a patient requires monitoring, make sure that the monitor is being observed (and that alarms are programmed appropriately) so that immediate action can be taken if necessary, should the rhythm change.

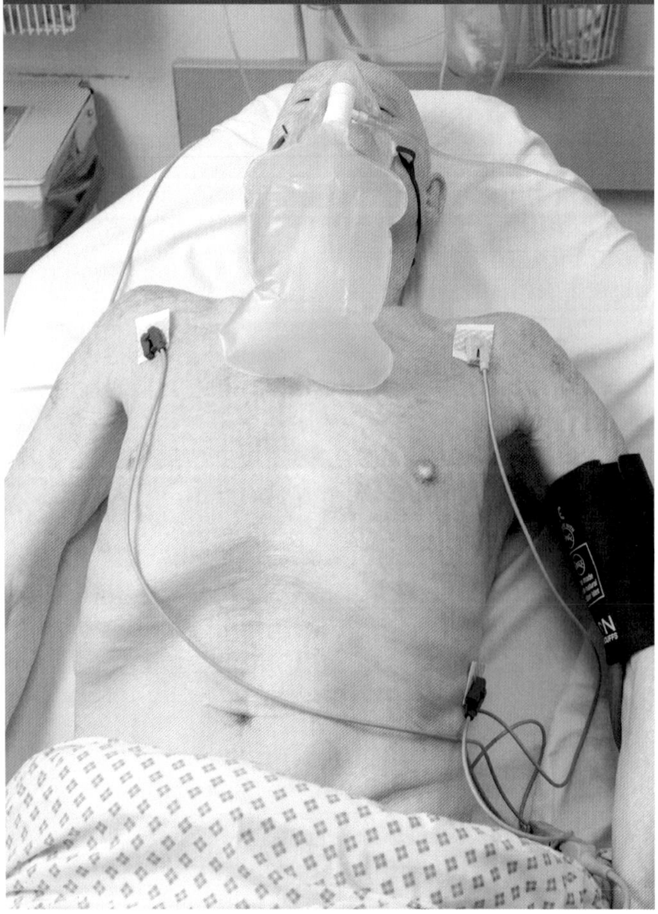

How to attach a monitor

Attach ECG electrodes to the patient using the positions shown in Figure 8.1. These will enable monitoring using 'modified limb leads' I, II and III. Make sure that the skin is dry, not greasy (use an alcohol swab and/or abrasive pad to clean), and either place the electrodes on relatively hair-free skin or shave off dense hair. Place electrodes over bone rather than muscle, to minimise interference in the ECG signal from muscle artefact. Different electrode positions may be used when necessary (e.g. trauma, recent surgery, skin disease).

Most ECG leads are colour-coded to help with correct connection.

The usual colours are:

Red for the **Right** arm lead
(usually placed over the right shoulder joint)

yeLLow for the **Left** arm lead
(usually placed over the left shoulder joint)

Green for the **leG** lead
(usually placed on the abdomen or lower left chest wall).

Begin by monitoring in modified lead II as this usually displays good amplitude sinus P waves and good amplitude QRS complexes, but switch to another lead if necessary to obtain the best ECG signal. Try to minimise muscle and movement artefact by explaining to patients what the monitoring is for and by keeping them warm and relaxed.

Figure 8.1   Electrode positions for ECG monitoring using modified limb leads

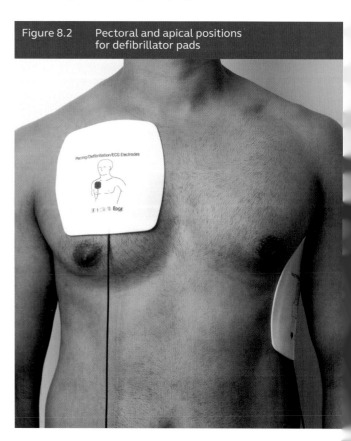

Figure 8.2   Pectoral and apical positions for defibrillator pads

Emergency monitoring

In an emergency, such as a collapsed patient, assess the cardiac rhythm as soon as possible by applying adhesive defibrillator pads, which can be used for monitoring and for shock delivery (Figure 8.2). Apply the pads in the conventional positions, beneath the right clavicle and in the left mid-axillary line. Use anterior and posterior positions as an alternative if the conventional positions cannot be used (e.g. permanent pacemaker in right pectoral position, chest wall trauma). Rapid application of manual defibrillator paddles also enables the cardiac rhythm to be determined rapidly. However in most UK healthcare environments paddles are no longer used.

Diagnosis from cardiac monitors

Use the ECG displays and printouts from monitors only for rhythm recognition. Do not attempt to interpret ST-segment abnormalities or other more sophisticated elements of the ECG from monitors. When an arrhythmia is detected on a monitor, record a rhythm strip whenever possible.

If the arrhythmia persists for long enough, record a 12-lead ECG. It may not be possible to identify an arrhythmia by looking at only one of the 12-leads on a monitor or rhythm strip. The heart is a three-dimensional organ and the 12-lead ECG examines the electrical signals from the heart in three dimensions. Sometimes, features that enable precise identification of cardiac rhythm are visible in only one or two leads of the 12-lead ECG and would not be seen on a rhythm strip recorded in any other lead (Figure 8.3). See the end of chapter for guidance on correct lead placement for the 12-lead ECG.

These recordings may assist with rhythm interpretation at the time but are also useful for later examination and planning of treatment in the longer term. Therefore effective management of any arrhythmia, including a cardiac arrest arrhythmia, includes recording and storing a good quality ECG, as well as interpretation and treatment of the rhythm at the time.

Valuable information about the nature and origin of a tachyarrhythmia can also be obtained by recording the response to treatment (e.g. carotid sinus massage, adenosine). Whenever possible, the effect of any such intervention should be documented on a continuous ECG recording, if possible using multiple leads (Figure 8.4).

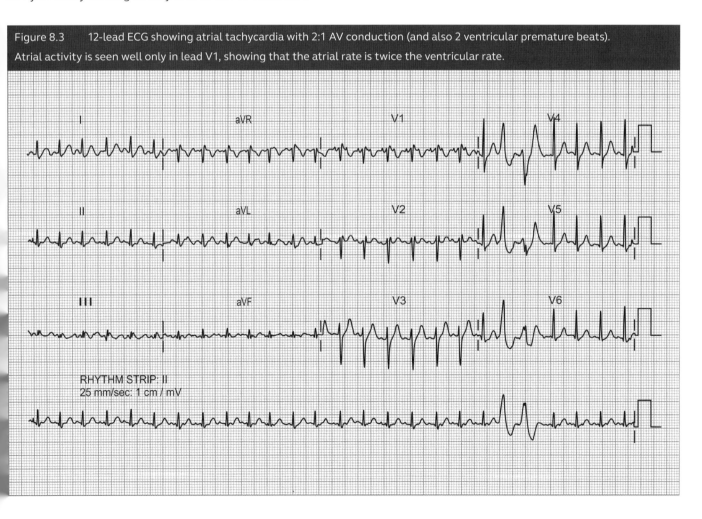

Figure 8.3   12-lead ECG showing atrial tachycardia with 2:1 AV conduction (and also 2 ventricular premature beats). Atrial activity is seen well only in lead V1, showing that the atrial rate is twice the ventricular rate.

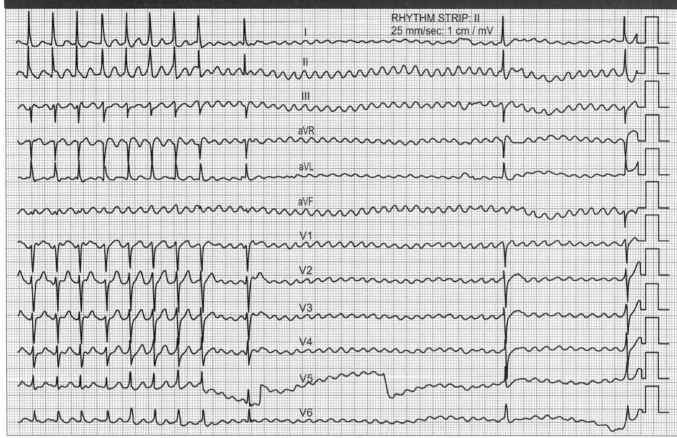

Figure 8.4   12-lead ECG showing initially a regular narrow-complex tachycardia.

Adenosine did not terminate the arrhythmia but caused transient AV block, showing clearly that the initial rhythm was atrial flutter with 2:1 AV conduction.

Basic electrocardiography

At rest, the cells of the heart's conducting system and myocardium are 'polarised'. A potential difference of approximately 90 mV is present between the inside of the cell (which is negatively charged) and the extracellular space. A sudden shift of ions across the cell membrane triggers depolarisation, generating the electrical signal that travels through the conducting system and triggers contraction of myocardial cells.

In normal sinus rhythm, depolarisation begins in a group of specialised 'pacemaker' cells, called the sino-atrial (SA) node, located close to the entry of the superior vena cava into the right atrium. A wave of depolarisation then spreads from the SA node through the atrial myocardium. This is seen on the ECG as the P wave (Figure 8.5). Atrial contraction is the mechanical response to this electrical impulse.

The transmission of this electrical impulse to the ventricles occurs through specialised conducting tissue (Figure 8.6). Firstly, there is slow conduction through the atrioventricular (AV) node, followed by rapid conduction to the ventricular myocardium by specialised conducting tissue (Purkinje fibres). The bundle of His carries these fibres from the AV node and then divides into right and left bundle branches, spreading out through the right and left ventricles respectively. Rapid conduction down these fibres ensures that the ventricles contract in a coordinated fashion.

Depolarisation of ventricular myocardium is seen on the ECG as the QRS complex (Figure 8.5). Ventricular contraction is the mechanical response to this electrical impulse.

Between the P wave and QRS complex is a small isoelectric segment, which largely represents the delay in transmission through the AV node. The normal sequence of atrial depolarisation followed by ventricular depolarisation (P wave followed by QRS complex) is sinus rhythm (Rhythm strip 1).

The T wave, which follows the QRS complex, represents recovery of the resting potential in the cells of the conducting system and ventricular myocardium (ventricular repolarisation). Because the normal conducting system transmits the depolarising impulse rapidly to both ventricles, the normal QRS complex is of relatively short duration (normal < 0.12 s).

When one of the bundle branches is diseased or damaged, rapid conduction to the corresponding ventricle is prevented. The depolarising impulse travels more rapidly down the other bundle branch to its ventricle and then more slowly, through ordinary ventricular myocardium to the other ventricle. This situation is called bundle branch block (Figure 8.6). Because depolarisation of both ventricles takes longer than normal it is seen on the ECG as a broad QRS complex (0.12 s or longer).

How to read a rhythm strip

Experience and expertise may be needed to identify some rhythm abnormalities with complete accuracy and confidence. However, a simple, structured approach to interpreting the rhythm on any ECG recording will define any rhythm in sufficient detail to enable you to choose the most appropriate immediate treatment.

Use the 6-stage system to analyse rhythm on an ECG:

1. Is there any electrical activity?

2. What is the ventricular (QRS) rate?

3. Is the QRS rhythm regular or irregular?

4. Is the QRS complex width normal ('narrow') or broad?

5. Is atrial activity present?

6. Is atrial activity related to ventricular activity and, if so, how?

Any cardiac rhythm can be described accurately (e.g. irregular narrow complex tachycardia, regular broad-complex bradycardia, etc.) using the first four steps and its immediate management can then be decided safely and effectively. Do not go further to steps 5 and 6 unless you are confident that you can see atrial activity.

1. Is there any electrical activity?

If you cannot see any electrical activity, check that the gain control is not too low and that the electrodes and leads are connected securely to both the patient and the monitor.

Check the patient: is a pulse present? If the patient is pulseless and there is still no activity on the ECG this is asystole (Rhythm strip 2). Atrial and ventricular asystole are often both present, resulting in a line with no deflections. A completely straight line usually indicates that a lead has become disconnected. During asystole the ECG usually shows slight undulation of the baseline, and may show electrical interference due to respiratory movement, or chest compression.

Atrial activity (usually P waves but occasionally atrial fibrillation (AF) or atrial flutter) may continue for a short time after the onset of ventricular asystole. The ECG will show the atrial activity but no QRS complexes – ventricular standstill (Rhythm strip 3). Recognition of this is important because pacing is more likely to achieve a cardiac output in this situation than in most cases of complete asystole (Chapter 10).

If the patient is pulseless and electrical activity is present, decide whether recognisable QRS complexes are present. If not, and the ECG shows rapid, bizarre, irregular deflections of random frequency and amplitude, this is ventricular defibrillation (VF) (Rhythm strip 4).

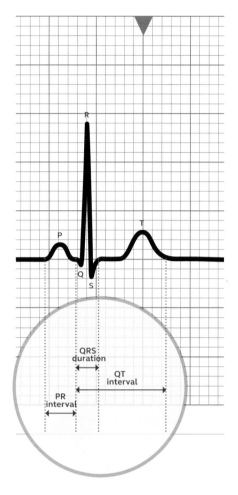

Figure 8.5 Components of the normal ECG signal

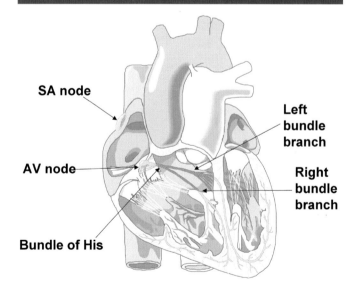

Figure 8.6 Electrical conduction in the heart

SA node

Left bundle branch

AV node

Right bundle branch

Bundle of His

In VF all co-ordination of electrical activity is lost. There is no effective ventricular contraction and no detectable cardiac output. People in VF do not remain conscious for more than a few seconds after its onset, so a rhythm that appears to be sustained VF in a conscious patient is likely to have some other explanation (e.g. artefact – Rhythm strip 23).

Ventricular fibrillation is sometimes classified as coarse (Rhythm strip 4) or fine (Rhythm strip 5) depending on the amplitude of the complexes. Do not spend time attempting to distinguish fine VF from coarse VF, or extremely fine VF from asystole during the 5 s rhythm check. If the rhythm appears to be VF give a shock, and if it appears to be asystole continue chest compressions (Chapter 6). For Rhythm strips 4 and 5 defibrillation should be attempted as they both clearly show VF.

If electrical activity is present and contains recognisable QRS complexes, continue with the following steps in rhythm analysis. If the patient is pulseless and there are recognisable complexes on the ECG that would be expected to produce a pulse, this is pulseless electrical activity (PEA) and requires immediate CPR and consideration of a possible reversible cause. Do not delay CPR whilst the cardiac rhythm is analysed further.

2. What is the ventricular (QRS) rate?

The normal heart rate (ventricular rate) at rest is 60–100 beats min^{-1}. A bradycardia has a heart rate slower than 60 min^{-1}. A tachycardia has a rate faster than 100 min^{-1}.

ECG paper is calibrated in mm, with bolder lines every 5 mm. Standard paper speed in the UK is 25 mm s^{-1}. One second is represented by 5 large squares (25 small squares).

The best way of estimating the heart rate is to count the number of cardiac cycles (R wave to R wave, including fractions) that occur in 6 s (30 large squares) and multiply by 10. This provides an estimate of heart rate, even when the rhythm is irregular. For example, if 19.6 cardiac cycles occur in 30 large squares the rate is 196 min^{-1} (Figure 8.7). For shorter rhythm strips count the number of cardiac cycles in 3 s (15 large squares) and multiply by 20.

3. Is the QRS rhythm regular or irregular?

This is not always as easy as it seems; at faster heart rates beat-to-beat variation during some irregular rhythms appears less obvious. Some rhythms may be regular in places but intermittent variation in R-R interval makes them irregular. Inspect an adequate length of rhythm strip carefully, measuring out each R-R interval and comparing it to others to detect any irregularity that is not obvious at first glance. Dividers are very useful for comparing the

R-R intervals. Alternatively, the position of two adjacent identical points in the cardiac cycle (such as the tips of the R waves) can be marked on a strip of paper; this can then be moved to another section of the rhythm strip. If the rhythm is regular the marks will align precisely with each pair of R waves.

If the QRS rhythm is irregular, decide:

- Is this totally irregular, with no recognisable pattern of R-R interval?
- Is the basic rhythm regular, with intermittent irregularity?
- Is there a recurring cyclical variation in the R-R intervals?

If there is a cyclical pattern, the relationship between the QRS complexes and the P waves requires careful analysis, as described below. If the R-R intervals are totally irregular (irregularly irregular) and the QRS complex is of constant morphology, the rhythm is most likely to be AF (Rhythm strip 6).

A regular underlying rhythm may be made irregular by extrasystoles (ectopic beats). Extrasystoles can arise from the atria or the ventricles, and the position in the heart from which they arise will determine their morphology on an ECG. If the QRS complex of ectopic beats is narrow (< 0.12 s), the beat is likely to have come from above the ventricular myocardium (i.e. from atrial muscle or the AV node). Broad-complex ectopic beats may be of ventricular origin or may be supraventricular ectopic beats with bundle branch block.

Broad-complex atrial premature beats can sometimes be identified by a preceding ectopic P wave. Some ventricular ectopic beats may be accompanied by a P wave occurring shortly after the QRS complex, caused by retrograde conduction from the ventricles to the atria. Ectopic beats that occur early (that is before the next regular sinus beat was due to occur) are referred to as premature beats (Rhythm strip 7).

A beat that arises from the AV node or from ventricular myocardium after a long pause, for example during sinus bradycardia or after sinus arrest, is referred to as an escape beat (Rhythm strip 8). This implies that the focus in the AV node or ventricle that generates this beat is acting as a back-up pacemaker, because the normal pacemaker

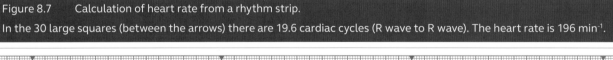

Figure 8.7   Calculation of heart rate from a rhythm strip.
In the 30 large squares (between the arrows) there are 19.6 cardiac cycles (R wave to R wave). The heart rate is 196 min^{-1}.

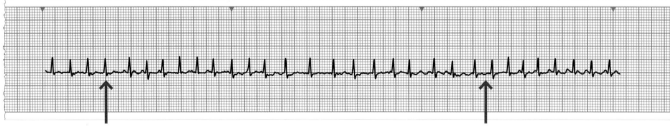

function of the sinus node is too slow or absent. Complete AV block is an escape rhythm in which the cells generating the ventricular rhythm are acting as a pacemaker because no atrial impulses are transmitted to the ventricles.

Ectopic beats may occur singly, in pairs (couplets) or in threes (triplets). If more than three ectopic beats occur in rapid succession, this is regarded as a tachyarrhythmia. An arrhythmia that occurs intermittently, interspersed with periods of normal sinus rhythm, is described as paroxysmal. When ectopic beats occur alternately with sinus beats for a sustained period this is called bigeminy. It may be referred to as atrial bigeminy or ventricular bigeminy, depending on whether the ectopic beats are atrial or ventricular in origin.

4. Is the QRS complex duration normal or prolonged?

The upper limit of normal for the QRS duration is 0.12 s (3 small squares). If the QRS width is less than this, the rhythm originates from above the bifurcation of the bundle of His and may be from the SA node, atria or AV node, but not from the ventricular myocardium. If the QRS duration is 0.12 s or more the rhythm may be coming from ventricular myocardium or may be a supraventricular rhythm, transmitted with aberrant conduction (i.e. bundle branch block).

5. Is atrial activity present?

Having defined the rhythm in terms of rate, regularity and QRS width, examine the ECG carefully for evidence of atrial activity. This may be difficult or impossible to identify, either because it is not visible or because atrial activity is partly or completely obscured by QRS complexes or T waves. Do not guess or try to convince yourself that you can identify atrial activity unless you are completely sure.

Depending on the nature of the arrhythmia and the ECG lead being examined, P waves may be present as positive deflections, negative deflections or biphasic deflections. When present, U waves may be mistaken for P waves. P waves may coincide with and cause distortion or variation of QRS complexes, ST-segments, or T waves. Whenever possible, recording of a 12-lead ECG may enable P waves to be identified in one or more leads, even if they cannot be seen clearly in the initial monitoring lead. Lead V1 is often useful for clear demonstration of some types of atrial activity including sinus P waves and AF. Sinus P waves are usually seen clearly in lead II.

Other types of atrial activity may be present. During atrial flutter, atrial activity is seen as flutter waves - an absolutely regular repetitive deflection with a 'saw-tooth' appearance, often at a rate of about 300 min[-1]. This is usually seen best in the inferior leads (II, III, aVF)(Figure 8.4).

During AF, circuits and waves of depolarisation travel randomly through both atria. There are no P waves. Atrial fibrillation waves may be seen as rapid deviations from the baseline of varying amplitude and duration, usually seen best in lead V1. In some patients this may be of such low amplitude that no definite atrial activity can be seen.

During a sustained tachycardia atrial activity may not be visible between the QRS complexes. If the rhythm is of atrial origin (e.g. atrial flutter or AF) it may be possible to reveal atrial activity by slowing the ventricular rate whilst recording an ECG, preferably in multiple leads. For example, if a regular tachycardia of 150 min[-1] is due to atrial flutter with 2:1 conduction it may not be possible to identify flutter waves with confidence. A transient increase in AV block by vagal stimulation or by an intravenous bolus of adenosine will demonstrate the flutter waves and identify the rhythm accurately (Figure 8.4).

The shape and direction of P waves help to identify the atrial rhythm. For example, sinus P waves are upright in leads II and aVF. If retrograde activation of the atria is taking place from the region of the AV node (i.e. the rhythm is junctional or ventricular in origin), the P waves will be inverted in leads II and aVF because atrial depolarisation travels in the opposite direction to normal.

The rate and regularity of P waves and flutter waves are assessed in the same way as the rate and regularity of QRS complexes. Suspected atrial flutter waves that are irregular are likely to be fibrillation waves.

6. Is atrial activity related to ventricular activity and, if so, how?

If there is a consistent interval between each P wave and the following QRS complex, it is likely that conduction between atrium and ventricle is intact and that ventricular depolarisation is triggered by atrial depolarisation.

Examine a long rhythm strip to make sure that variation in the PR interval is not missed. Occasionally conduction between atria and ventricles is reversed (i.e. ventricular depolarisation is followed by retrograde conduction through the AV node and then by atrial depolarisation); the P wave occurs soon after the QRS complex. It may sometimes be difficult to distinguish between this situation and the presence of a very long PR interval.

In other circumstances careful inspection will detect no relationship between the timing of P waves and of QRS complexes. This will indicate that atrial and ventricular depolarisation is arising independently, sometimes referred to as atrioventricular dissociation. Examples of this include:

- Complete (third-degree) AV block, where a normal sinus rate (or AF) in the atria is accompanied by a regular bradycardia arising below the AV node.

- Some examples of ventricular tachycardia (VT) in which regular broad QRS complexes are present and regular P waves can be seen at a different, slower rate, out of phase with the QRS complexes.

Difficulty may arise when the relationship between the P waves and the QRS complexes varies in a recurring pattern. This may be misinterpreted as atrioventricular dissociation. This is seen most commonly in one form of second-degree AV block (called Wenckebach or Mobitz I AV block).

Examine a long rhythm strip carefully for recurring patterns and plot and compare the timing of P waves and QRS complexes. In complete AV block, the QRS rhythm is usually completely regular.

In AF, the atrial activity is completely irregular, so there is no identifiable relationship between this atrial activity and the irregular ventricular rhythm that results from it. If AF is accompanied by a completely regular ventricular rhythm with a slow rate this is likely to be due to complete AV block in the presence of AF in the atria.

In atrial flutter there may be a consistent relationship between the flutter waves and the QRS complexes, giving rise to 1:1, 2:1, 3:1 conduction etc. In some instances, there is a varying relationship, producing an irregular QRS rhythm; this is atrial flutter with variable AV conduction.

Cardiac arrest rhythms

The rhythms seen during cardiac arrest can be classified into 3 groups:

1. shockable rhythms: Ventricular fibrillation (VF) and pulseless ventricular tachycardia (pVT)

2. asystole

3. pulseless electrical activity (PEA).

Extreme bradycardia and, rarely, very fast supraventricular tachyarrhythmia may also cause such a severe fall in cardiac output to cause the clinical features of cardiac arrest.

Ventricular fibrillation

The characteristic appearance of VF (Rhythm strip 4) is usually easy to recognise, and this is the only rhythm that does not need the systematic rhythm analysis described earlier in this chapter. When a monitor appears to show VF, check the patient immediately to establish whether this is VF requiring immediate defibrillation, or whether the appearance is due to artefact (Rhythm strip 23). If the patient is conscious or has a pulse, the rhythm is not VF.

Two rhythm abnormalities may resemble VF in some circumstances, since both produce an irregular, broad-complex, fast rhythm:

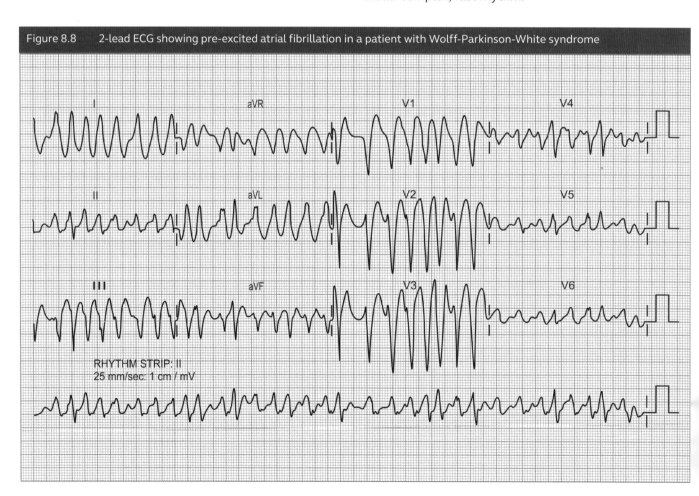

Figure 8.8   2-lead ECG showing pre-excited atrial fibrillation in a patient with Wolff-Parkinson-White syndrome

RHYTHM STRIP: II
25 mm/sec: 1 cm / mV

One is polymorphic VT (Rhythm strip 12). This may cause cardiac arrest and, when it does, the immediate treatment is the same as for VF, so failure to distinguish this immediately from VF would not lead to inappropriate treatment. However, it is important to document polymorphic VT and to recognise it so that, following immediate resuscitation, the causes can be identified and corrected and appropriate treatment given to prevent recurrence and greatly reduce the risk of sudden death.

The second possible source of confusion is pre-excited AF. This can occur in the presence of an 'accessory pathway' connecting atrial and ventricular muscle in the Wolff-Parkinson-White (WPW) syndrome. Some of these accessory pathways can conduct very rapidly, transmitting atrial impulses to the ventricles, sometimes at 300 min^{-1} or faster. This produces an irregular broad complex tachycardia (Figure 8.8) that does not usually resemble VF but might be mistaken for polymorphic VT. Left untreated, this rhythm may lead to VT or VF causing cardiac arrest. If pre-excited AF itself causes clinical cardiac arrest, the correct treatment is immediate defibrillation (as for any broad-complex pulseless tachycardia) so misinterpretation as VT or VF would not lead to inappropriate treatment. Again, the importance of documenting and recognising the rhythm is to ensure that the patient receives appropriate specialist referral without delay for treatment to protect them against the risk of recurrence of this potentially dangerous arrhythmia.

Ventricular tachycardia

Ventricular tachycardia may cause loss of cardiac output resulting in cardiac arrest, particularly at faster rates or in the presence of structural heart disease (e.g. impaired left ventricular function, severe left ventricular hypertrophy, aortic stenosis). VT may degenerate suddenly into VF. Pulseless VT is treated in the same way as VF – by immediate defibrillation.

In the presence of a cardiac output (i.e. palpable pulse), treatment of VT follows the broad-complex tachycardia algorithm described in Chapter 11. The QRS morphology may be monomorphic or polymorphic. In monomorphic VT (Rhythm strip 10), the rhythm is regular (or almost regular). The rate during VT may be anything from 100 to 300 min^{-1}, rarely faster. It is unusual to see more than slight variation in heart rate during any single episode of VT (other than in response to anti-arrhythmic drug therapy). Atrial activity may continue independently of ventricular activity; the identification of P waves, dissociated from QRS complexes during broad complex tachycardia, confirms the rhythm as VT. Occasionally these atrial beats may be conducted to the ventricles, causing capture beats or fusion beats (Rhythm strip 11).

A capture beat produces a single normal-looking QRS complex during monomorphic VT, without otherwise interrupting the arrhythmia. In a fusion beat, a wave of depolarisation travelling down from the AV node occurs simultaneously with a wave of depolarisation travelling up from the ventricular focus producing the arrhythmia. This results in a hybrid QRS complex caused by fusion of the normal QRS complex with the complex of the monomorphic VT.

In the presence of bundle branch block, a supraventricular tachycardia (SVT) will produce a broad-complex tachycardia. After myocardial infarction, most broad-complex tachycardia will be ventricular in origin. The safest approach is to regard all broad-complex tachycardia as VT until, or unless, proved otherwise.

One important type of polymorphic VT is torsade de pointes (TdP) in which the axis of the electrical activity changes in a rotational way so that the overall appearance of the ECG on a rhythm strip produces a sinusoidal pattern (Rhythm strip 12). This arrhythmia usually arises in patients with a prolonged QT interval. This can occur as an inherited condition in some families (long QT syndromes). In some people it is caused by drugs, including some anti-arrhythmic drugs, and it may occur less commonly as a manifestation of myocardial ischaemia or other myocardial disease.

Many patients with TdP are also hypokalaemic and/or hypomagnesaemic. It is important to recognise TdP because effective treatment (prevention of recurrent episodes) will require removal of any predisposing causes (i.e. drugs), treatment with intravenous magnesium and/or potassium, and may also require the use of overdrive pacing.

Drugs that prolong QT interval (including amiodarone) should be avoided in patients with TdP. This arrhythmia can itself cause cardiac arrest (in which case it is treated by defibrillation) and it can also degenerate into VF.

Asystole

The ECG features of asystole have been described already (Rhythm strip 2). If the rhythm appears to be VF, give a shock, and if it appears to be asystole continue chest compressions (Chapter 6).

Pulseless electrical activity

The term pulseless electrical activity (PEA) does not refer to a specific cardiac rhythm. It defines the clinical absence of cardiac output despite electrical activity that would normally be expected to produce a cardiac output.

Potentially treatable causes include severe fluid depletion or blood loss, cardiac tamponade, massive pulmonary embolism and tension pneumothorax.

Peri-arrest arrhythmias

These are defined according to heart rate (bradyarrhythmia, tachyarrhythmia or arrhythmia with a normal rate), as this will dictate initial treatment (Chapter 11). In an unstable patient, concentrate on early treatment to prevent deterioration, rather than on prolonged attempts to identify the precise rhythm.

Bradyarrhythmia

A bradycardia is present when the ventricular (QRS) rate is < 60 min^{-1} (Rhythm strip 13). Bradycardia may be a physiological state in very fit people or during sleep, or may be an expected result of treatment (e.g. with a beta blocker). Pathological bradycardia may be caused by malfunction of the SA node or from partial or complete failure of atrioventricular conduction. Some patients with these rhythm abnormalities may need treatment with an implanted pacemaker (Rhythm strip 14).

The emergency treatment of most bradycardia is with atropine and/or cardiac pacing (Chapter 10). Occasionally it may be necessary to use sympathomimetic drugs such as isoprenaline or adrenaline. The need for treatment depends on the haemodynamic effect of the arrhythmia and the risk of developing asystole, rather than the precise ECG classification of the bradycardia. Extreme bradycardia may sometimes precede cardiac arrest and this may be prevented by prompt and appropriate treatment of the bradycardia. In this context the most important bradyarrhythmia is acquired complete heart block (see below).

Heart block: first-degree atrioventricular block

The PR interval is the time between the onset of the P wave and the start of the QRS complex (whether this begins with a Q wave or R wave). The normal PR interval is 0.12–0.20 s. First-degree atrioventricular (AV) block is present when the PR interval is > 0.20 s and is a common finding (Rhythm strip 15). It represents a delay in conduction through the AV junction (the AV node and/or bundle of His). In some instances this may be physiological (for example in trained athletes). There are many other causes of first-degree AV block, including primary disease (fibrosis) of the conducting system, various types of structural heart disease, ischaemic heart disease and use of drugs that delay conduction through the AV node. First-degree AV block rarely causes any symptoms and as an isolated finding rarely requires treatment.

Heart block: second-degree atrioventricular block

Second-degree AV block is present when some, but not all, P waves are conducted to the ventricles, resulting in absence of a QRS complex after some P waves. There are two types:

Mobitz Type I AV block (also called Wenckebach AV block)

The PR interval shows progressive prolongation after each successive P wave until a P wave occurs without a resulting QRS complex. Usually the cycle is then repeated (Rhythm strip 16). Any condition that delays AV conduction can produce Wenckebach AV block. In some situations this may be physiological, for example in highly trained athletes with high vagal tone. Outside that setting Wenckebach AV block is usually pathological. Its many causes include acute myocardial infarction (especially inferior infarction). If asymptomatic, this rhythm does not usually require immediate treatment. The need for treatment is dictated by the effect of the bradyarrhythmia on the patient and the risk of developing more severe AV block or asystole.

Mobitz Type II AV block

There is a constant (often prolonged) PR interval in the conducted beats but some of the P waves are not followed by QRS complexes. This may occur randomly, without any consistent pattern. People with Mobitz II AV block have an increased risk of progression to complete AV block and asystole.

2:1 and 3:1 AV block

The term 2:1 AV block describes the situation in which alternate P waves are followed by a QRS complex (Rhythm strip 17). 2:1 AV block may be due to Mobitz I or Mobitz II AV block and it may be difficult to distinguish which it is from the ECG appearance. If bundle branch block is present as well as 2:1 block (broad QRS complexes) this is likely to be Mobitz II block. 3:1 AV block (Rhythm strip 18) is less common and is a form of Mobitz II AV block. Immediate decisions about treatment of these rhythms (see algorithm for treatment of bradycardia, Chapter 11) will be determined by the effect of the resulting bradycardia on the patient. After identifying and providing any necessary immediate treatment continue ECG monitoring and arrange expert cardiology assessment.

Heart block: third-degree atrioventricular block

In third-degree (complete (CHB)) AV block, there is no relationship between P waves and QRS complexes; atrial and ventricular depolarisation arises independently from separate 'pacemakers' (Rhythm strip 19). The site of the 'pacemaker' stimulating the ventricles will determine the ventricular rate and QRS width. A 'pacemaker' site in the AV node or proximal bundle of His may have an intrinsic rate of 40–50 min^{-1} or sometimes higher and may produce a narrow QRS complex. A 'pacemaker' site in the distal His-Purkinje fibres or ventricular myocardium will produce broad QRS complexes, often have a rate of 30–40 min^{-1} or less, and is more likely to stop abruptly, resulting in asystole.

Escape rhythms

If the normal cardiac 'pacemaker' (SA node) fails, or operates abnormally slowly, cardiac depolarisation may be initiated from a subsidiary 'pacemaker' in atrial myocardium, AV node, conducting fibres or ventricular myocardium. The resulting escape rhythm will be slower than the normal sinus rate. As indicated above, subsidiary 'pacemakers' situated distally in the conducting system tend to produce slower heart rates than those situated more proximally. Thus a ventricular escape rhythm will usually be slower than a junctional rhythm arising from the AV node or bundle of His.

The term idioventricular rhythm is used to describe a rhythm arising from ventricular myocardium. This includes ventricular escape rhythms seen in the presence of complete AV block. The term accelerated idioventricular rhythm is used to describe an idioventricular rhythm with a normal heart rate (usually faster than the sinus rate but not fast enough to be VT). This type of rhythm is observed quite frequently after successful thrombolysis or primary percutaneous coronary intervention for acute myocardial infarction (a 'reperfusion arrhythmia'). Accelerated idioventricular rhythms do not usually present a serious risk unless they cause haemodynamic compromise or develop into VT or VF, which is uncommon. The QRS complex of an idioventricular rhythm will be broad (i.e. 0.12 s or greater), whereas a junctional rhythm may be narrow or broad, depending on whether conduction to the ventricles occurs normally, or with bundle branch block.

Agonal rhythm

Agonal rhythm occurs in dying patients. It is characterised by the presence of slow, irregular, wide ventricular complexes, often of varying morphology (Rhythm strip 20). An agonal rhythm does not usually generate a palpable pulse. This rhythm is seen commonly during the later stages of unsuccessful resuscitation attempts. The complexes slow inexorably and often become progressively broader before progressing to asystole.

Tachyarrhythmia

A pathological tachycardia may arise from atrial myocardium, the AV junction or ventricular myocardium. When a tachycardia arises from tissue situated above the bifurcation of the bundle of His, it is described as supraventricular (Rhythm strip 21). The QRS complexes will be narrow if ventricular depolarisation occurs normally, but will be broad if bundle branch block is present. Sinus tachycardia is not an arrhythmia and usually represents a response to some other physiological or pathological state (e.g. exercise, anxiety, blood loss, pain, fever etc).

Narrow-complex tachycardia

This results from a supraventricular tachycardia with normal conduction to the ventricles (Rhythm strip 21). QRS complexes may be regular in many rhythms or may be irregular in the presence of atrial fibrillation or variably conducted atrial flutter. Many tachycardias with narrow QRS complexes have a favourable prognosis, but the outlook will vary with individual clinical circumstances.

These rhythms may be tolerated poorly by patients with structural heart disease and may provoke angina, especially in patients with coronary artery disease.

Atrial fibrillation

Atrial fibrillation is the most common sustained arrhythmia encountered in clinical practice. It is characterised by disorganised electrical activity in the atria. No recognisable P waves or coordinated atrial activity can be seen in any lead (Rhythm strip 6). The baseline is irregular and chaotic atrial activity is best seen in lead V1 where the atrial waveform is irregular in both amplitude and frequency. The QRS rhythm is irregularly irregular (i.e. the R-R interval varies in random fashion from beat to beat). The ventricular rate will depend on the refractory period of the AV junction. In the absence of drug treatment or pre-existing disease affecting the AV node, the resulting ventricular rate will be rapid, usually 120–180 min^{-1} or faster.

Common causes of AF include hypertension, obesity, alcohol excess and structural heart disease. In coronary heart disease AF usually occurs as a result of left ventricular impairment (acute or chronic) and not as a direct result of ischaemia of the atrial myocardium.

Atrial flutter

In atrial flutter, atrial activity is seen on the ECG as flutter waves at a rate of about 300 min^{-1} (Rhythm strip 22). These are usually best seen in the inferior leads II, III and aVF where they have a 'saw-tooth' appearance (Figure 8.4).

The ventricular rate depends on AV conduction but there is often 2:1 (Rhythm strip 9) or 3:1 conduction (often referred to as atrial flutter with 2:1 or 3:1 block). If conduction is constant the ventricular rhythm will be regular, but variable conduction causes an irregular ventricular rhythm. Like AF, atrial flutter is often, but not always, associated with underlying disease. Atrial flutter usually arises in the right atrium, so is a recognized complication of diseases that affect the right heart, including chronic obstructive pulmonary disease, major pulmonary embolism, complex congenital heart disease and chronic congestive heart failure of any cause.

Broad-complex tachycardia

Broad-complex tachycardia may be:

- a tachycardia arising in the ventricle below the bifurcation of the bundle of His (i.e. VT – Rhythm strip 10), or

- a supraventricular tachycardia conducted aberrantly (right or left bundle branch block) to the ventricles.

The clinical consequences depend on:

- the heart rate during the arrhythmia

- the presence or absence of structural heart disease or coronary disease

- the duration of the arrhythmia.

Ventricular tachycardia may degenerate into VF, especially if the VT is very fast (e.g. 200 min^{-1} or faster) or if the myocardium is unstable as a consequence of acute ischaemia or infarction, or in the presence of electrolyte abnormality (hypokalaemia or hypomagnesaemia).

The safest approach is to treat all broad-complex tachycardia as ventricular tachycardia unless there is good evidence that it is supraventricular in origin. Patients with WPW syndrome have accessory pathways connecting atrial and ventricular myocardium. Some atrioventricular conduction occurs through these pathways as well as through the AV node (resulting in pre-excitation). This results in widening of the QRS complexes by so-called

delta waves (Figure 8.9). In the presence of such an accessory pathway that bypasses the AV node, AF may result in a ventricular rate that is so fast that cardiac output decreases dramatically. The ECG appearances are of a very rapid, irregular, broad complex tachycardia that usually shows variability in the width of QRS complexes (Figure 8.8).

This rhythm may be misdiagnosed as 'irregular VT', polymorphic VT or possibly as VF. Overall the rhythm is more organised than ventricular fibrillation (it lacks the random chaotic activity of variable amplitude).

The QT interval

When identifying and treating rhythm abnormalities it is important to recognise likely underlying causes that may influence choice of effective treatment. These may be identified from clinical assessment (e.g. heart failure), laboratory tests (e.g. electrolyte abnormality) or from the ECG. Prolongation of the QT interval predisposes people to ventricular arrhythmia, in particular TdP and VF.

The QT interval is measured from the start of the QRS complex to the end of the T wave. It can be difficult to measure accurately, mainly because it may be difficult to identify the end of the T wave. This may be especially difficult when prominent U waves are present, merging with the end of the T wave. U waves can be a feature of

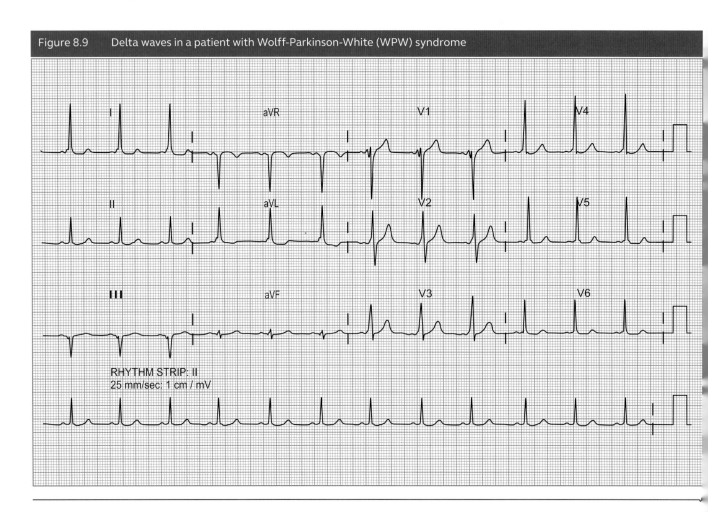

Figure 8.9   Delta waves in a patient with Wolff-Parkinson-White (WPW) syndrome

RHYTHM STRIP: II
25 mm/sec: 1 cm / mV

some abnormalities (e.g. hypokalaemia) and some types of inherited cardiac conditions but may be present in some healthy people with normal hearts.

The duration of the QT interval may also vary between different leads of the same 12-lead ECG. This may partly reflect variation in amplitude and direction of the T wave, making it more difficult to measure in some leads than others. Lead II is usually recommended for QT measurement, with leads I and V5 as other options, but your choice of lead may be dictated by the lead that best allows you to identify the end of the T wave.

The QT interval varies slightly with age and with gender and is usually slightly longer in the presence of bundle branch block. The QT interval is affected substantially by heart rate. The QT interval shortens as the heart rate increases. A correction can be made to allow for this, using the measured QT interval and heart rate to calculate the corrected QT interval (QTc). The normal range quoted for QTc varies slightly. It is reasonable to consider a QTc in men normal up to 0.43 s and in women normal up to 0.45 s. A QTc in a man > 0.45 s or in a woman > 0.47 s can be regarded as definitely prolonged. A QTc of 0.5 s or more indicates a high risk of cardiac arrest and sudden death.

Many modern ECG machines measure the QT interval and calculate the QTc automatically. These measurements are accurate only if the ECG recording is of good quality. Most ECG machines cannot distinguish between T waves and U waves. Always look at the recording and make sure that the quoted measurements are not obviously inaccurate. If in doubt seek expert help with interpretation.

Abnormality of the QT interval can be seen in various situations. A shortened QT interval may be seen with hypercalcaemia and digoxin treatment. Hypokalaemia, hypomagnesaemia, hypocalcaemia, hypothermia, myocarditis and in some instances myocardial ischaemia can all cause QT prolongation. There is also a long list of drugs that may prolong the QT interval, including class I and class III anti-arrhythmic drugs.

There are several genetic abnormalities in which the QT interval is abnormal or there is abnormality of ventricular repolarisation (principally the long QT, short QT and Brugada syndromes). The repolarisation abnormality places them at risk of ventricular arrhythmia and sudden death. These people require expert assessment to identify whether treatment is needed to reduce this risk. For some effective treatment will include an implantable cardioverter-defibrillator to treat any episode of VF or VT immediately. It is especially important that patients with long QT syndromes are not given any drug that may cause further QT prolongation.

Further reading

European Society of Cardiology Clinical Practice Guidelines: https://www.escardio.org/Guidelines/Clinical-Practice-Guidelines

08: Summary learning

A systematic approach to ECG rhythm analysis allows accurate assessment of any rhythm abnormality sufficiently to enable safe, effective immediate treatment.

ECG recordings of any rhythm abnormality and of the ECG in sinus rhythm provide valuable diagnostic information and help the correct choice of longer-term treatment.

Accurate monitoring of cardiac rhythm is essential for any patient at high risk of developing life-threatening arrhythmia.

Accurate monitoring of the cardiac rhythm is essential in the management of cardiac arrest.

My key take-home messages from this chapter are:

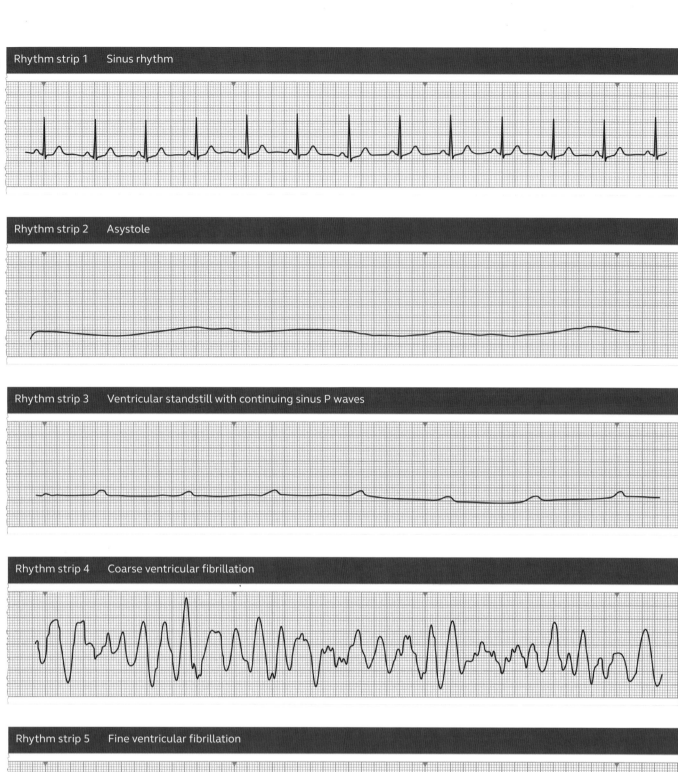

Rhythm strip 1   Sinus rhythm

Rhythm strip 2   Asystole

Rhythm strip 3   Ventricular standstill with continuing sinus P waves

Rhythm strip 4   Coarse ventricular fibrillation

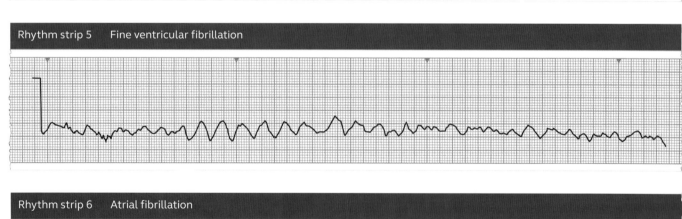

Rhythm strip 5   Fine ventricular fibrillation

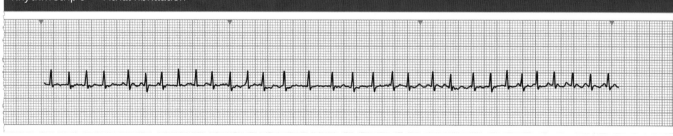

Rhythm strip 6   Atrial fibrillation

Rhythm strip 7   Ventricular premature beat

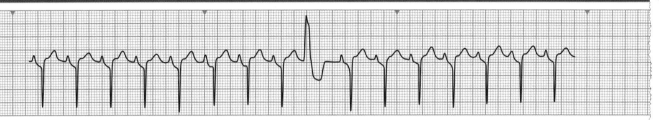

Rhythm strip 8   Junctional escape beat

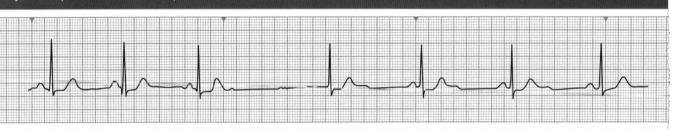

Rhythm strip 9   Atrial flutter with 2:1 AV conduction

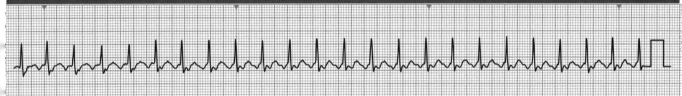

Rhythm strip 10   Monomorphic ventricular tachycardia

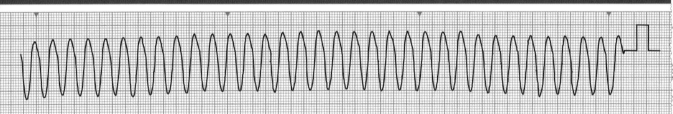

Rhythm strip 11   Ventricular tachycardia with capture beats and fusion beats

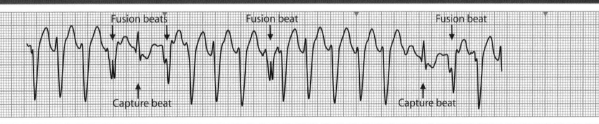

Fusion beats   Fusion beat   Fusion beat

Capture beat   Capture beat

Rhythm strip 12   Torsade de pointes polymorphic ventricular tachycardia

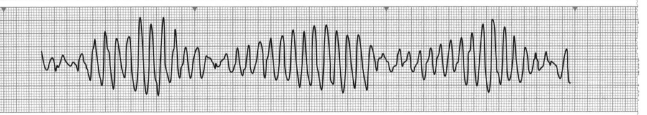

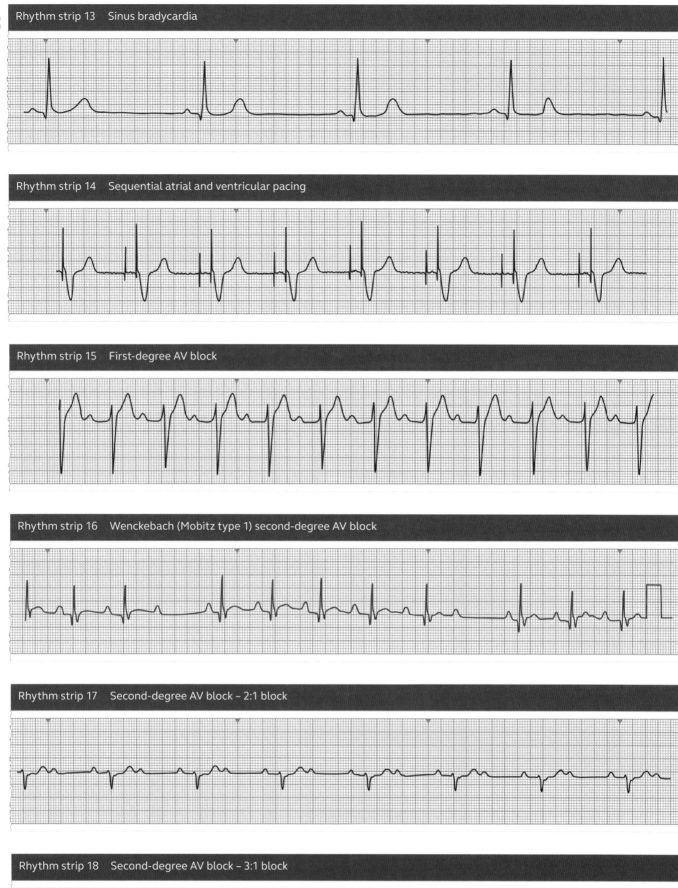

Rhythm strip 13   Sinus bradycardia

Rhythm strip 14   Sequential atrial and ventricular pacing

Rhythm strip 15   First-degree AV block

Rhythm strip 16   Wenckebach (Mobitz type 1) second-degree AV block

Rhythm strip 17   Second-degree AV block – 2:1 block

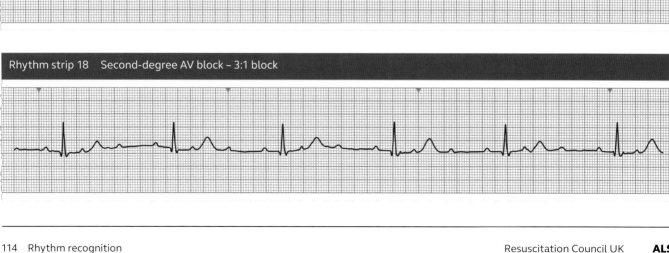

Rhythm strip 18   Second-degree AV block – 3:1 block

Rhythm strip 19   Third-degree (complete) AV block

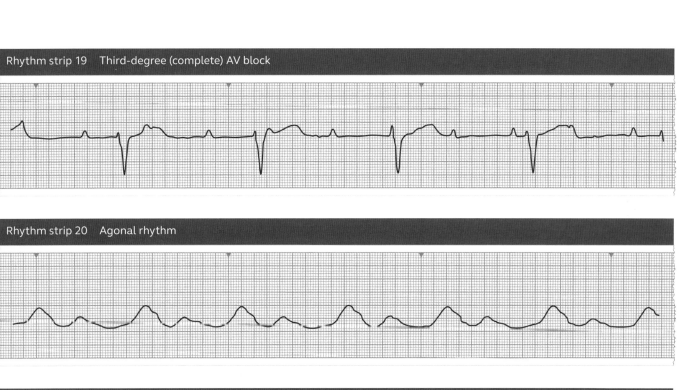

Rhythm strip 20   Agonal rhythm

Rhythm strip 21   Regular narrow-complex tachycardia ('supraventricular tachycardia')

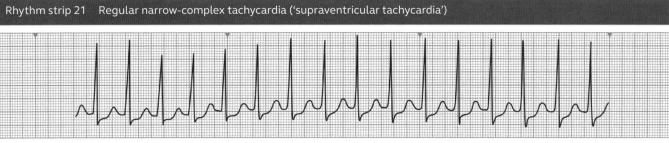

Rhythm strip 22   Atrial flutter with high-degree AV block causing extreme bradycardia (heart rate approximately 20 min⁻¹).

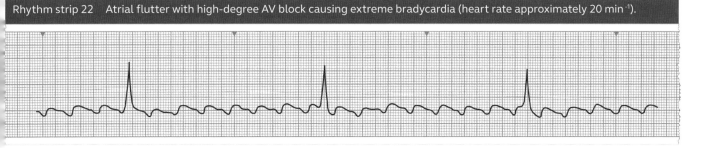

Rhythm strip 23a   Artefact. A brief period of recurrent artefact that was misinterpreted as 'intermittent VF'

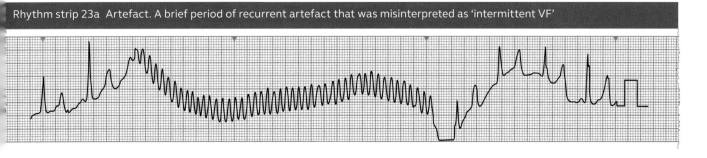

Rhythm strip 23b   Artefact from same patient. Artefact is seen superimposed on uninterrupted, regular QRS complexes, demonstrating that this could not be VF.

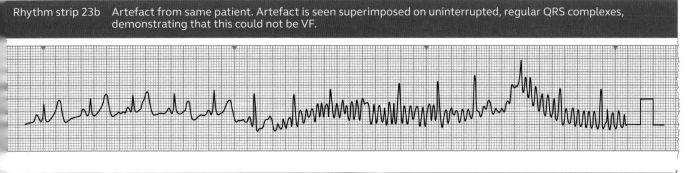

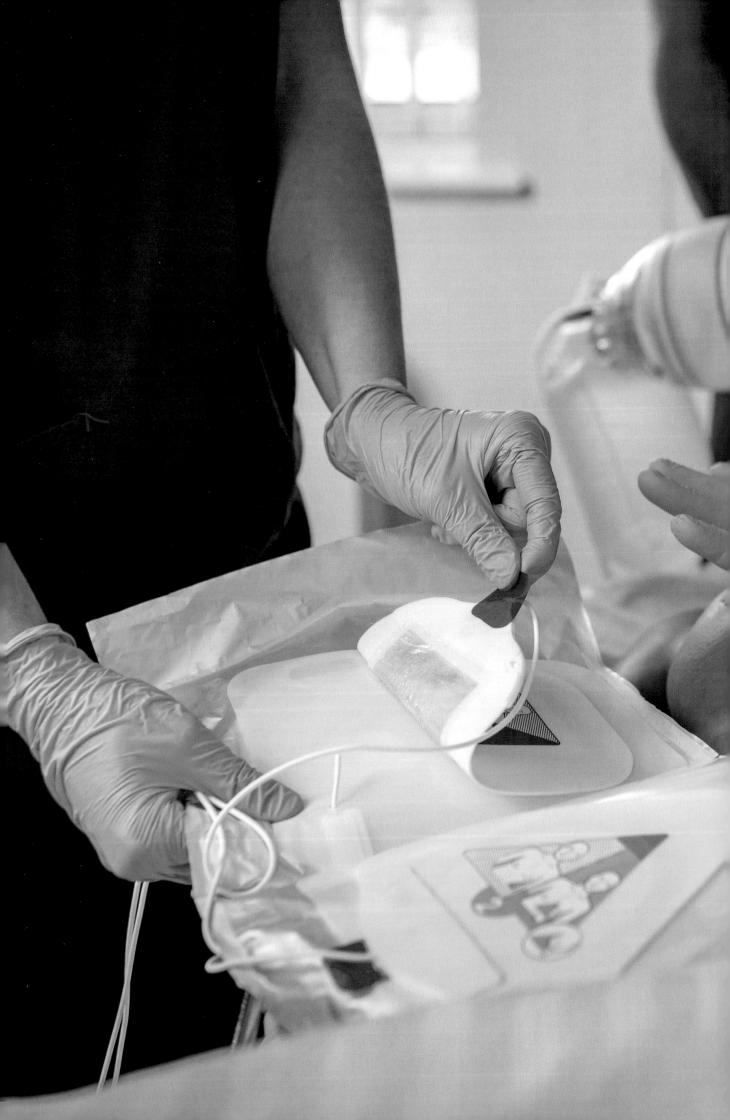

Defibrillation

In this chapter

Probability of successful defibrillation

Mechanism of defibrillation

Factors affecting defibrillation success

Shock energies

Safety during defibrillation

Automated external defibrillators (AEDs) and sequence for use

Manual defibrillation and sequence for use

Defibrillation with an AED in children

Synchronised cardioversion

Implanted electronic devices (IEDs)

The learning outcomes will enable you to:

Understand how to safely deliver a shock with an AED or manual defibrillator

Understand how to minimise pauses in chest compressions during defibrillation

Introduction

Following the onset of ventricular fibrillation or pulseless ventricular tachycardia (VF/pVT), cardiac output ceases – early successful defibrillation with return of spontaneous circulation (ROSC) is essential for a good outcome. Defibrillation is a key link in the Chain of Survival and is one of the few interventions proven to improve outcome from VF/pVT cardiac arrest.

The probability of successful defibrillation

There are several factors that need to be taken into account:

1. Time from onset to delivery of shock. Early defibrillation is one of the most important factors in determining survival from cardiac arrest. In the absence of bystander CPR, for every minute that passes between collapse and attempted defibrillation, mortality increases by 7–10%. The shorter the interval between the onset of VF/pVT and delivery of the shock, the greater the chance of successful defibrillation and survival.

2. Continuous, uninterrupted chest compressions. Clinical studies have shown that even short interruptions in chest compressions (e.g. to deliver rescue breaths or perform rhythm analysis) significantly reduce the chances of successful defibrillation. Animal studies show that even if defibrillation is successful, these short interruptions are associated with post-resuscitation myocardial dysfunction and reduced survival. Analysis of CPR performance following both out-of-hospital and in-hospital cardiac arrest has shown that significant interruptions are common and every effort should be made to minimise interruptions. The aim should be to ensure that chest compressions are performed continuously throughout the resuscitation attempt, and both the number and duration of pauses limited to only enable specific planned interventions.

3. The duration of the interval between stopping chest compressions and delivering the shock is called the pre-shock pause. The duration of the pre-shock pause is related inversely to the chance of successful defibrillation; one study has shown that every 5-second increase in the pre-shock pause almost halves the chance of successful defibrillation (defined by the absence of VF 5 s after shock delivery). Consequently, defibrillation must always be performed quickly and efficiently in order to maximise the chances of successful resuscitation.

If there is any delay in obtaining a defibrillator, and while the defibrillator pads are applied, start chest compressions and ventilation immediately. When bystander CPR is given the decrease in survival is more gradual and averages 3–4% per min from collapse to defibrillation. Bystander CPR doubles survival from witnessed cardiac arrest.

Mechanism of defibrillation

Defibrillation is the passage of an electrical current of sufficient magnitude across the myocardium to depolarise a critical mass of cardiac muscle simultaneously, enabling the natural pacemaker tissue to resume control. To achieve this, all defibrillators have three features in common:

- a power source capable of providing direct current

- a capacitor that can be charged to a pre-determined energy level

- two electrodes which are placed on the patient's chest, either side of the heart, across which the capacitor is discharged.

Successful defibrillation is defined as the absence of VF/pVT at 5 s after shock delivery, although the ultimate goal is ROSC.

Factors affecting defibrillation success

Defibrillation success depends on sufficient current being delivered to the myocardium. However, the delivered current is difficult to determine because it is influenced by transthoracic impedance (electrical resistance) and electrode position. Furthermore, much of the current is diverted along non-cardiac pathways in the thorax and, as a result, as little as 4% reaches the heart.

Transthoracic impedance

Current flow is inversely proportional to transthoracic impedance; however, biphasic defibrillators can measure the transthoracic impedance and adjust the energy delivered to compensate. Their efficacy is therefore independent of transthoracic impedance (impedance compensation).

Ensure good contact between self-adhesive pads and the patient's skin. This may be compromised when:

- A transdermal drug patch is on the patient's chest. If it is in the area where self-adhesive pads would be applied, remove the patch and dry the skin. If this is likely to delay defibrillation, place the pads in an alternative position that avoids the patch (see below).

- The patient has a very hairy chest. This is only a problem if the self-adhesive pads do not stick to the chest. Defibrillation should not be delayed if a razor is not to hand immediately. In very hairy patients, a bi-axillary electrode position may enable more rapid defibrillation.

Electrode position

No human studies have evaluated the electrode position as a determinant of ROSC or survival from cardiac arrest due to a shockable rhythm. Transmyocardial current during defibrillation is likely to be maximal when the

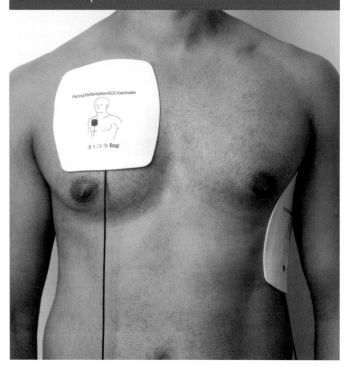

Figure 9.1a Standard electrode pectoral and apical positions for defibrillation

electrodes are placed so that the area of the heart that is fibrillating lies directly between them (i.e. ventricles in VF/pVT, atria in atrial fibrillation (AF)). Therefore, the optimal electrode position may not be the same for ventricular and atrial arrhythmias.

When attempting to defibrillate a patient in VF/pVT, the standard procedure is to place one electrode to the right of the upper sternum below the clavicle. The apical pad is placed in the left mid-axillary line, approximately level with the V6 ECG electrode. This position should be clear of any breast tissue. It is important that this electrode is placed sufficiently laterally (Figures 9.1a, b, c, d).

Although the electrodes are marked positive and negative, each can be placed in either position. Other acceptable pad positions include:

- One electrode anteriorly, over the left precordium, and the other electrode on the back behind the heart, just inferior to the left scapula (antero-posterior).

- One electrode placed in the mid-axillary line, approximately level with the V6 ECG electrode or female breast and the other electrode on the back, just inferior to the right scapula (postero-lateral).

- Each electrode on the lateral chest walls, one on the right and the other on the left side (bi-axillary).

More patients are presenting with implantable medical devices (e.g. permanent pacemaker, implantable cardioverter defibrillator (ICD)). Medic Alert bracelets are recommended for these patients. These devices may be damaged during defibrillation if current is discharged through electrodes placed directly over the device. Place the electrode away from the device (at least 10–15 cm) or use an alternative electrode position (anterior-lateral, anterior-posterior) as described above.

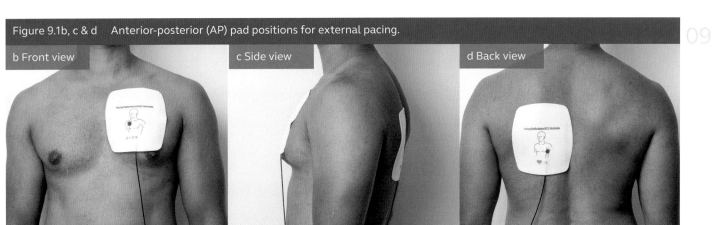

Figure 9.1b, c & d   Anterior-posterior (AP) pad positions for external pacing.

b Front view

c Side view

d Back view

CPR or defibrillation first?

In any unwitnessed cardiac arrest, those responding should provide high-quality, uninterrupted CPR while a defibrillator is retrieved, attached and charged. Attempt defibrillation as soon as possible; a period of CPR (e.g. 2–3 min) before rhythm analysis and shock delivery is not recommended.

Shock sequence

The optimal shock strategy for any survival end-point is unknown. There is no conclusive evidence that a single shock strategy increases rate of ROSC or reduces recurrence of VF compared with three stacked shocks, but given that outcome is improved by minimising interruptions to chest compressions, single shocks are recommended for most situations. The importance of early, uninterrupted chest compressions is emphasised throughout these guidelines, together with minimising the duration of pre-shock and post-shock pauses.

- Continue CPR while a defibrillator is retrieved and applied; as soon as the defibrillator is available, assess the rhythm and attempt defibrillation when indicated.

- Continue chest compressions during charging of the defibrillator. During compressions, ensure all rescuers stand clear other than the individual performing chest compressions.

- When defibrillating ensure that the total interruption to chest compressions is less than 5 s and after defibrillation immediately resume chest compressions.

- Immediately after a shock do not delay CPR for rhythm re-analysis or a pulse check.

- Continue CPR (30 compressions: 2 ventilations) for 2 min until rhythm re-analysis is undertaken and another shock is given (if indicated). Even if the defibrillation attempt is successful, it takes time until the post-shock circulation is established and a pulse is not usually palpable with a perfusing rhythm immediately after defibrillation.

- Patients can remain pulseless for over 2 min. The duration of asystole before ROSC can be longer than 2 min in as many as 25% of successful shocks.

Witnessed and monitored VF/pVT cardiac arrest

If a patient has a monitored and witnessed cardiac arrest in the catheter laboratory, coronary care unit, a critical care area, or whilst monitored after cardiac surgery, and a manual defibrillator is rapidly available:

- Confirm cardiac arrest and shout for help.

- If the initial rhythm is VF/pVT, give up to three quick successive (stacked) shocks.

- Rapidly check for a rhythm change and, if appropriate check for a pulse and other signs of ROSC after each defibrillation attempt.

- Start chest compressions and continue CPR for 2 min if the third shock is unsuccessful.

This three-shock strategy may also be considered for an initial, witnessed VF/pVT cardiac arrest if the patient is already connected to a manual defibrillator although these circumstances are rare. There are no data supporting a three-shock strategy in any of these circumstances, but it is unlikely that chest compressions will improve the already very high chance of ROSC when defibrillation occurs early in the electrical phase, immediately after onset of VF/pVT.

Shock energies

A range of defibrillation energy levels have been recommended by manufacturers and previous guidelines, ranging from 120–360 J. In the absence of any clear evidence for the optimal initial and subsequent energy levels, any energy level within this range is acceptable for the initial shock, followed by a fixed or escalating strategy up to maximum output of the defibrillator.

For subsequent shocks, there remains no evidence to support either a fixed or escalating energy protocol, although an escalating protocol may be associated with a lower incidence of refibrillation. Both strategies are acceptable; however, if the first shock is not successful and the defibrillator is capable of delivering shocks of higher energy it is reasonable to increase the energy for subsequent shocks. With manual defibrillators it is also appropriate to consider escalating the shock energy in patients when refibrillation occurs.

Safety

Attempted defibrillation should be undertaken without risk to members of the resuscitation team. This is achieved best by using self-adhesive electrodes, which minimise the possibility of anyone touching the electrode during electrical discharge. Be wary of wet surroundings or clothing – wipe any water from the patient's chest before attempted defibrillation. No part of any person should make direct or indirect contact with the patient. Do not hold intravenous infusion equipment or the patient's trolley during shock delivery. The operator must ensure that everyone is clear of the patient before delivering a shock.

There is no evidence that continuous chest compressions during shock delivery increases the chance of achieving ROSC. Furthermore, the latex gloves routinely available and used by healthcare professionals do not provide sufficient protection from the electric current, therefore a shock is delivered only when everyone is clear of contact with the patient.

Safe use of oxygen during defibrillation

In an oxygen-enriched atmosphere sparking from poorly applied defibrillator paddles can cause a fire and significant burns to the patient. The use of self-adhesive electrodes is far less likely to cause sparks than manual paddles – no fires have been reported in association with the use of self-adhesive electrodes. The following are recommended as good practice:

- Take off any oxygen mask or nasal cannulae and place them at least 1 m away from the patient's chest.

- Leave the ventilation bag connected to the tracheal tube or supraglottic airway device; no increase in oxygen concentration occurs in the zone of defibrillation, even with an oxygen flow of 15 L min^{-1}.

- Alternatively, disconnect the ventilation bag from the tracheal tube or supraglottic airway device and remove it at least 1 m from the patient's chest during defibrillation.

If the patient is connected to a ventilator, for example in the operating room or critical care unit, leave the ventilator tubing (breathing circuit) connected to the tracheal tube unless chest compressions prevent the ventilator from delivering adequate tidal volumes. In this case, the ventilator is usually substituted by a ventilation bag, which can be left connected or detached and removed to a distance of at least 1 m. Ensure that the disconnected ventilator tubing is kept at least 1 m from the patient or, better still, switch the ventilator to standby during the period of the resuscitation attempt; modern ventilators generate high oxygen flows when left disconnected. During normal use, when connected to a tracheal tube, oxygen from a ventilator in the critical care unit will be vented from the main ventilator housing well

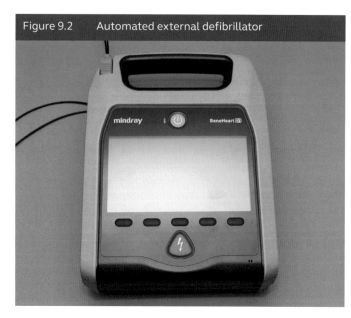

Figure 9.2   Automated external defibrillator

away from the defibrillation zone. Patients in the critical care unit may be dependent on positive end expiratory pressure (PEEP) to maintain adequate oxygenation; during cardioversion, when the spontaneous circulation potentially enables blood to remain well oxygenated, it is particularly appropriate to leave the critically ill patient connected to the ventilator during shock delivery.

Automated external defibrillators

Automated external defibrillators (AEDs) are sophisticated, reliable, computerised devices that use voice and visual prompts to guide lay rescuers and healthcare professionals to attempt defibrillation safely in cardiac arrest patients (Figure 9.2).

Advances in technology, particularly with respect to battery capacity, and software arrhythmia analysis, have enabled the mass production of relatively cheap, reliable and easily operated portable defibrillators. Shock-advisory defibrillators have ECG-analysis capability but can usually be manually over-ridden by healthcare providers capable of rhythm recognition.

Automated rhythm analysis

Automated external defibrillators have microprocessors that analyse several features of the ECG, including frequency and amplitude. Some AEDs are programmed to detect spontaneous movement by the patient.

Automated external defibrillators have been tested extensively against libraries of recorded cardiac rhythms and in many trials in adults and children. They are extremely accurate in rhythm analysis. Although AEDs are not designed to deliver synchronised shocks, all AEDs will also recommend shocks for VT if the rate and R-wave morphology exceed preset values.

In-hospital use of AEDs

When patients sustain cardiac arrest in unmonitored hospital beds and in outpatient departments, several minutes may elapse before a resuscitation team arrives with a defibrillator. There are no published randomised trials comparing in-hospital use of AEDs with manual defibrillators, and it has been shown that an AED can be used successfully before the arrival of the hospital resuscitation team. Rescuers who are not comfortable with rapid rhythm assessment and shock delivery during CPR should use an AED.

AEDs should therefore be considered for areas of the hospital where there is a risk of delayed defibrillation because of the time taken for a resuscitation team to attend or where staff have no rhythm recognition skills or where they use defibrillators infrequently.

In hospital areas where there is rapid access to manual defibrillation, either from trained staff or a resuscitation team, use manual defibrillation in preference to an AED. Ensure that an effective system for training and retraining is in place.

Healthcare providers with a duty to perform CPR should be trained, equipped, and authorised to perform defibrillation, and sufficient numbers should be trained to enable the goal of providing the first shock within 3 min of collapse anywhere in the hospital. Hospitals should monitor collapse-to-first shock intervals.

Public access defibrillation (PAD) programmes

Public access defibrillation (PAD) and first responder AED programmes may increase the number of patients who receive bystander CPR and early defibrillation, thus improving survival from out-of-hospital cardiac arrest. Public access AED programmes are most effective when implemented in public places with a high density and movement of citizens such as airports, railway stations, bus terminals, sport facilities, shopping malls, and offices where cardiac arrests are usually witnessed and trained CPR providers can quickly be on scene. Resuscitation Council UK and British Heart Foundation have published a guide to AEDs which provides information on how they can be deployed in the community. Registration of AEDs for public access, and the use of mobile apps so that dispatchers can direct CPR providers to a nearby AED, may also help to optimise response.

Sequence for use of an AED
(or shock-advisory defibrillator)

It is critically important that CPR providers pay attention to AED voice prompts and follow them without any delay.

1. Make sure the patient, any bystanders, and you are safe.

2. If the patient is unresponsive and not breathing normally:
    –   ask someone to call for an ambulance or the resuscitation team and collect the AED. If you are on your own, do this yourself.

3. Start CPR according to the guidelines (Chapter 5).

4. As soon as the AED arrives, switch it on and follow the voice/visual directions (for pad placement and rhythm analysis).

5A. If a shock IS advised:
    –   ensure that nobody touches the patient
    –   push the shock button as directed
    –   continue as directed by the voice/visual prompts.

5B. If NO shock is advised:
    –   immediately resume CPR using a ratio of 30 compressions to 2 rescue breaths
    –   continue as directed by the voice/visual prompts.

6. Continue to follow the AED prompts until:
    –   qualified help (e.g. ambulance or resuscitation team) arrives and takes over
    –   the patient starts to breathe normally, or
    –   you become exhausted.

Notes: The carrying case with the AED must contain strong scissors for cutting through clothing and a disposable razor for shaving excessive chest hair in order to obtain good electrode contact. If ALS providers are using an AED they should, where the defibrillator functionality enables, switch to manual mode.

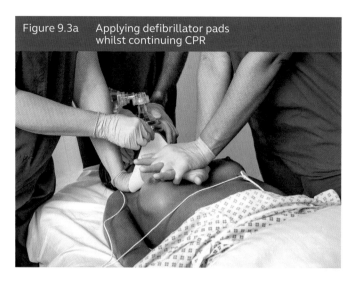

Figure 9.3a   Applying defibrillator pads whilst continuing CPR

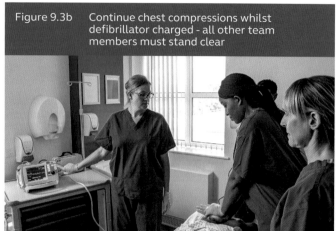

Figure 9.3b   Continue chest compressions whilst defibrillator charged - all other team members must stand clear

Manual defibrillation

Manual defibrillators have several advantages over AEDs. They enable the operator to diagnose the rhythm and deliver a shock rapidly without having to wait for rhythm analysis. This minimises the interruption in chest compressions. Manual defibrillators often have additional functions, such as the ability to deliver synchronised shocks, and external pacing facilities. The main disadvantage of these devices is that the operator has to be skilled in ECG rhythm recognition; therefore in comparison with AEDs, extra training is required.

Sequence for use of a manual defibrillator

This sequence is an integral part of the ALS algorithm in Chapter 6.

1. Confirm cardiac arrest – check for signs of life or, if trained to do so, normal breathing and pulse simultaneously.

2. Call the resuscitation team.

3. Perform uninterrupted chest compressions while applying self-adhesive defibrillation/monitoring pads (Figure 9.3a) – one below the right clavicle and the other in the V6 position in the midaxillary line.

4. Plan actions before pausing CPR for rhythm analysis and communicate these to the team.

5. Stop chest compressions; confirm VF/pVT from the ECG. This pause in chest compressions should be brief and no longer than 5 s.

6. Resume chest compressions immediately; warn all rescuers other than the individual performing the chest compressions to "stand clear" (Figure 9.3b) and remove any oxygen delivery device as appropriate.

7. The designated person selects the appropriate energy on the defibrillator and presses the charge button. Choose an energy setting of at 120 to 150 J for the first shock, the same or a higher energy for subsequent shocks, or follow the manufacturer's guidance for the particular defibrillator.

8. Ensure that the rescuer giving the compressions is the only person touching the patient.

9. Once the defibrillator is charged and the safety check is complete, tell the rescuer doing the chest compressions to "stand clear" (Figure 9.3c); when clear, give the shock (Figure 9.3d).

10. After shock delivery immediately restart CPR using a ratio of 30:2, starting with chest compressions. Do not pause to reassess the rhythm or feel for a pulse. This pause in chest compressions should be brief and no longer than 5 s.

11. Continue CPR for 2 min; the team leader prepares the team for the next pause in CPR.

12. Pause briefly to check the monitor.

13. If VF/pVT, repeat steps 6–12 above and deliver a second shock.

14. If VF/pVT persists repeat steps 6–8 above and deliver a third shock. Resume chest compressions immediately. Give adrenaline 1 mg IV and amiodarone 300 mg IV while performing a further 2 min CPR. Withhold adrenaline if there are signs of ROSC during CPR.

15. Repeat this 2 min CPR – rhythm/pulse check – defibrillation sequence if VF/pVT persists.

16. Give further adrenaline 1 mg IV after alternate shocks (i.e. approximately every 3–5 min).

17. If organised electrical activity compatible with a cardiac output is seen during a rhythm check, seek evidence of ROSC (check for signs of life, a central pulse and end-tidal CO_2 if available):
    – If there is ROSC, start post-resuscitation care.
    – If there are no signs of ROSC, continue CPR and switch to the non-shockable algorithm.

18. If asystole is seen, continue CPR and switch to the non-shockable algorithm.

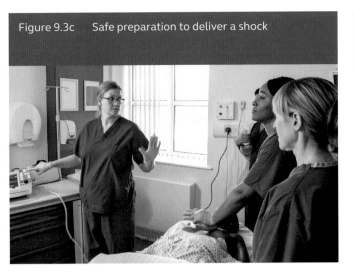

Figure 9.3c   Safe preparation to deliver a shock

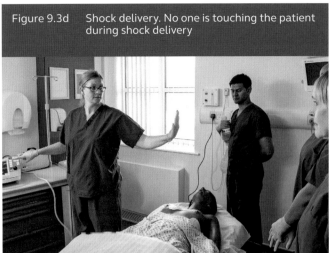

Figure 9.3d   Shock delivery. No one is touching the patient during shock delivery

Synchronised cardioversion

If electrical cardioversion is used to convert atrial or ventricular tachyarrhythmias, the shock must be synchronised with the R wave of the ECG (VF and pVT do not require synchronised shocks). By avoiding the relative refractory period in this way, the risk of inducing VF is minimised. Conscious patients must be anaesthetised or sedated before synchronised cardioversion is attempted. Most manual defibrillators incorporate a switch that enables the shock to be triggered by the R wave on the electrocardiogram. Electrodes are applied to the chest wall and cardioversion is achieved in the same way as attempted defibrillation, but the operator must anticipate the slight delay between pressing the buttons and the discharge of the shock when the next R wave occurs.

If synchronisation fails, choose another lead and/or adjust the amplitude. In a peri-arrest patient with VT, if synchronisation fails give an unsynchronised shock to avoid delay in restoring sinus rhythm.

With some defibrillators, the synchronised mode has to be reset if a second or subsequent shocks are required. Other machines remain in the synchronised mode; be careful not to leave the synchronisation switch in the 'on' position following use as this will inhibit discharge of the defibrillator when it is next used for treating VF/pVT. Energy doses for cardioversion are discussed in Chapter 11.

Implanted electronic devices

When a patient needs external defibrillation, effective measures to try to restore life take priority over concerns about any implanted device such as a pacemaker, implantable cardioverter-defibrillator, implantable event recorder or neurostimulator. Current resuscitation guidelines are followed, but awareness of the presence of an implanted device allows some additional measures to optimise outcome.

Cardiac pacemakers and implantable cardioverter-defibrillators

If the patient has an implanted electronic device in the chest wall, choose the position for defibrillator electrode placement carefully. Cardiac pacemakers and implantable cardioverter-defibrillators (ICDs) are usually implanted in the pectoral region, more commonly on the left than the right. Some people may have subcutaneous ICDs (S-ICDs), which are wholly subcutaneous, with a subcutaneous electrode running parallel to the sternum and the generator usually in a left lateral position.

Although modern electronic devices are designed to resist damage by external defibrillation currents, there is a remote possibility of damage when a shock is delivered through a defibrillation pad placed over, or close to, these implanted devices. There is also a theoretical risk of damage to the patient's myocardium due to excess current flow. This may elevate pacing thresholds or damage the myocardium at the electrode-tissue interface.

To minimise this risk, place the defibrillator electrodes away from the pacemaker or ICD generator (> 8 cm) without compromising effective defibrillation. If necessary place the pads in the antero-posterior, postero-lateral or bi-axillary position as described above. In people with S-ICDs (or with other devices in a left lateral position) place the external defibrillator electrodes in the antero-posterior position.

An implanted ICD gives no warning when it delivers a shock. On sensing a shockable rhythm, an ICD will discharge approximately 40 J (approximately 80 J for subcutaneous devices) through an internal pacing wire embedded in the right ventricle. The precise number of shocks that may be delivered in this situation will vary from one person/device to another, and is often up to eight, sometimes more.

The ICD will re-start its discharge sequence if it detects even brief apparent cessation of the tachyarrhythmia (including transient slowing of heart rate below the rate programmed to trigger shocks). This could result in the patient receiving a large number of shocks, causing pain and distress.

A ring magnet placed over the ICD will disable the defibrillation function in these circumstances (Chapter 10). Deactivation of an ICD in this way does not disable the ability of the device to act as a pacemaker if it has that capability.

During cardiorespiratory arrest in a shockable rhythm, external defibrillation should be attempted in the usual way if the ICD has not delivered a shock, or if its shocks have failed to terminate the arrhythmia.

Following successful resuscitation from cardiac arrest, interrogation of a pacemaker or ICD (by a cardiac physiologist from a pacemaker service) may provide valuable information about the rhythm behaviour that led to the cardiac arrest, as well as providing an opportunity to check lead thresholds and device function.

Implantable event recorders (also known as implantable loop recorders and implantable cardiac monitors)

These small devices (about the size of a computer memory stick) are used to record the heart's rhythm at the time of an event such as transient loss of consciousness. They are usually implanted under the skin on the anterior chest wall, overlying the heart, but occasionally may be placed in the axilla. They have no connected leads or other attachments and do not deliver any treatment. They present no risk to those giving CPR and no known risk to the patient during defibrillation. As with other devices there is a remote possibility of damage to the device itself by a high-energy shock if a defibrillator pad is placed directly over or close to the device, so careful pad placement (as far away from the device as possible without compromising effective defibrillation) is recommended.

If a person with an implantable event recorder suffers cardiorespiratory arrest, and CPR achieves ROSC, as soon as is clinically appropriate arrange to have the device interrogated (usually by a cardiac physiologist from a pacemaker service) because it may have recorded valuable information about the cardiac rhythm that initiated the arrest.

Implantable neurostimulators

Neurostimulators may be implanted subcutaneously in positions similar to those used for pacemakers and are similar in appearance. They are attached to the 'target' part of the nervous system by a lead, similar to a pacemaker lead. They present no known or likely risk to the patient or to those giving CPR. Similar principles to those used for ICDs are applied with these devices. Some manufacturers advise a minimum distance of 10–15 cm from the implanted device (between the edge of the implanted device and the edge of the defibrillator electrode).

Internal defibrillation

Internal defibrillation using paddles applied directly across the ventricles requires considerably less energy than that used for external defibrillation. For biphasic shocks, use 10–20 J, delivered directly to the myocardium through internal paddles. Monophasic shocks require approximately double these energy levels. Do not exceed 50 J when using internal defibrillation – failure to defibrillate at these energy levels requires myocardial optimisation before defibrillation is attempted again.

09: **Summary learning**

For the patient in VF/pVT, early defibrillation is the only effective means of restoring a spontaneous circulation.

When using a defibrillator, minimise interruptions to chest compressions.

Follow the manufacturer's guidance for shock energies.

For manual defibrillators, consider escalating energy levels for refractory and recurrent VF.

My key take-home messages from this chapter are:

Further reading

A guide to automated external defibrillators (AEDs). Resuscitation Council UK and British Heart Foundation. December 2019.

https://www.resus.org.uk/library/publications/publication-guide-automated-external-defibrillators

Cardiovascular implanted electronic devices in people towards the end of life, during cardiopulmonary resuscitation and after death. Guidance from the Resuscitation Council UK, British Cardiovascular Society and National Council for Palliative Care. March 2015.

https://www.resus.org.uk/library/publications/publication-cardiovascular-implanted-electronic-devices

Soar J, Berg KM, Andersen LW, et al. Advanced life support: 2020 International Consensus on Cardiopulmonary Resuscitation and Emergency Cardiovascular Care Science With Treatment Recommendations. Resuscitation 2020;156:A80–A119.

Soar J, Böttiger BW, Carli P, Couper K, Deakin CD, Djärv T, Lott C, Olasveengen TM, Paal P, Pellis T, Perkins GD, Sandroni C, Nolan JP. European Resuscitation Council Guidelines 2021: Advanced Life Support. Resuscitation. 2021;161.

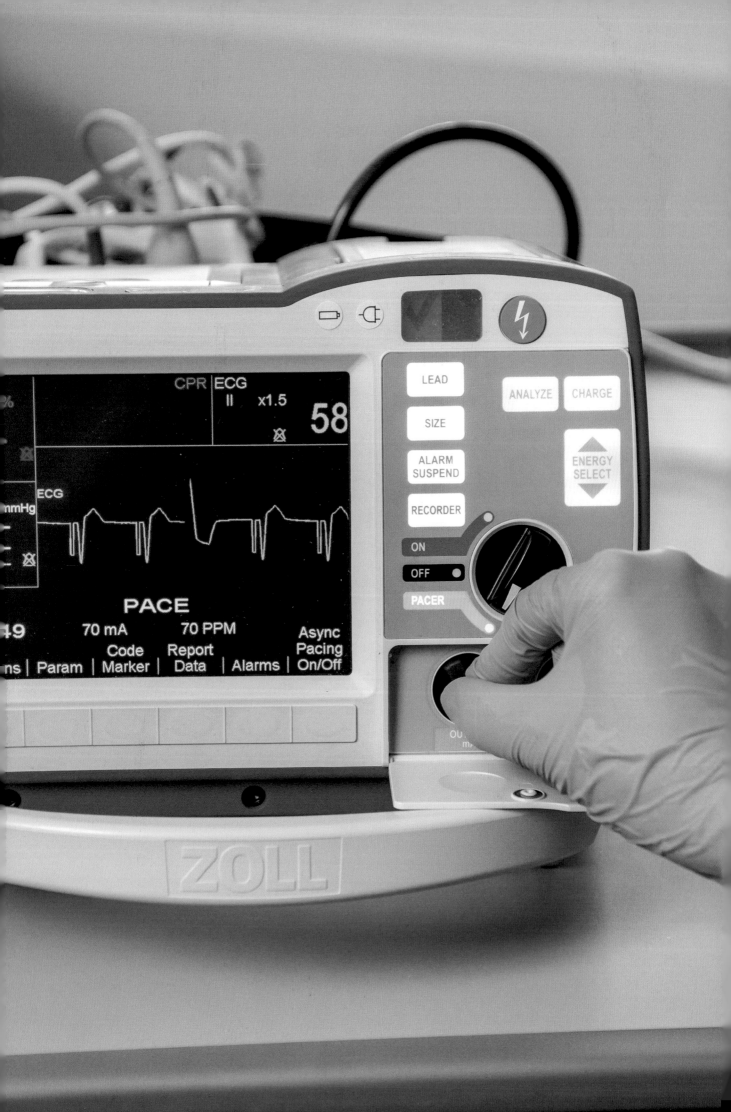

Cardiac pacing

In this chapter

Formation and transmission of the heart's spontaneous electrical signals

Ways in which failure of these may result in a need for cardiac pacing

Different methods of delivering cardiac pacing in various clinical settings

How to recognise failure of cardiac pacing and reasons for it

Safe and effective delivery of CPR for people who have implanted pacemakers or implanted cardioverter-defibrillators (ICDs)

Consideration of the need for ICD implantation in people resuscitated from cardiac arrest in a shockable rhythm

Actions needed after the death of a person with an implanted electronic device

The learning outcomes will enable you to:

Understand the indications for cardiac pacing in the peri-arrest setting

Use percussion pacing

Apply non-invasive, transcutaneous electrical pacing

Describe the problems that may occur with temporary transvenous pacing and how to correct them

Manage patients with implanted permanent pacemakers and cardioverter defibrillators in peri-arrest and cardiac arrest settings, and after death

Introduction

In some cardiac arrest or peri-arrest settings, use of cardiac pacing can be life-saving. Non-invasive pacing may be used to maintain cardiac output temporarily while expert help to deliver longer-term treatment is obtained. Non-invasive pacing can be established rapidly and as an ALS provider you should be able to achieve this.

The ALS provider does not need to have a detailed technical knowledge of permanent pacemakers and implanted cardioverter defibrillators (ICDs) but needs to be able to recognise when one of these devices is present, when they are failing, and how the presence of an implanted device may influence the management of a cardiac arrest.

Formation and failure of the heart's electrical signal

The electrical signal that stimulates each normal heartbeat arises in the sino-atrial (SA) node, which can be regarded as the heart's natural pacemaker. This depolarizes spontaneously and regularly, generating an electrical signal without any external stimulus. This behaviour is called 'automaticity', and any cardiac tissue that has this ability is capable of initiating a heartbeat and behaving as a 'pacemaker'. Different parts of the conducting system generate spontaneous signals at different rates (Figure 10.1). The fastest 'pacemaker' will generate the cardiac rhythm and slower natural pacemakers will only take over if the faster ones slow down or stop working. For example, in sinus arrest or extreme sinus bradycardia the atrioventricular (AV) node may take over and provide a junctional escape rhythm and in complete atrioventricular block (complete heart block – CHB) the escape rhythm arises from ventricular myocardium or from conducting tissue below the atrioventricular node.

Figure 10.1	Cardiac conducting system

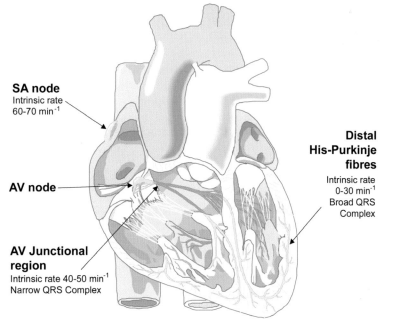

SA node
Intrinsic rate
60-70 min^{-1}

Distal His-Purkinje fibres
Intrinsic rate
0-30 min^{-1}
Broad QRS Complex

AV node

AV Junctional region
Intrinsic rate 40-50 min^{-1}
Narrow QRS Complex

When CHB occurs at the level of the AV node, the most rapid automatic activity arises from cells immediately below the block and these become the new pacemaker. The heart rate produced by these cells is usually relatively fast (often about 50 min⁻¹). The resulting escape rhythm tends to be relatively stable and relatively unlikely to fail suddenly, and cause asystole.

The QRS complexes resulting from this type of block are narrow because the impulse is transmitted to the ventricles rapidly through an intact bundle of His and bundle branches. This situation may be seen complicating acute inferior myocardial infarction. In this setting, narrow-complex CHB often may not require pacing because the heart rate is not especially slow and the risk of asystole is usually low. Assess the patient (ABCDE) to identify the effect of the bradycardia and any need for treatment.

Complete heart block can occur lower in the conducting system. Examples of causes include:

- degenerative conducting tissue fibrosis
- extensive anteroseptal myocardial infarction affecting all the fibres of the bundle branches
- cardiomyopathies
- calcific valve disease.

Any automatic activity arising below this block in the distal Purkinje fibres or myocardium is likely to be slow and unreliable. In this situation, the resulting QRS complexes are broad, since the impulse passes slowly through ventricular muscle rather than rapidly through the conducting system. This escape rhythm is unreliable and may fail transiently, leading to syncope (Stokes-Adams attack), or fail completely, causing ventricular standstill and cardiac arrest. Broad-complex CHB requires cardiac pacing, and the occurrence of long ventricular pauses (> 3 s) makes this need urgent, as it implies a risk of asystole. The possible risk of more severe AV block and asystole should always be considered in a person who has presented with syncope and has any ECG evidence of conduction delay (e.g. long PR interval or bundle branch block). Start ECG monitoring and obtain expert assessment for all such patients.

In the peri-arrest setting, pacemakers are used when the heart rate is too slow or unreliable, and not responding to the treatment described in the peri-arrest algorithm for bradycardia (Chapter 11). Pacing will be effective only if the heart is able to respond to the pacing stimulus. In the setting of cardiac arrest the presence of P waves makes this more likely. Pacing is rarely successful in asystole in the absence of P waves and should not be attempted routinely in this situation.

The pacing stimulus may be mechanical, as in percussion pacing, or electrical, as in transcutaneous and transvenous pacing.

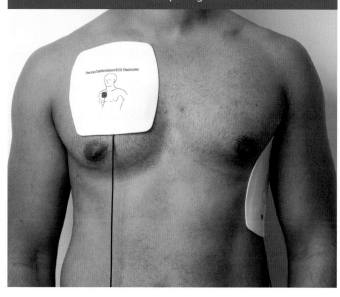

Figure 10.2a Conventional pectoral and apical pad positions can be used for pacing and for defibrillation

If a pacing stimulus induces an immediate QRS complex this is referred to as 'capture'. Check that this electrical activity seen on the ECG is accompanied by mechanical activity that produces a palpable pulse.

Methods of pacing

Methods of pacing may be classified as:

Non-invasive

- Percussion pacing ('fist pacing')
- Transcutaneous pacing

Invasive

- Temporary transvenous pacing (internal temporary transvenous/externalised permanent trans-venous, endocardial systems or surgical epicardial systems)
- Permanent pacing (using an implanted pacemaker)

Transcutaneous pacing does not, however, provide reliable ventricular stimulation, and should be used for as briefly as possible (until resolution/more reliable pacing can be established) and with monitoring to ensure there is a regular pulse.

Implanted devices that deliver pacing include pacemakers implanted for the treatment of bradycardia, biventricular pacemakers implanted for the treatment of heart failure (cardiac resynchronisation therapy) and implanted cardioverter defibrillators (ICDs), which also have a pacemaker function.

Non-invasive pacing

Percussion pacing

When bradycardia is so profound that it causes clinical cardiac arrest, percussion pacing (often called 'fist pacing') can be used in preference to CPR because it may

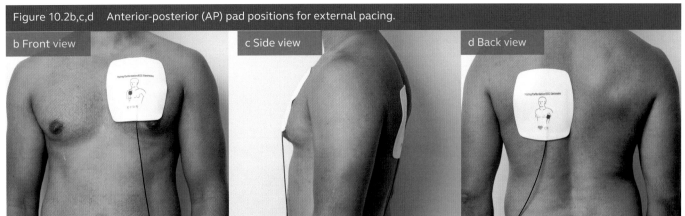

Figure 10.2b,c,d Anterior-posterior (AP) pad positions for external pacing.

10

b Front view

c Side view

d Back view

produce an adequate cardiac output with less trauma to the patient. It is more likely to be successful when ventricular standstill is accompanied by continuing P wave activity (Chapter 8).

How to perform percussion pacing

1. With the side of a closed fist deliver repeated firm thumps to the praecordium, just lateral to the lower left sternal edge.

2. Raise the hand about 20 cm above the chest before each thump.

3. Monitor the ECG and assess whether a QRS complex is generated by each thump.

4. If possible a second person should check whether a pulse is generated by each QRS complex.

5. If initial thumps do not produce a QRS complex try using slightly harder thumps.

6. If this still fails to produce a QRS complex move the point of contact around the praecordium until a site is found that produces repeated ventricular stimulation.

Percussion pacing is not as reliable as electrical pacing in stimulating QRS complexes. If percussion does not produce a regular pulse promptly, regardless of whether or not it generates QRS complexes, start CPR immediately.

Like CPR, percussion pacing is an emergency measure that is used to try to maintain circulation to vital organs. In this way it may enable either recovery of a spontaneous cardiac rhythm or initiation of transcutaneous or transvenous pacing.

Transcutaneous pacing

Compared with transvenous pacing, non-invasive transcutaneous pacing has the following advantages:

- It can be established very quickly.

- It is widely available.

- It is easy to perform and requires a minimum of training.

- It can be initiated by healthcare providers including nurses, paramedics and doctors, while waiting for expert help to establish transvenous pacing.

The major disadvantage of transcutaneous pacing in the conscious patient is discomfort. The pacing impulse stimulates painful contraction of chest wall muscles as well as causing some direct discomfort. Many defibrillators also can deliver transcutaneous pacing.

Most transcutaneous pacing systems are capable of demand pacing in which the device detects spontaneous QRS complexes and delivers a pacing stimulus only when it is needed.

How to perform transcutaneous pacing

1. Avoid delay, but pay careful attention to technique in order to increase the chance of success.

2. If necessary, use scissors or a razor to quickly remove excess chest hair from the skin where the electrode (pad) is to be applied.

3. Make sure that the skin is dry.

4. If necessary attach ECG monitoring electrodes and leads – these are needed with some transcutaneous pacing devices. If in any doubt, attach both monitoring electrodes and leads as a default.

5. Position the pads in the 'conventional' right pectoral and apical positions if possible (Figure 10.2a). For right pectoral and apical positions place one pad over the right pectoral muscle, just below the clavicle. Place the apical pad in the left mid-axillary line, overlying the V6 ECG electrode position. Apply this pad to the chest wall, not over breast tissue. If this is prevented (e.g. by chest trauma or an implanted device in this position) anterior-posterior (A-P) pad positions can be used.

6. For A-P positions (Figure 10.2b–d) place the anterior pad on the left anterior chest wall, beside the sternum, overlying the V2 and V3 ECG electrode positions. Place the posterior pad between the lower part of the left scapula and the spine, at the same horizontal level on the trunk as the anterior pad. These precise positions may not be optimal for cardioversion of atrial tachyarrhythmia, for which the anterior pad is best placed overlying the right sternal border.

7. If you are using a pacing device that is not capable of defibrillation, use A-P positions for the pacing electrode pads so that defibrillator pads can still be applied in the right pectoral and apical positions.

8. Make sure that you are familiar with the device that you are using and that you know how to operate it. Different transcutaneous pacing devices have different operational features. For example, some

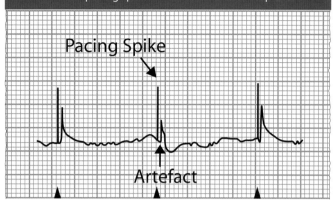

Figure 10.3a Transcutaneous pacing. ECG appearance of pacing spikes without ventricular capture

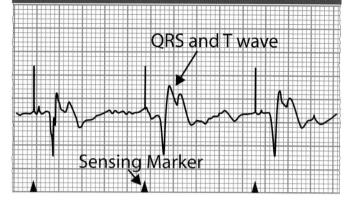

Figure 10.3b Transcutaneous pacing. ECG shows ventricular capture after each pacing spike

require the operator to increase the current delivered with each pacing stimulus until electrical capture is achieved, whilst others use a constant current that cannot be adjusted and a longer pulse duration (duration of the pacing stimulus) than other devices.

9. Most transcutaneous pacing devices pace the heart in demand mode. The pacemaker will be inhibited if it detects a spontaneous QRS complex. However, if there is movement artefact on the ECG this may inhibit the pacemaker. Avoid causing movement artefact as far as possible. If artefact still appears to be inhibiting the pacemaker, switch the device to deliver fixed-rate pacing.

10. Select an appropriate pacing rate. This will usually be in the range 60–90 min^{-1} for adults, but in some circumstances (e.g. complete AV block with an idioventricular rhythm at 50 min^{-1}) a slower pacing rate of 40 or even 30 min^{-1} may be appropriate in order to deliver pacing only during sudden ventricular standstill or more extreme bradycardia.

11. If the pacing device has an adjustable energy output set this at its lowest value and turn on the pacemaker. Gradually increase the output while observing the patient and the ECG. As the current is increased the muscles of the chest wall will contract with each impulse and a pacing 'spike' will appear on the ECG (Figure 10.3a). Increase the current until each pacing spike is followed immediately by a QRS complex, indicating electrical capture (typically with a current of 50–100 mA). This means that the pacing stimuli are causing depolarisation of the ventricles (Figure 10.3b).

12. Check that the apparent QRS complex is followed by a T wave. Occasionally, artefact generated by the pacing current travelling through the chest may look like a QRS complex, but such artefact will not be followed by a T wave (Figure 10.3).

13. If the highest current setting is reached and electrical capture has not occurred, try changing the electrode positions. Continued failure to achieve electrical capture may indicate non-viable myocardium, but other conditions (e.g. severe hyperkalaemia) may prevent successful pacing.

14. Having achieved electrical capture with the pacemaker, check that each paced QRS complex is followed by a pulse. A palpable pulse confirms a mechanical response of the heart (i.e. contraction of the myocardium) to the paced QRS complex. Good electrical capture that fails to generate a pulse constitutes pulseless electrical activity (PEA). This may be due to severe myocardial failure but consider other possible causes of PEA in these circumstances.

15. Warn conscious patients that they are likely to experience considerable discomfort during transcutaneous pacing. Be ready to give them intravenous analgesia and/or sedation as required, especially if prolonged transcutaneous pacing is needed. If sedation is used, reassess the patient frequently (ABCDE) because sedative drugs may suppress respiratory effort.

16. If necessary, provide good-quality chest compressions. These can be given and other manual contact with the patient maintained as necessary with transcutaneous electrodes in place. There is no hazard from transcutaneous pacing to people who are in contact with the patient. However, there is no benefit in trying to deliver transcutaneous pacing during chest compressions, so it is best to turn off the pacemaker whilst CPR is in progress.

17. When transcutaneous pacing produces an adequate cardiac output seek expert help immediately to arrange emergency transvenous pacing.

Invasive pacing

Temporary transvenous pacing

It is rarely appropriate to try to attempt to insert a transvenous pacing wire during a cardiac arrest. In this setting, use non-invasive pacing to attempt to achieve a cardiac output, and then seek expert help with transvenous pacing. Failure of an existing temporary transvenous pacing system may cause cardiac arrest, particularly when the patient is pacing-dependent.

Temporary transvenous pacing systems can fail in three ways:

1. High threshold

When a temporary pacing lead is inserted the usual aim is to position its tip in the apex of the right ventricle, where it is least likely to be displaced. After positioning the lead, it is used to pace the heart. The pacing 'threshold' is measured by gradually reducing the voltage delivered by the pacemaker to determine the minimum voltage needed to stimulate the ventricle. The usual aim is to achieve a threshold of < 1.0 V at the time of lead insertion. Higher thresholds suggest that the electrode is not making satisfactory contact with the myocardium, so there may be a need to reposition the lead.

It is usual to pace the heart with a 3–4 V stimulus, well above the initial pacing threshold. Over the first days and weeks after insertion of a pacing lead (temporary or permanent) a transient rise in the threshold can be expected.

Check the threshold on temporary pacing leads at least daily to make sure that the output of the pacemaker Is well above the threshold. If not, loss of capture may occur. This is seen on the ECG as a pacing spike without a subsequent QRS complex. Loss of capture may be intermittent, so any apparent 'missed beat' of this nature should prompt a repeat check of the pacing threshold, as should introduction of some classes of anti-arrhythmic drugs.

If loss of capture occurs because of a high threshold, increase the output of the pacemaker immediately to well above the threshold. A sudden increase in pacing threshold may be caused by lead displacement, so obtain a chest x-ray and seek expert help, as repositioning of the lead may be needed.

2. Connection failure

Most temporary transvenous pacing leads are bipolar. One electrode is at the tip of the lead and the second is about 1 cm proximal to the tip. Each electrode is connected by the lead to separate connectors at the other end, outside the patient. These are usually inserted into sockets at one end of a connecting cable that in turn is connected to the terminals of the pacemaker. Make sure that all connections between the lead and the pacemaker are making good, secure contact that is unlikely to be lost easily, for example by minor movement of the lead or cable.

Failure of any of these connections will prevent delivery of the pacing stimulus to the heart, seen on the ECG as absence of a pacing spike. This may be intermittent and symptomless, or may be sudden and total and may result in syncope or cardiac arrest in asystole. When pacing failure is accompanied by loss of the pacing spike on the ECG, check all connections immediately. Check that the pacemaker has not been turned off inadvertently and check that its batteries are not depleted. Try another pacing box. If the problem remains unresolved another possible explanation is a fracture of a wire within its insulation. This usually causes intermittent pacing failure and the fracture is more likely to be in the connecting cable than in the pacing lead. If this is suspected change the connecting cable immediately.

3. Lead displacement

The tip of an endocardial transvenous ventricular pacing lead is usually positioned in the apex of the right ventricle. There should be enough slack in the lead to allow for changes in patient posture and deep inspiration, but not so much as to encourage displacement of the lead tip. The tip of a pacing lead can perforate the wall of the right ventricle and enter the pericardium with little or no apparent change in position on chest radiography. Very rarely, this may cause cardiac tamponade, so consider this possibility if a patient with a recently implanted pacing lead suffers cardiac arrest with pulseless electrical activity. Perforation of the right ventricle may also be suspected if the ECG shows ST-elevation.

When displacement or perforation occurs, the ECG will still show a pacing spike, but there is likely to be intermittent or complete loss of capture of the pacing stimulus (when the pacing spike is not followed by a QRS complex). When a pacing lead displaces but remains in the right ventricle it may trigger ventricular extrasystoles or more serious ventricular arrhythmia, including VT and VF. When transvenous pacing fails, there is a risk of ventricular standstill. This may be relatively short-lived and cause syncope, or prolonged and cause cardiac arrest in asystole. In this situation use non-invasive pacing until effective transvenous pacing can be re-established.

Cardiovascular implanted electronic devices

This term refers mainly to implanted pacemakers and implantable cardioverter-defibrillators (ICDs). Occasionally, a permanent pacing system may be used with an externalised generator box, potentially providing a more stable temporary pacing solution. In the event of cardiac arrest, these should be managed as an implanted permanent pacemaker. Detailed guidance and quality standards for the management of these devices towards the end of life, during cardiac arrest and after death have been published by Resuscitation Council UK, the British Cardiovascular Society and the National Council for Palliative Care (see 'Further reading' below).

Implanted permanent pacemakers

Problems with permanent pacing systems failing are rare, because the connections between pacing electrodes and the pacemaker are much more secure. Lead displacement may occur as an early complication in the first few days after implantation, but becomes progressively less likely thereafter and rarely occurs more than 4–6 weeks after implantation. Occasional fracture of a permanent pacing lead may occur, usually following trauma such as a fall on to an outstretched arm on the side of the pacemaker. This may cause permanent or intermittent loss of the pacing spike.

When assessing a patient using the ABCDE approach check (during 'E') for the presence of an implanted device. These devices are usually implanted below the

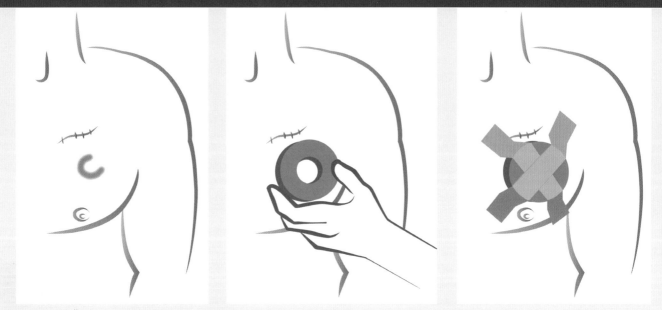

clavicle, often but not always on the left side. If a device is identified consider whether it is a pacemaker or an ICD and in the case of a pacemaker try to establish whether it was implanted as treatment for bradyarrhythmia or as treatment for heart failure. Be aware also that leadless pacemakers now exist. These are implanted transvenously, entirely within the right ventricle and will not be detectable on clinical examination.

If a patient with an implanted subcutaneous pacemaker or ICD has a cardiac arrest or requires cardioversion, place defibrillation pads > 8 cm from the device.

Devices that are implanted below the left clavicle usually present no problem with the use of standard defibrillator pad positions. If a device has been implanted below the right clavicle or just below the left axilla, use A-P positions for defibrillation or cardioversion if possible.

Biventricular pacing systems

The traditional reason for implantation of a permanent pacemaker was treatment of bradycardia, caused mostly by malfunction of atrioventricular conduction or the sino-atrial node. Over several years there has been increasing use of biventricular pacemakers as 'cardiac resynchronisation therapy' in patients with heart failure. Many of these patients do not need pacing for bradycardia. The aim of these devices is to improve cardiac efficiency by resynchronising contraction of the ventricles. These pacemakers require the same precautions during defibrillation and cardioversion as any other pacemaker, but failure of a pacemaker that has been inserted for this purpose will not usually cause any major change in heart rate or any dangerous rhythm abnormality. Some biventricular pacing systems also incorporate an ICD function (see below).

Implantable cardioverter-defibrillators

These devices resemble large implanted pacemakers. Unlike a simple pacemaker, the primary function of an ICD is to terminate a life-threatening tachyarrhythmia.

A 'simple' ICD can deliver a shock when it detects VF or fast VT. Many of these devices are programmed also to deliver critically timed pacing stimuli to attempt to terminate VT that is not especially fast and is unlikely in itself to cause cardiac arrest, resorting to defibrillation only if the VT accelerates or degenerates into VF. Most ICDs can function as demand pacemakers in the event of bradycardia and some devices will also deliver biventricular pacing for heart failure, as well as delivering defibrillation if required.

National and international guidelines define indications for ICD implantation. These include indications for their use in 'primary prevention' in people who have not experienced cardiac arrest but are at high risk of VF or VT causing sudden cardiac death. ICDs may improve survival in selected patients after major myocardial infarction, selected patients with heart failure and in some people with certain types of inherited cardiac condition.

ICDs are implanted usually in the pectoral region in a similar subcutaneous position to pacemakers. Though these devices may seem complex, the means by which they sense changes in cardiac rhythm is relatively simple, depending mainly on automated detection of very rapid heart rates (from an ECG signal). Consequently, ICDs may occasionally misdiagnose an arrhythmia, or misinterpret other electrical signals, and deliver inappropriate shocks, which are very unpleasant for a conscious patient. If necessary, to prevent inappropriate shocks, ICDs can be disabled temporarily by holding or taping a ring magnet on the skin overlying the device (Figure 10.4). This will also prevent the ICD from recognising and shocking VF and VT. Seek urgent expert help if ICD malfunction is suspected.

If a patient with an ICD has a cardiac arrest that is not terminated by the ICD, deliver CPR in the usual way. It is believed that chest compressions can be delivered without major risk to the rescuer, even if the ICD delivers an internal shock to the patient during chest compressions. However, there have been rare reports of shocks from an ICD causing transient myalgia and paraesthesia in the arms of a person delivering chest compressions. If a shockable cardiac arrest rhythm is present and is not terminated by the ICD, use external defibrillation in a standard way, taking the same precautions with choice of defibrillator pad positions as in a patient with an implanted pacemaker. During CPR, if an ICD delivers repeated inappropriate shocks that are impeding delivery of high- quality CPR consider deactivating the ICD using a ring magnet as above. Do not delay or interrupt CPR while locating or positioning a magnet for this purpose.

Consider the possible requirement for ICD implantation in any patient who has been resuscitated from cardiac arrest in a shockable rhythm outside the context of proven acute ST-segment elevation myocardial infarction. All such patients should be referred before discharge from hospital for assessment by a cardiologist with expertise in heart rhythm disorders.

Implanted electronic devices – management after death

When a person dies with an active ICD in place arrange for its deactivation (usually done by a cardiac physiologist) as soon as is reasonably practicable. An ICD must be deactivated prior to its removal from the body or performance of an autopsy. Any implanted electronic devices (including pacemakers, ICDs, event ('loop') recorders and neurostimulators) must be removed prior to cremation.

Further reading

Brignole (M, Auricchio A, Baron-Esquivias G, Bordachar P et al. The Task Force on cardiac pacing and resynchronization therapy of the European Society of Cardiology. Developed in collaboration with the European Heart Rhythm Association (EHRA). 2013 ESC Guidelines on cardiac pacing and cardiac resynchronization therapy. Europ Heart J 2013; 34: 2281–2329.

Kusumoto FM, Schoenfeld MH, Barrett C, et al. 2018 ACC/AHA/HRS Guideline on the Evaluation and Management of Patients With Bradycardia and Cardiac Conduction Delay: A Report of the American College of Cardiology/American Heart Association Task Force on Clinical Practice Guidelines and the Heart Rhythm Society. J Am Coll Cardiol 2019;74:e51-e156.

National Institute for Clinical Health & Excellence 2014. Technology appraisal 324. Dual chamber pacemakers for symptomatic bradycardia due to sick sinus syndrome without atrioventricular block (part review of technology appraisal guidance 88). www.nice.org.uk.

Priori SG, Blomstrom-Lundqvist C (Co-chairs). The Task Force for the Management of Patients with Ventricular Arrhythmias and the Prevention of Sudden Cardiac Death of the European Society of Cardiology (ESC). 2015 ESC Guidelines for the management of patients with ventricular arrhythmias and the prevention of sudden cardiac death. Eur Heart J 2015: doi:10.1093/eurheartj/ehv316. www.escardio.org

10: Summary learning

Non-invasive pacing can be delivered by an ALS provider and is the immediate treatment for severe bradyarrhythmia that is a potential risk to a patient who does not respond to initial drug treatment.

Non-invasive pacing is a temporary, emergency measure to be used briefly until either a stable and effective spontaneous rhythm returns, or a competent person establishes transvenous pacing.

During resuscitation attempts in patients with implanted pacemakers and ICDs deliver CPR in the usual way, taking care not to place external defibrillator pads over or close to an implanted device.

Consider the possible need for an ICD in patients resuscitated from cardiac arrest in VT or VF, in whom there is a possible risk of recurrence and refer accordingly.

Active ICDs should be deactivated as soon as practicable after a person's death. Remove all implanted electronic devices before cremation.

My key take-home messages from this chapter are:

Pitcher D, Soar J, Hogg K, et al. Cardiovascular implanted electronic devices in people towards the end of life, during cardiopulmonary resuscitation and after death: guidance from Resuscitation Council UK, British Cardiovascular Society and National Council for Palliative Care Heart 2016;102: A1–A17.

Soar J, Böttiger BW, Carli P, Couper K, Deakin CD, Djärv T, Lott C, Olasveengen TM, Paal P, Pellis T, Perkins GD, Sandroni C, Nolan JP. European Resuscitation Council Guidelines 2021: Advanced Life Support. Resuscitation. 2021;161.

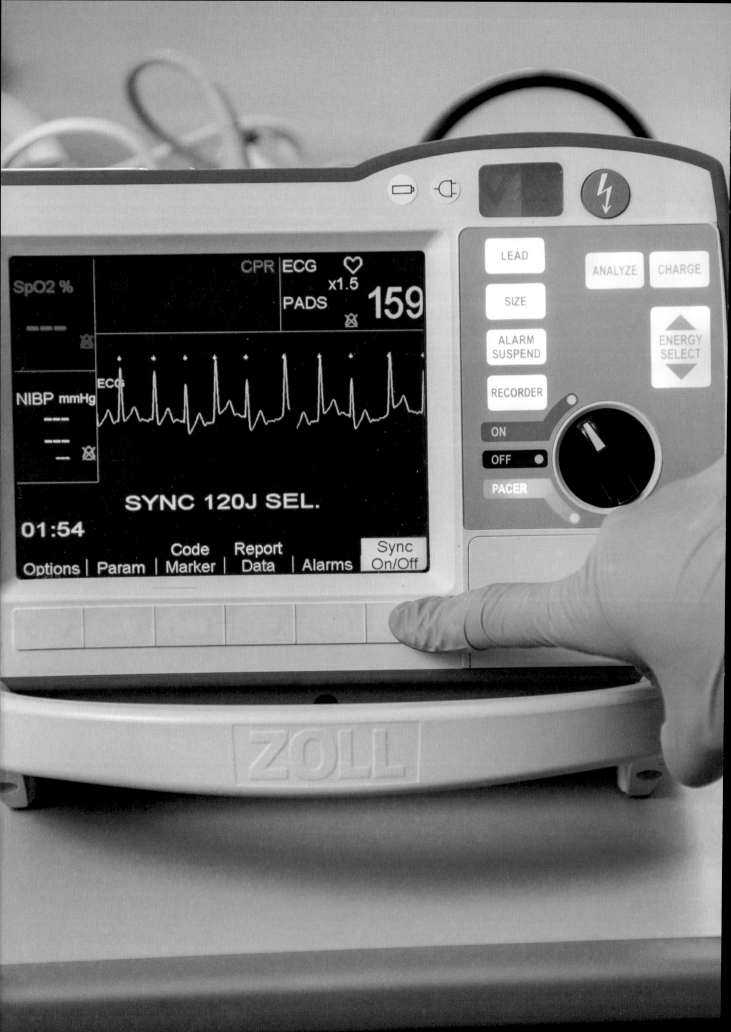

Peri-arrest arrhythmias

In this chapter

Arrhythmias that may lead to cardiac arrest or recurrent cardiac arrest

Assessment of a patient with an arrhythmia or suspected arrhythmia

Life-threatening features indicating a need for urgent treatment

Immediate treatment of cardiac arrhythmia by non-specialists

Tachyarrhythmia and bradyarrhythmia algorithms

When to seek specialist/expert help

The learning outcomes will enable you to:

Understand the importance of arrhythmias that may precede or follow a cardiac arrest

Assess peri-arrest arrhythmias

Understand the principles of treating peri-arrest arrhythmias

Introduction

Rhythm abnormalities that occur in the 'peri-arrest' period may be considered in two main categories:

1. Arrhythmias that may lead to cardiac arrest

Many rhythm abnormalities occur without causing cardiac arrest. Although arrhythmias are a relatively common complication of acute myocardial infarction (AMI) they are common also in patients with other cardiac abnormalities and in people who do not have coronary disease or structural heart disease. Untreated, some of these arrhythmias may lead to cardiac arrest or to avoidable deterioration in the patient's condition. Others require no immediate treatment.

2. Arrhythmias that occur after initial resuscitation from cardiac arrest

These often indicate that the patient's condition is still unstable and that there is a risk of deterioration or further cardiac arrest.

You should be able to recognise common arrhythmias, know how to assess whether they require immediate treatment and know when to call for expert help. Arrhythmias may be categorised by heart rate as tachyarrhythmias, bradyarrhythmias and arrhythmias with a normal heart rate. Most peri-arrest arrhythmias will fall into the first two categories, so the remainder of this chapter will focus on these. However, some arrhythmias with a normal rate may indicate a potentially treatable risk of cardiac arrest (e.g. hypokalaemia), so any arrhythmia or suspected arrhythmia should be assessed carefully in the context of the individual circumstances at the time. The treatment algorithms described in this section have been designed to enable the non-specialist ALS provider to treat a patient effectively and safely in an emergency; for this reason, they have been kept as simple as possible. If patients are not acutely ill there may be treatment options, including the use of drugs (oral or parenteral), that will be less familiar to the non-expert. In this situation you should, whenever possible, seek advice from cardiologists or other senior specialists with the appropriate expertise.

Sequence of actions to take in all arrhythmias

A   B   C   D   E

When an arrhythmia is present or suspected, start by assessing the patient using the ABCDE approach, including early ECG monitoring (Chapter 8). Assess the patient specifically for life-threatening features (see below). Clinical assessment is of limited value in identifying the precise rhythm abnormality. Whenever possible, record a 12-lead ECG at the earliest opportunity. This will help to identify the precise rhythm, either before treatment or retrospectively if necessary, with the help of an expert. Insert an intravenous cannula. If hypoxaemia is present give oxygen, aiming for an SpO_2 of 94–98% (88–92% in COPD).

For any patient with an arrhythmia or suspected arrhythmia assess and document:

1. the condition of the patient (presence or absence of adverse features)
2. the heart rate (bradycardia, tachycardia or normal heart rate)
3. the nature of the arrhythmia.

Life-threatening features

The presence or absence of life-threatening symptoms and/or signs will dictate the urgency and choice of treatment for most arrhythmias. The following features indicate that a patient is unstable and at risk of deterioration, whether entirely or partly because of the arrhythmia:

- **Shock** – hypotension (systolic blood pressure < 90 mmHg), pallor, sweating, cold extremities, confusion or impaired consciousness.

- **Syncope** – transient loss of consciousness because of global reduction in blood flow to the brain.

- **Heart failure** – pulmonary oedema and/or raised jugular venous pressure (with or without peripheral oedema and liver enlargement).

- **Myocardial ischaemia** – typical ischaemic chest pain and/or evidence of myocardial ischaemia on a 12-lead ECG.

- **Extremes of heart rate** – in addition to the above features it may be appropriate to consider extremes of heart rate as life-threatening features in themselves, requiring more urgent assessment and treatment than less extreme tachycardia or bradycardia with no life-threatening features.

A. Extreme tachycardia: when heart rate increases, diastole is shortened to a greater degree than systole.

Rhythm abnormalities that cause very fast heart rates (e.g. > 150 min^{-1}) reduce cardiac output dramatically (because diastole is very short and the heart does not have time to fill properly) and reduce coronary blood flow (because this mostly occurs during diastole), potentially causing myocardial ischaemia. The faster the heart rate, the less well it will be tolerated.

B. Extreme bradycardia: in general, the slower the bradycardia the less well it will be tolerated and heart rates below 40 min^{-1} are often tolerated poorly.

This is especially so when people have severe heart disease and cannot compensate for the bradycardia by increasing stroke volume. Some people with very severe heart disease require faster than normal heart rates to maintain cardiac output, and even a 'normal' heart rate may be inappropriately slow for them.

Treatment options

Depending on the presence or absence of life-threatening features and the nature of the arrhythmia, choose one of four options for immediate treatment:

1. no treatment needed
2. simple clinical intervention (e.g. vagal manoeuvres, percussion pacing)
3. pharmacological (drug treatment)
4. electrical (cardioversion for tachyarrhythmia or pacing for bradyarrhythmia).

Most drugs act more slowly and less reliably than electrical treatments, so electrical treatment is usually the preferred treatment for an unstable patient with life-threatening features.

If a patient develops an arrhythmia as a complication of some other condition (e.g. infection, AMI, heart failure), make sure that the underlying condition is assessed and treated appropriately, involving relevant experts if necessary.

Subsequent monitoring and treatment

After successful treatment of an arrhythmia continue to monitor the patient until you are confident that the risk of further arrhythmia is low. Remember always to record a 12-lead ECG after successful treatment of an arrhythmia because this may show abnormalities (or absence of abnormalities) that will be important in planning future management. Correct all reversible factors that may predispose to further arrhythmia. Ensure that appropriate further expert help and advice is obtained at the most appropriate time for the patient.

Tachyarrhythmia

If the patient has life-threatening features

These imply that the patient's condition is unstable and that they are at risk of deterioration. If this appears to be because of the tachyarrhythmia, attempt to correct this using synchronised cardioversion (Figure 11.1).

In people with otherwise normal hearts, adverse signs and symptoms are uncommon if the heart rate is < 150 min^{-1} (so correction of the rhythm by cardioversion may be of limited benefit). However, people with impaired cardiac function, structural heart disease or other serious medical conditions (e.g. severe lung disease) may be symptomatic and unstable during arrhythmias with heart rates between 100–150 min^{-1} (so may be more likely to benefit from rhythm correction by cardioversion).

If cardioversion fails to terminate the arrhythmia, and adverse features persist, give amiodarone 300 mg IV over 10–20 min and attempt further synchronised cardioversion. The loading dose of amiodarone can be followed by an infusion of 900 mg over 24 h, given into a large vein (preferably via central venous catheter).

Synchronised cardioversion

Carry out cardioversion under conscious sedation or general anaesthesia, administered by a healthcare professional competent in the technique. Ensure that the defibrillator is set to deliver a synchronised shock. This delivers the shock to coincide with the R wave. An unsynchronised shock could coincide with a T wave and cause ventricular fibrillation (VF).

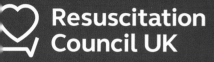

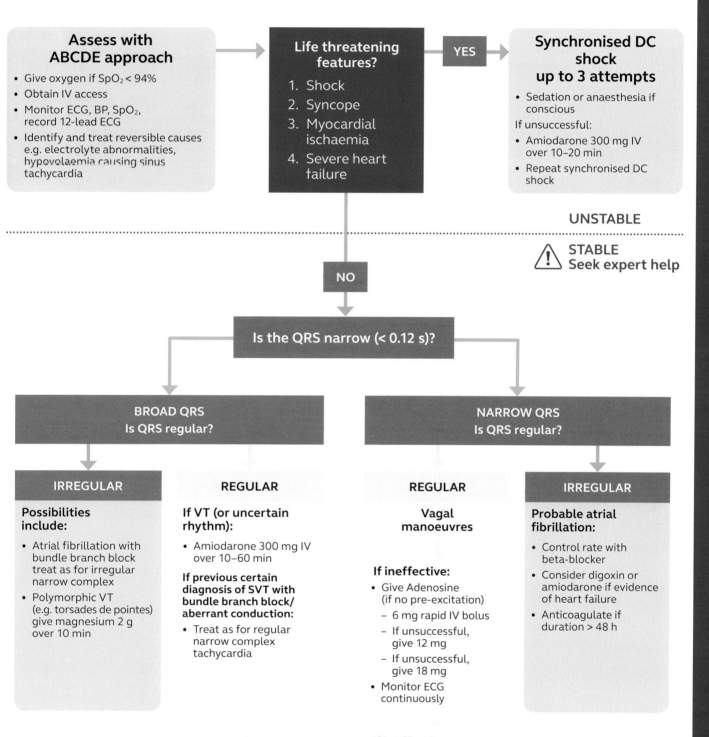

Adult tachycardia

Assess with ABCDE approach
- Give oxygen if $SpO_2 < 94\%$
- Obtain IV access
- Monitor ECG, BP, SpO_2, record 12-lead ECG
- Identify and treat reversible causes e.g. electrolyte abnormalities, hypovolaemia causing sinus tachycardia

Life threatening features?
1. Shock
2. Syncope
3. Myocardial ischaemia
4. Severe heart failure

YES

Synchronised DC shock up to 3 attempts
- Sedation or anaesthesia if conscious

If unsuccessful:
- Amiodarone 300 mg IV over 10–20 min
- Repeat synchronised DC shock

UNSTABLE

⚠ **STABLE** Seek expert help

NO

Is the QRS narrow (< 0.12 s)?

BROAD QRS Is QRS regular?

NARROW QRS Is QRS regular?

IRREGULAR

Possibilities include:
- Atrial fibrillation with bundle branch block treat as for irregular narrow complex
- Polymorphic VT (e.g. torsades de pointes) give magnesium 2 g over 10 min

REGULAR

If VT (or uncertain rhythm):
- Amiodarone 300 mg IV over 10–60 min

If previous certain diagnosis of SVT with bundle branch block/ aberrant conduction:
- Treat as for regular narrow complex tachycardia

REGULAR

Vagal manoeuvres

If ineffective:
- Give Adenosine (if no pre-excitation)
  - 6 mg rapid IV bolus
  - If unsuccessful, give 12 mg
  - If unsuccessful, give 18 mg
- Monitor ECG continuously

If ineffective:
- Verapamil or beta-blocker

IRREGULAR

Probable atrial fibrillation:
- Control rate with beta-blocker
- Consider digoxin or amiodarone if evidence of heart failure
- Anticoagulate if duration > 48 h

If ineffective:
- Synchronised DC shock up to 3 attempts
- Sedation or anaesthesia if conscious

For a broad-complex tachycardia start with 120–150 J and increase in increments if this fails. For atrial fibrillation (AF) start at the maximum defibrillator output. Atrial flutter and regular narrow-complex tachycardia will often be terminated by lower-energy shocks: start with 70–120 J. For atrial fibrillation and flutter use anteroposterior defibrillator pad positions when it is practicable to do so.

When delivering the shock, press the shock button and keep it pressed until after the shock has occurred – there may be a slight delay before the shock is delivered. If a second shock is needed, remember to reactivate the synchronisation switch if necessary.

If the patient has no life-threatening features

If there are no life-threatening features consider firstly whether or not any treatment is necessary. If treatment is needed consider using drug treatment in the first instance. Seek expert to help with the diagnosis. Assess the ECG and measure the QRS duration. If the QRS duration is 0.12 s (3 small squares at ECG paper speed 25 mm s^{-1}) or more this is a broad-complex tachycardia. If the QRS duration is < 0.12 s it is a narrow-complex tachycardia.

A B C D E

Following any drug therapy, continue to reassess the patient (ABCDE) and monitor heart rate and rhythm to assess the response to treatment. Some anti-arrhythmic drugs cause myocardial depression, which may cause or worsen heart failure or hypotension, and in some cases an anti-arrhythmic drug may cause other tachyarrhythmia or provoke severe bradycardia.

Broad-complex tachycardia

Broad-complex tachycardia (QRS ≥ 0.12 s) may be ventricular in origin or may be a supraventricular rhythm with aberrant conduction (i.e. bundle branch block).

In a person with adverse features due to the arrhythmia the distinction will not affect the immediate treatment needed. Attempt synchronised cardioversion as described above.

If a patient has a broad-complex tachycardia but no adverse features, next determine whether the rhythm is regular or irregular.

Regular broad-complex tachycardia

A regular broad-complex tachycardia may be ventricular tachycardia (VT) or a supraventricular rhythm with bundle branch block. The safest approach is to treat all broad-complex tachycardia as VT unless there has been a previous certain diagnosis of SVT with bundle branch block. Treat with amiodarone 300 mg IV over 20–60 min, followed by an infusion of 900 mg over 24 h. If the broad complex tachycardia persists after the initial 300 mg

dose of amiodarone, synchronised cardioversion may be considered but such a decision should be deferred to an expert. If a regular broad-complex tachycardia is known to be a supraventricular arrhythmia with bundle branch block and the patient is stable, use the treatment strategy recommended for narrow-complex tachycardia (below).

Irregular broad-complex tachycardia

This is most likely to be AF with bundle branch block, but careful examination of a 12-lead ECG (if necessary by an expert) may provide confident identification of the rhythm. Other possible causes are AF with ventricular pre-excitation (in patients with Wolff-Parkinson-White (WPW) syndrome), or polymorphic VT (e.g. torsade de pointes), but polymorphic VT is unlikely to be present without adverse features. Seek expert help with the assessment and treatment of irregular broad-complex tachyarrhythmia.

Treat torsade de pointes VT by stopping immediately all drugs known to prolong the QT interval. Correct electrolyte abnormalities, especially hypokalaemia. Give magnesium sulfate 2 g IV over 10 min. Obtain expert help, as other treatment (e.g. overdrive pacing) may be indicated to prevent relapse once the arrhythmia has been corrected. If adverse features develop, which is common, arrange immediate synchronised cardioversion. If the patient becomes pulseless, attempt defibrillation immediately (ALS algorithm).

Narrow-complex tachycardia

Examine the ECG to determine if the rhythm is regular or irregular. Regular narrow-complex tachycardias include sinus tachycardia, paroxysmal supraventricular tachycardia, and atrial flutter with regular AV conduction (usually 2:1).

An irregular narrow-complex tachycardia is most likely to be AF, or sometimes atrial flutter with variable AV conduction ('variable block').

Regular narrow-complex tachycardia

Sinus tachycardia

Sinus tachycardia is not an arrhythmia. This is a common physiological response to stimuli such as exercise or anxiety. In a sick patient it may occur in response to many conditions including pain, infection, anaemia, blood loss, and heart failure. Treatment is directed at the underlying cause. Trying to slow sinus tachycardia that has occurred in response to most of these situations will usually make the situation worse. Do not attempt to treat sinus tachycardia with cardioversion or anti-arrhythmic drugs.

Paroxysmal supraventricular tachycardia

Paroxysmal supraventricular tachycardia (SVT) causes a regular, narrow-complex tachycardia, often with no clearly visible atrial activity on the ECG. The heart rate is usually well above the upper limit of sinus rate at rest (100 min⁻¹). It is usually benign, unless there is additional, co-incidental, structural heart disease or coronary disease, but it may cause symptoms that the patient finds frightening. Paroxysmal SVT can occur in patients with the WPW syndrome but is still usually benign, unless there is additional structural heart disease.

Atrial flutter with regular AV conduction (often 2:1 block)

This produces a regular narrow-complex tachycardia. It may be difficult to see atrial activity and identify flutter waves on the ECG with confidence, so the rhythm may be indistinguishable, at least initially from paroxysmal SVT.

Typical atrial flutter has an atrial rate of about 300 min⁻¹, so atrial flutter with 2:1 conduction produces a tachycardia of about 150 min⁻¹. Much faster rates (160 min⁻¹ or more) are unlikely to be caused by atrial flutter with 2:1 conduction. Regular tachycardia with slower rates (125–150 min⁻¹) may be caused by atrial flutter with 2:1 conduction, usually when the rate of the atrial flutter has been slowed by drug therapy.

Treatment of regular narrow-complex tachyarrhythmia

If the patient has life-threatening features and is at risk of deterioration because of the tachyarrhythmia, perform synchronised cardioversion. In this situation it is reasonable to attempt vagal manoeuvres (see below) or to give intravenous adenosine (see below) to a patient with a regular narrow-complex tachyarrhythmia while preparations are being made for synchronised cardioversion. However, do not delay electrical cardioversion if these treatments fail to terminate the arrhythmia.

In the absence of life-threatening features:

1. Start with vagal manoeuvres. Carotid sinus massage or the Valsalva manoeuvre will terminate up to a quarter of episodes of paroxysmal SVT. Record an ECG (preferably 12-lead) during each manoeuvre. If the rhythm is atrial flutter with 2:1 conduction, transient slowing of the ventricular response will often occur and reveal flutter waves.

2. If the arrhythmia persists and is not atrial flutter, give adenosine 6 mg as a very rapid intravenous bolus followed by a flush. Use a relatively large cannula and large (e.g. antecubital) vein. Warn the patient that they will feel unwell and probably experience chest discomfort for a few seconds after the injection. Record an ECG (preferably 12-lead) during the injection. If the ventricular rate slows transiently, but then speeds up again, look for atrial activity, such as atrial flutter or other atrial tachycardia, and treat accordingly. If there is no response (i.e. no transient slowing or termination of the tachyarrhythmia) to adenosine 6 mg, give a 12 mg bolus. If there is no response give an 18 mg bolus. When using an 18 mg bolus dose consider the individual patient's ability to tolerate the side effects of adenosine. Apparent lack of response to adenosine will be likely if the bolus is given too slowly or into a peripheral vein.

3. Vagal manoeuvres or adenosine will terminate almost all paroxysmal SVTs within seconds. Failure to terminate a regular narrow-complex tachycardia with adenosine suggests an atrial tachycardia such as atrial flutter (unless the adenosine has been injected too slowly or into a peripheral vein).

4. If adenosine is contraindicated, or fails to terminate a regular narrow-complex tachycardia without demonstrating that it is atrial flutter, consider giving verapamil 2.5–5 mg intravenously over 2 min or a beta-blocker such as metoprolol (2.5–15 mg given IV in 2.5 mg bolus doses).

5. If the narrow-complex tachycardia persists, consider synchronised cardioversion. In the conscious patient this will require anaesthesia.

Rapid narrow-complex tachycardia with no pulse

Rarely, a very rapid (usually > 250 min⁻¹) narrow-complex tachycardia can impair cardiac output to such an extent that the pulse may be impalpable and consciousness impaired or lost. If the patient is pulseless and unconscious, this situation is pulseless electrical activity (PEA) and you should start CPR. As the arrhythmia is potentially treatable by DC shock, the most appropriate treatment is immediate synchronised cardioversion. This is an exception to the non-shockable branch of the ALS algorithm (Chapter 6).

Irregular narrow-complex tachycardia

An irregular narrow-complex tachycardia is most likely to be AF with a rapid ventricular response or, less commonly, atrial flutter with variable AV conduction. Record a 12-lead ECG to identify the rhythm.

If the patient has life-threatening features and is at risk of deterioration because of the tachyarrhythmia, perform synchronised cardioversion. In the absence of contraindications, start anticoagulation prior to cardioversion, initially with low-molecular-weight heparin or unfractionated heparin (see below), at the earliest opportunity. Do not allow this treatment to delay cardioversion.

If there are no life-threatening features, immediate treatment options include:

- rate control by drug therapy
- rhythm control using drugs to achieve chemical cardioversion
- rhythm control by synchronised cardioversion
- treatment to prevent complications (e.g. anticoagulation).

Obtain expert help to determine the most appropriate treatment for the individual patient. The longer a person remains in AF the greater is the likelihood of atrial thrombus developing. In general, people who have been in AF for > 48 h should not be treated by cardioversion (electrical or chemical) until they have been fully anticoagulated for at least 3 weeks, or unless trans-oesophageal echocardiography has detected no evidence of atrial thrombus.

If the clinical situation dictates that cardioversion is needed more urgently, give either low- molecular-weight heparin in therapeutic dose or an intravenous bolus injection of unfractionated heparin followed by a continuous infusion to maintain the activated partial thromboplastin time (APTT) at 1.5–2 times the reference control value. Continue heparin therapy and commence oral anticoagulation after successful cardioversion. Seek expert advice on the duration of anticoagulation, which should be a minimum of 4 weeks, often substantially longer.

If the aim is to control heart rate, the usual drug of choice is a beta-blocker. Diltiazem may be used in patients in whom beta-blockade is contraindicated or not tolerated; however, in the UK it is available only as an oral formulation. Digoxin may be used in patients with heart failure but takes longer than beta-blockers to act.

Amiodarone may also be used for rate control and can also be used to attempt chemical cardioversion (see below). Magnesium is also used for rate control but the data supporting this are limited. When possible, seek expert help in selecting the best choice of treatment for rate control in each individual patient.

If the duration of AF is < 48 h and rhythm control is considered the appropriate strategy, chemical cardioversion may be appropriate. Seek expert help with the use of drugs such as propafenone or flecainide. Do not use propafenone or flecainide in the presence of heart failure, left ventricular impairment or ischaemic heart disease, or a prolonged QT interval. Amiodarone (300 mg intravenously over 20–60 min followed by 900 mg over 24 h) may be used to attempt chemical cardioversion but is less often effective and takes longer to act. Electrical cardioversion remains an option in this setting and will restore sinus rhythm in more patients than chemical cardioversion.

Seek expert help if a patient (with known or previously undiagnosed WPW syndrome) presents with pre-excited AF. Avoid using adenosine, diltiazem, verapamil, or digoxin in patients with pre-excited AF or atrial flutter as these drugs block the AV node and may cause a relative increase in pre-excitation.

Bradyarrhythmia

Bradycardia is defined as a resting heart rate of < 60 min^{-1}. It may be:

- physiological (e.g. in athletes or during sleep)
- cardiac in origin (e.g. atrioventricular block or sinus node disease)
- non-cardiac in origin (e.g. vasovagal, hypothermia, hypothyroidism, hyperkalaemia)
- drug-induced (e.g. beta-blockade, diltiazem, digoxin, amiodarone).

Assess a patient with bradycardia using the ABCDE approach. Consider the possible cause of the bradycardia and look for adverse signs (Figure 11.2). Treat any reversible causes of bradycardia identified in the initial assessment.

If the patient has life-threatening features

If adverse features are present start to treat the bradycardia. Initial treatment is usually pharmacological. Pacing is used for people in whom initial pharmacological treatment is ineffective or inadequate and those at risk of asystole.

Pharmacological treatment for bradycardia

If adverse features are present give atropine 500 mcg IV and, if necessary, repeat every 3–5 min to a total of 3 mg. Doses of atropine of < 500 mcg can cause paradoxical slowing of the heart rate. In healthy volunteers a dose of 3 mg produces the maximum achievable increase in resting heart rate. Use atropine cautiously in the presence of acute myocardial ischaemia or myocardial infarction; the resulting increase in heart rate may worsen ischaemia or increase the size of the infarct.

If bradycardia with adverse signs persists despite atropine, consider cardiac pacing. If pacing cannot be achieved promptly, consider the use of second-line drugs. Seek expert help to select the most appropriate choice.

In some clinical settings second-line drugs may be appropriate before the use of cardiac pacing. For example, consider giving intravenous glucagon if a beta-blocker or calcium channel blocker is a likely cause of the bradycardia. Consider using digoxin-specific antibody fragments for bradycardia caused by digoxin toxicity.

Consider using aminophylline (100–200 mg by slow IV injection) for bradycardia complicating acute inferior wall myocardial infarction, spinal cord injury or cardiac transplantation. Do not give atropine to patients with cardiac transplants. Their hearts are denervated and will not respond to vagal blockade by atropine, which may cause paradoxical sinus arrest or high-grade AV block.

Other options for second-line drug therapy include infusion of isoprenaline (starting dose 5 mcg min^{-1}), adrenaline (2–10 mcg min^{-1}), or dopamine (2.5–10 mcg kg^{-1} min^{-1}).

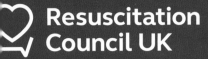

Adult bradycardia

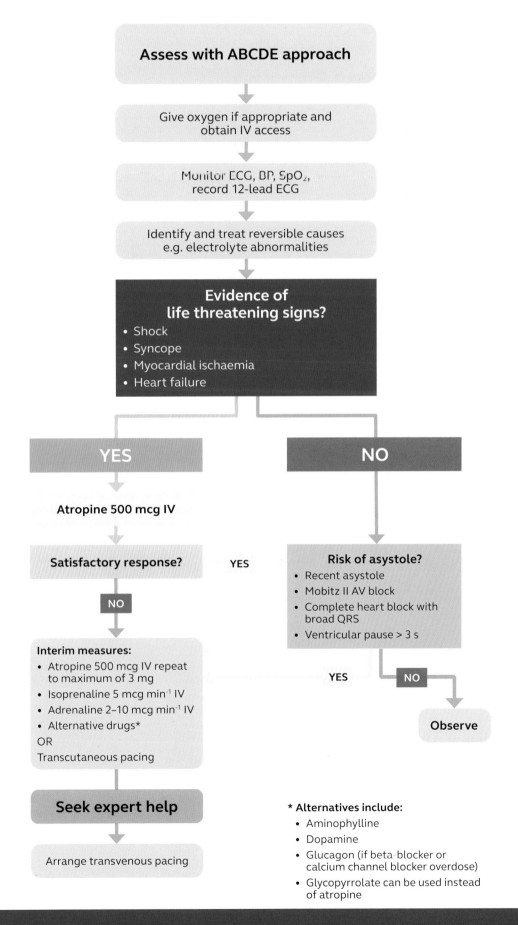

Assess with ABCDE approach

Give oxygen if appropriate and
obtain IV access

Monitor ECG, BP, SpO₂,
record 12-lead ECG

Identify and treat reversible causes
e.g. electrolyte abnormalities

**Evidence of
life threatening signs?**

- Shock
- Syncope
- Myocardial ischaemia
- Heart failure

YES

NO

Atropine 500 mcg IV

Satisfactory response?   YES

NO

Interim measures:
- Atropine 500 mcg IV repeat
  to maximum of 3 mg
- Isoprenaline 5 mcg min⁻¹ IV
- Adrenaline 2–10 mcg min⁻¹ IV
- Alternative drugs*
OR
Transcutaneous pacing

Seek expert help

Arrange transvenous pacing

Risk of asystole?
- Recent asystole
- Mobitz II AV block
- Complete heart block with
  broad QRS
- Ventricular pause > 3 s

YES   **NO**

Observe

* Alternatives include:
- Aminophylline
- Dopamine
- Glucagon (if beta-blocker or
  calcium channel blocker overdose)
- Glycopyrrolate can be used instead
  of atropine

Cardiac pacing for bradycardia

For a patient with bradycardia and adverse features, if there is no response to atropine or if atropine is contraindicated, initiate transcutaneous pacing immediately (Chapter 10).

In the presence of life-threatening, extreme bradycardia use percussion pacing as an interim measure until transcutaneous pacing is achieved. Give repeated rhythmic thumps with the side of a closed fist over the left lower edge of the sternum at a rate of 50–70 min⁻¹ to try to stimulate the heart with each thump.

Transcutaneous pacing can be painful and may fail to achieve effective electrical 'capture' (i.e. a QRS complex after each pacing stimulus) or fail to achieve a mechanical response (i.e. palpable pulse). Check for electrical capture on the monitor or ECG and, when achieved, check whether it is producing a pulse.

A B C D E

Reassess the patient's condition (ABCDE).

Use analgesia and sedation as necessary to control pain and distress. Remember that sedation may compromise respiratory effort, so continue to reassess the patient at frequent intervals. Attempt to identify the cause of the bradyarrhythmia.

Seek expert help to assess the need for temporary transvenous pacing and to initiate this when appropriate. Consider temporary transvenous pacing (or early permanent pacemaker implantation as appropriate) if there is documented recent asystole (ventricular standstill of > 3 s), Mobitz type II AV block, or complete CHB AV block (especially with broad QRS or initial heart rate < 40 min⁻¹).

If the patient has NO life-threatening features

For a patient with bradycardia who has no life-threatening features and no high risk of progression to asystole, do not initiate immediate treatment. Continue to monitor the patient and assess them to identify the cause of the bradycardia. If the cause is physiological or easily reversible (e.g. by stopping suppressant drug therapy) no further treatment may be needed. Seek expert help with further assessment and treatment of people with other causes of bradycardia.

11: Summary learning

Arrhythmias occurring after resuscitation from cardiac arrest and ROSC may need treatment to stabilise the patient and prevent recurrence of cardiac arrest.

In other settings some arrhythmias require prompt treatment to prevent deterioration (including progression to cardiac arrest) and others do not require immediate treatment.

The urgency for treatment and the best choice of immediate treatment is determined by the condition of the patient (presence or absence of life-threatening features) and by the nature and cause of the arrhythmia.

Assessment of a patient with an arrhythmia should follow the ABCDE approach.

Whenever possible the arrhythmia should be documented on a 12-lead ECG.

My key take-home messages from this chapter are:

Further reading

Brugada J, Katritsis DG, Arbelo E, et al. 2019 ESC Guidelines for the management of patients with supraventricular tachycardia. The Task Force for the management of patients with supraventricular tachycardia of the European Society of Cardiology (ESC). Eur Heart J 2020;41:655-720.

Kusumoto FM, Schoenfeld MH, Barrett C, et al. 2018 ACC/AHA/ HRS Guideline on the Evaluation and Management of Patients With Bradycardia and Cardiac Conduction Delay: A Report of the American College of Cardiology/American Heart Association Task Force on Clinical Practice Guidelines and the Heart Rhythm Society. J Am Coll Cardiol 2019;74:e51-e156.

Hindricks G, Potpara T, Dagres N, et al. 2020 ESC Guidelines for the diagnosis and management of atrial fibrillation developed in collaboration with the European Association of Cardio-Thoracic Surgery (EACTS). Eur Heart J 2020.

Soar J, Böttiger BW, Carli P, Couper K, Deakin CD, Djärv T, Lott C, Olasveengen TM, Paal P, Pellis T, Perkins GD, Sandroni C, Nolan JP. European Resuscitation Council Guidelines 2021: Advanced Life Support. Resuscitation. 2021;161.

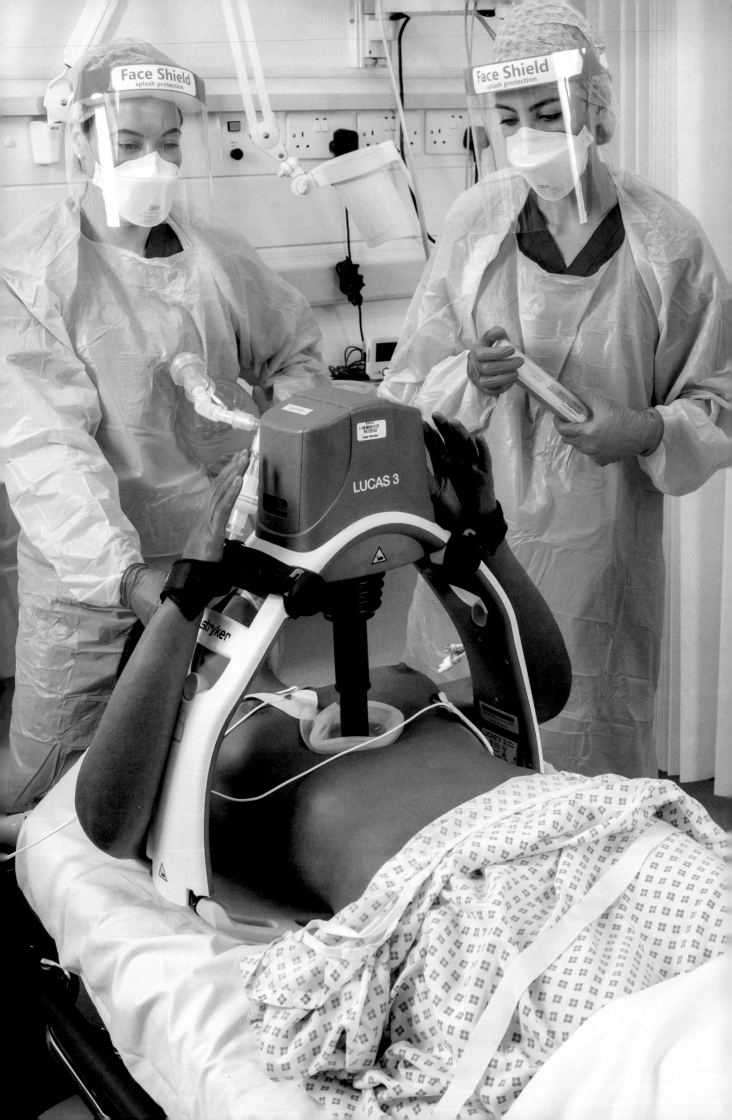

Resuscitation in special circumstances

In this chapter

Life-threatening electrolyte disorders

Dialysis

Sepsis

Toxins (poisoning)

Hypoxia

Asthma

Anaphylaxis

Pregnancy

Traumatic cardiorespiratory arrest

Perioperative cardiac arrest (including after cardiac surgery)

Drowning

Accidental hypothermia

Hyperthermia

Obesity

The learning outcomes will enable you to:

Use the ABCDE approach for early recognition and treatment to prevent cardiac arrest

Consider the modifications required before and after cardiac arrest in special circumstances

Introduction

Resuscitation needs to be modified in specific circumstances. Early recognition of signs and symptoms and effective treatment will often prevent cardiac arrest.

These conditions account for a large proportion of cardiac arrests in younger patients with no co-existing disease. It is essential to ask for expert help early for most of these conditions because they can require specialist interventions.

A B C D E

Survival in all these conditions still relies on using the ABCDE approach to help prevent cardiac arrest. If cardiac arrest does occur, high-quality CPR with minimal interruption and treatment of reversible causes are still the most important interventions.

When cardiac arrest occurs, ALS may require tailoring according to the specific circumstances and need to treat an underlying cause, including the need for a prolonged resuscitation attempt. In those settings where it is feasible, extracorporeal support with veno-arterial extracorporeal membrane oxygenation (VA-ECMO) should be considered for selected patients when standard ALS measures are failing.

Life-threatening electrolyte disorders

Electrolyte abnormalities can cause cardiac arrhythmias or cardiorespiratory arrest. Life-threatening arrhythmias are most commonly associated with potassium disorders, particularly hyperkalaemia, and less commonly with disorders of serum calcium and magnesium.

Consider starting treatment in life-threatening electrolyte disorders before laboratory results are available. Electrolyte values for definitions are quoted as a guide to clinical decision-making. The precise values that trigger treatment decisions will depend on the patient's clinical condition and rate of change of electrolyte values.

Prevention of electrolyte disorders

Treat life-threatening electrolyte abnormalities before cardiac arrest occurs.

Remove precipitating factors (e.g. drugs, diet) and monitor electrolyte concentrations to prevent recurrence of the abnormality.

Monitor renal function in patients at risk of electrolyte disorders (e.g. patients with acute and chronic kidney disease, heart failure) and avoid combinations of drugs that may exacerbate electrolyte disorders.

Review renal replacement therapy (e.g. haemodialysis) regularly to avoid inappropriate electrolyte shifts during treatment.

Potassium disorders

Potassium homeostasis

Extracellular potassium concentration is tightly regulated between 3.5–5.0 mmol L^{-1}. A large concentration gradient normally exists between intracellular and extracellular fluid compartments. This potassium gradient across cell membranes contributes to the excitability of nerve and muscle cells, including the myocardium. Evaluation of serum potassium must take into consideration the effects of changes in serum pH. When serum pH decreases (acidaemia), serum potassium increases because potassium shifts from the cellular to the vascular space; a process that is reversed when serum pH increases (alkalaemia). Anticipate the effects of pH changes on serum potassium during therapy for hyperkalaemia or hypokalaemia.

Hyperkalaemia

Hyperkalaemia is the most common electrolyte disorder associated with cardiac arrest and occurs in up to 10% of hospitalised patients. Acute hyperkalaemia is more likely than chronic hyperkalaemia to cause life-threatening cardiac arrhythmias or cardiac arrest. Hyperkalaemia is usually caused by increased potassium release from cells or impaired excretion by the kidneys.

Definition of hyperkalaemia

There is no universal definition. We have defined hyperkalaemia as a serum potassium concentration > 5.5 mmol L^{-1}; in practice, hyperkalaemia is a continuum. As the potassium concentration increases above 5.5 mmol L^{-1}, the risk of adverse events increases and the need for urgent treatment increases. Severe hyperkalaemia has been defined as a serum potassium concentration > 6.5 mmol L^{-1}.

Causes of hyperkalaemia

The main causes of hyperkalaemia are:

- **Renal failure** (i.e. acute kidney injury or chronic kidney disease).
- **Drugs** (e.g. angiotensin converting enzyme inhibitors (ACE-I), angiotensin II receptor antagonists (ARB), potassium sparing diuretics, non-steroidal anti-inflammatory drugs, beta-blockers, trimethoprim).
- **Tissue breakdown** (e.g. rhabdomyolysis, tumour lysis, haemolysis).
- **Metabolic acidosis** (e.g. renal failure, diabetic ketoacidosis).
- **Endocrine disorders** (e.g. Addison's disease).
- **Diet** (may be sole cause in patients with advanced chronic kidney disease).
- **Spurious** – pseudo-hyperkalaemia describes the finding of a raised serum (clotted blood) potassium value, when the actual value in plasma (non-clotted blood) is normal. The clotting process releases potassium from cells and platelets. The most common cause is a prolonged transit time to the laboratory or poor storage conditions.

The risk of hyperkalaemia is even greater when there is a combination of factors.

Recognition of hyperkalaemia

Exclude hyperkalaemia in all patients with an arrhythmia or cardiac arrest. Patients can present with weakness progressing to flaccid paralysis, paraesthesia, or depressed deep tendon reflexes. Most patients will have ECG abnormalities at a serum potassium concentration > 6.7 mmol L^{-1}. The use of a blood gas analyser that measures potassium helps reduce delays in recognition. The effect of hyperkalaemia on the ECG depends on the absolute serum potassium concentration as well as the rate of increase (Figure 12.1).

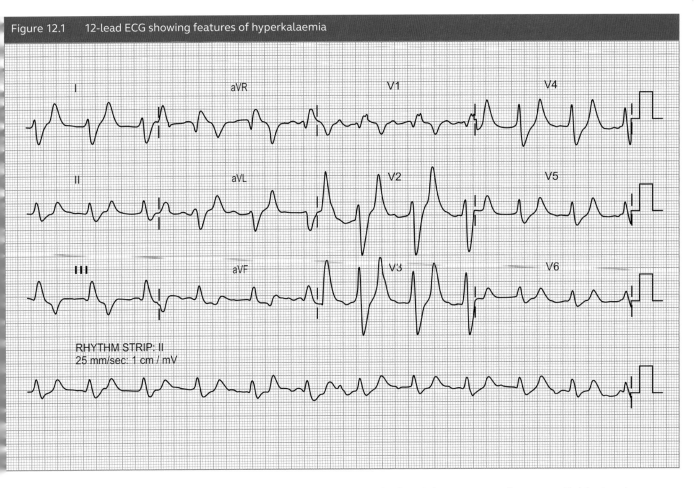

Figure 12.1   12-lead ECG showing features of hyperkalaemia

ECG changes with hyperkalaemia are usually progressive and include:

- first degree heart block (prolonged PR interval > 0.2 s)
- flattened or absent P waves
- tall, peaked (tented) T waves (i.e. T wave larger than R wave in more than one lead)
- ST-segment depression
- S and T wave merging (sine wave pattern)
- widened QRS (> 0.12 s)
- ventricular tachycardia
- bradycardia.

Cardiac arrest may occur with any presenting rhythm (PEA, ventricular fibrillation/pulseless ventricular tachycardia (VF/pVT), asystole).

Treatment of hyperkalaemia

The five key steps in treating hyperkalaemia are:

1. cardiac protection
2. shifting potassium into cells
3. removing potassium from the body
4. monitoring serum potassium and glucose concentration
5. prevention of recurrence.

When hyperkalaemia is strongly suspected (e.g. in the presence of ECG changes), start life-saving treatment even before laboratory results are available. Involve expert help from renal or intensive care teams at an early stage, especially for those patients who might require renal replacement therapy (e.g. haemodialysis).

The main risks associated with the treatment of hyperkalaemia are:

- Hypoglycaemia following insulin-glucose administration (usually occurs within three hours of treatment, but may occur up to six hours after the infusion ends). Monitor blood glucose and treat hypoglycaemia promptly.
- Tissue necrosis secondary to extravasation of intravenous calcium salts. Ensure secure vascular access prior to administration.
- Rebound hyperkalaemia after the effect of drug treatment has worn off (i.e. within 4–6 h). Continue to monitor serum potassium for a minimum of 24 h after an episode.

Patient not in cardiac arrest

Assess patient:

- use the ABCDE approach and correct any abnormalities, obtain IV access
- check serum potassium
- record a 12-lead ECG.

Treatment is determined according to severity of hyperkalaemia. Approximate values are provided to guide treatment.

Mild elevation (5.5–5.9 mmol L^{-1}):

- Address cause of hyperkalaemia to correct and avoid further rise in serum potassium (e.g. drugs, diet).

- If treatment is indicated, remove potassium from the body: potassium binders or cation-exchange resins e.g. calcium resonium 15–30 g, or sodium polystyrene sulfonate 15–30 g given either orally or by retention enema (onset in > 4 h). These options are only for short term use.

Moderate elevation (6.0–6.4 mmol L^{-1}) without ECG changes:

Shift potassium intracellularly with glucose/insulin: 10 units short-acting insulin and 25 g glucose IV over 15–30 min (onset in 15–30 min; maximal effect at 30–60 min; duration of action 4–6 h; monitor blood glucose). Follow up with 10% glucose infusion at 50 mL h^{-1} for 5 h in patients with a pre-treatment blood glucose < 7 mmol L^{-1}. Remove potassium from the body (see above; consider dialysis guided by clinical setting).

Severe elevation (≥ 6.5 mmol L^{-1}) without ECG changes:

- seek expert help

- give glucose/insulin (see above)

- give salbutamol 10–20 mg nebulised (onset in 15–30 min; duration of action 4–6 h)

- remove potassium from the body. Consider dialysis, sodium zirconium cyclosilicate (SZC, e.g. 5-10 g three times daily for up to 72 h) and/or patiromer

- consider commencement of continuous cardiac monitoring.

Severe elevation (≥ 6.5 mmol L^{-1}) with toxic ECG changes:

- Seek expert help.

- Protect the heart with calcium salts: 6.8 mmol Ca^{2+} via 10 mL 10% calcium chloride IV over 2–5 min (6.8 mmol Ca^{2+} /10 mL) or 30 mL 10% calcium gluconate over 15 min (2.26 mmol Ca^{2+} / 10 mL) to antagonise the toxic effects of hyperkalaemia at the myocardial cell membrane. This protects the heart by reducing the risk of VF/pVT but does not lower serum potassium (onset in 1–3 min).

- Use shifting agents (glucose/insulin and salbutamol).

- Remove potassium from the body (see above; consider dialysis at outset or if refractory to medical treatment).

- Start continuous cardiac monitoring. If hyperkalaemia persists or ECG appearances are not improved further IV calcium administration may be required.

Modifications to cardiopulmonary resuscitation associated with hyperkalaemia

The following modifications to standard ALS guidelines are recommended in the presence of severe hyperkalaemia during CPR:

- Confirm hyperkalaemia using a blood gas analyser if available.

- Protect the heart: give 10 mL calcium chloride 10% IV by rapid bolus injection. Consider repeating dose if cardiac arrest is prolonged or refractory.

- Shift potassium into cells: give glucose/insulin: 10 units short-acting insulin and 25 g glucose IV by rapid injection. Monitor blood glucose.

- Give sodium bicarbonate: 50 mmol (50 mL of 8.4% solution) IV by rapid injection (if severe acidosis or renal failure). Avoid mixing with calcium chloride as may cause a precipitate.

- Remove potassium from body: consider dialysis for hyperkalaemic cardiac arrest resistant to medical treatment. Several dialysis modalities have been used safely and effectively in cardiac arrest, but this may only be available in specialist centres. Consider the use of a mechanical chest compression device if prolonged CPR is needed.

Hypokalaemia

Hypokalaemia is the most common electrolyte disorder in clinical practice. It is seen in up to 20% of hospitalised patients. Hypokalaemia increases the incidence of arrhythmias and sudden cardiac death (SCD). The risk is increased further in patients with pre-existing heart disease and in those treated with digoxin.

Definition of hypokaleamia

Hypokalaemia is defined as a serum potassium level < 3.5 mmol L^{-1}. Severe hypokalaemia is defined as a serum potassium level < 2.5 mmol L^{-1} and may be associated with symptoms.

Causes of hypokalaemia

The main causes of hypokalaemia include:

- gastrointestinal loss (e.g. diarrhoea)

- drugs (e.g. diuretics, laxatives, steroids)

- renal losses (e.g. renal tubular disorders, diabetes insipidus, dialysis)

- endocrine disorders (e.g. Cushing's syndrome, hyperaldosteronism)

- metabolic alkalosis

- magnesium depletion

- poor dietary intake.

Treatment strategies used for hyperkalaemia may also induce hypokalaemia.

Table 12.1   Calcium and magnesium disorders

Disorder	Causes	Presentation	ECG	Treatment
Hypercalcaemia Total Calcium* > 2.6 mmol L⁻¹	Primary or tertiary hyperparathyroidism	Confusion	Short QT interval	Fluid replacement IV Furosemide 1 mg kg⁻¹ IV Hydrocortisone 200–300 mg IV Pamidronate 30–90 mg IV Treat underlying cause
	Malignancy	Weakness	Prolonged QRS Interval	
	Sarcoidosis	Abdominal pain	Flat T waves	
	Drugs	Hypotension	AV block	
		Arrhythmias	Cardiac arrest	
		Cardiac arrest		
Hypocalcaemia Total Calcium* < 2.1 mmol L⁻¹	Chronic renal failure	Paraesthesia	Prolonged QT interval	Calcium chloride 10% 10–40 mL IV 1–2 g 50% Magnesium sulfate (2–4 mL: 4–8 mmol) IV if necessary
	Acute pancreatitis	Tetany	T wave inversion	
	Calcium channel blocker overdose	Seizures	Heart block	
	Toxic shock syndrome	AV- block	Cardiac arrest	
	Rhabdomyolysis	Cardiac arrest		
	Tumour lysis syndrome			
Hypermagnesaemia Magnesium > 1.1 mmol L⁻¹	Renal failure	Confusion	Prolonged PR and QT intervals	Consider treatment when magnesium > 1.75 mmol L⁻¹ Calcium chloride 10% 5–10 mL IV repeated if necessary Ventilatory support if necessary Saline diuresis – 0.9% saline with furosemide 1 mg kg⁻¹ IV Haemodialysis
	Iatrogenic	Weakness	T wave peaking	
		Respiratory depression	AV block	
		AV-block	Cardiac arrest	
		Cardiac arrest		
Hypomagnesaemia Magnesium < 0.6 mmol L⁻¹	GI loss	Tremor	Prolonged PR and QT Intervals	Severe or symptomatic: 2 g 50% magnesium sulfate (4 mL; 8 mmol) IV over 15 min Torsade de pointes: 2 g 50% magnesium sulfate (4 mL; 8 mmol) IV over 1–2 min Seizure: 2 g 50% magnesium sulfate (4 mL; 8 mmol) IV over 10 min
	Polyuria	Ataxia	ST-segment depression	
	Starvation	Nystagmus	T wave inversion	
	Alcoholism	Seizures	Flattened P waves	
	Malabsorption	Arrhythmias – torsade de pointes	Increased QRS duration	
		Cardiac arrest	Torsade de pointes	

* A normal total calcium is about 2.2–2.6 mmol L⁻¹. A normal ionised calcium is about 1.1–1.3 mmol L⁻¹. Interpret calcium values cautiously. Seek expert help if not sure. Total calcium depends on serum albumin values and will need to be corrected for low albumin values (corrected total calcium). Ionised calcium values are often measured by blood gas machines. Do not confuse ionised calcium, total calcium, and corrected calcium values.

Recognition of hypokalaemia

Exclude hypokalaemia in every patient with an arrhythmia or cardiac arrest. In dialysis patients, hypokalaemia may occur at the end of a haemodialysis session or during treatment with peritoneal dialysis.

As serum potassium concentration decreases, the nerves and muscles are predominantly affected, causing fatigue, weakness, leg cramps, constipation. In severe cases (serum potassium < 2.5 mmol L⁻¹), rhabdomyolysis, ascending paralysis and respiratory difficulties may occur.

ECG features of hypokalaemia are:

* U waves
* T wave flattening
* ST-segment changes
* arrhythmias, especially if patient is taking digoxin.

Cardiac arrest may occur with any presenting rhythm (PEA, VF/pVT, asystole).

Treatment of hypokaleamia

This depends on the severity of hypokalaemia and the presence of symptoms and ECG abnormalities. Gradual replacement of potassium is preferable, but in an emergency, IV potassium is required. The maximum recommended IV dose of potassium is 20 mmol h⁻¹, but more rapid infusion (e.g. 2 mmol min⁻¹ for 10 min, followed by 10 mmol over 5–10 min) is indicated for unstable arrhythmias when cardiac arrest is imminent.

Continuous ECG monitoring is essential during IV infusion and the dose should be titrated after repeated sampling of serum potassium levels. Rapid replacement of potassium should be conducted via central venous access when available.

Many patients who are potassium deficient are also deficient in magnesium. Magnesium is important for potassium uptake and for the maintenance of intracellular potassium values, particularly in the myocardium. Repletion of magnesium stores will facilitate more rapid correction of hypokalaemia and is recommended in severe cases of hypokalaemia.

Calcium and magnesium disorders

The recognition and management of calcium and magnesium disorders is summarised in Table 12.1.

Dialysis

Patients receiving long-term haemodialysis are a high-risk group for out-of-hospital cardiac arrest, occurring up to 20 times more frequently than in the general population. Arrests on a dialysis unit are predominantly witnessed, and most occur during treatment. Risk factors include electrolyte disturbances, fluid volume shifts, and medical co-morbidities. Risks of cardiac arrest can be minimised by ensuring patients adhere to dietary and fluid restrictions, and that dialysis prescriptions are carefully managed. Survival-to-discharge after an arrest in a dialysis unit is comparable to arrests in other hospital areas.

Resuscitation should follow the standard ALS algorithm with the following modifications.

- Assign a trained dialysis nurse to operate the haemodialysis (HD) machine.
- Stop dialysis and return the patient's blood volume with a fluid bolus.
- Disconnect from the dialysis machine (unless defibrillation-proof) in accordance with the International Electrotechnical Committee (IEC) standards.
- Leave dialysis access open to use for drug administration.
- Dialysis may be required in the early post-resuscitation period.
- Provide prompt management of hyperkalaemia.
- Avoid excessive potassium and volume shifts during dialysis.

Sepsis

Sepsis is a common cause of acute deterioration and accounts for 48 000 deaths annually in the United Kingdom. Consider sepsis in any deteriorating patient who has clinical suspicion of infection. Cardiorespiratory arrest associated with sepsis has a poor survival rate. Early recognition and treatment of sepsis is key to improving outcomes and preventing cardiac arrest.

Definition of sepsis

Sepsis is life-threatening organ dysfunction caused by a dysregulated host response to infection: common sources include the chest, abdomen, urinary tract, skin and soft tissues. Sepsis is differentiated from the appropriate and normal (homeostatic) response of the body to pathogens by new or progressive organ failure which may be quantified by the Sequential Organ Failure Assessment (SOFA) score. A SOFA score ≥ 2 reflects an overall mortality risk of ~10% in a hospital patient.
Septic shock (sepsis requiring vasopressors to maintain a MAP ≥ 65 mmHg and a serum lactate > 2 mmol L^{-1} despite adequate fluid resuscitation) has a 40% mortality.

Treatment of sepsis

Supportive care based on the ABCDE approach while controlling the source of infection is critical to prevent shock, multiple-organ failure and cardiorespiratory arrest. Once immediately life-threatening problems have been addressed, initial resuscitation in patients with sepsis is covered by the Surviving Sepsis Campaign guidelines (https://www.sccm.org/SurvivingSepsisCampaign/Home) and in NICE Guideline 51 (https://www.nice.org.uk/guidance/ng51).

Escalation of treatment

Timely achievement of the 'Hour 1' care bundle following recognition of sepsis will frequently be sufficient to prevent organ dysfunction. Ask for senior assistance urgently at any time life is clearly immediately threatened, or if any of the following persist after initial appropriate fluid resuscitation:

- hypotension
- oliguria
- acute confusion
- lactate > 2 mmol L^{-1}.

Cardiac arrest and sepsis

Treat cardiac arrest in a patient with sepsis or suspected sepsis according to standard ALS guidelines. Correct hypoxia and hypovolaemia, and look for other potentially reversible causes using the 4 Hs and 4Ts approach.

HOUR 1 CARE BUNDLE

Action 1: Give high-flow oxygen

Hypotension, disordered capillary beds, and microthrombi compromise oxygen delivery to tissues. Give high flow oxygen via non-rebreather mask with resevoir during initial resuscitation and consider tracheal intubation in patients with signs of fatigue or severe cardiorespiratory compromise. Once reliable SpO_2 monitoring is in place, aim for a SpO_2 of 94–98%.

Action 2: Take blood cultures

Send at least one set of blood cultures and any other fluid/tissue samples to identify the source of infection (e.g. sputum) before starting antibiotic therapy. If a presumed source of infection is amenable to control (e.g. removal of an infected cannula or abscess drainage). Source control is an essential part of initial sepsis management.

Action 3: Give broad-spectrum antibiotics

Give appropriate intravenous antibiotics as soon as possible, and always within the first hour, according to local prescribing guidelines. Delays in giving antibiotics are directly linked to poor outcome.

Action 4: Initiate fluid resuscitation

Circulatory shock, resulting from a combination of vasodilatation and hypovolaemia (due to leaky capillaries), is the most common form of organ dysfunction in sepsis. Give fluid challenges in divided boluses of 250–500 mL of crystalloid to a maximum volume of 30 mL kg^{-1} body weight in patients with hypotension, serum lactate > 2 mmol L^{-1}, or other signs of circulatory dysfunction such as low urine output. If the mean arterial pressure is < 65 mmHg despite repeated fluid challenges treatment escalation and starting vasopressor therapy should be considered early.

Action 5: Measure lactate

Lactic acid is a product of anaerobic metabolism. While elevated lactate is not specific to sepsis, it does indicate circulatory compromise and can be used to predict outcome. An initially high lactate which decreases with fluid challenges can be used to guide ongoing resuscitation.

Action 6: Measure urine output

Accurate hourly measurement of urine output can therefore guide further fluid challenges and the need for critical care input.

Toxins (poisoning)

Poisoning is an infrequent cause of cardiac arrest, but remains a leading cause in those younger than 40 years. It is also a common cause of non-traumatic coma in this age group. Self-poisoning with therapeutic or recreational drugs is the main reason for hospital admission. Drug toxicity can also be caused by inappropriate dosing and drug interactions. Accidental poisoning is commonest in children.Homicidal poisoning is uncommon. Industrial accidents, warfare or terrorism may cause chemical, biological, radiological or nuclear (CBRN) exposure.

Prevention of cardiac arrest

Assess and treat the patient using the ABCDE approach. Airway obstruction and respiratory arrest secondary to a decreased conscious level is a common cause of death after self-poisoning (benzodiazepines, alcohol, opioids, tricyclics, barbiturates). Early tracheal intubation of unconscious patients by trained personnel can decrease the risk of aspiration. Drug-induced hypotension usually responds to IV fluids, but occasionally vasopressor support (e.g. noradrenaline infusion) is required. Hypertensive emergencies may be managed with benzodiazepines, vasodilators and alpha antagonists. Measure electrolytes (particularly potassium), blood glucose and arterial blood gases. Retain samples of blood and urine for analysis. Patients with severe poisoning should be cared for in a critical care setting.

Modifications to resuscitation

- Ensure your personal safety and wear appropriate personal protective equipment (PPE).
- Avoid mouth-to-mouth rescue breaths in the presence of chemicals such as cyanide, hydrogen sulphide, corrosives and organophosphates.
- Treat life-threatening tachyarrhythmias with cardioversion, according to the peri-arrest arrhythmia guidelines (Chapter 11). This includes correction of electrolyte, glucose and acid-base abnormalities.
- Once resuscitation has started, try to identify the toxin(s). Relatives, friends and ambulance crews can provide useful information. Examination of the patient may reveal diagnostic clues such as odours, needle marks, pupil size, and signs of corrosion in the mouth. These may align with known syndromes caused by specific toxins to narrow the differential diagnosis.
- Measure the patient's temperature because hypo- or hyperthermia can occur after drug overdose.
- Provide standard basic and advanced life support if cardiac arrest occurs.
- Be prepared to continue resuscitation for a prolonged period, particularly in young patients, as the poison

may be metabolised or excreted during extended resuscitation measures. Consider extracorporeal life support (ECLS).

- There is an increase in the use of new 'designer drugs' that can have actions similar to stimulants or depressants. In addition to supportive and symptomatic treatment expert advice will be required. Remember that multiple toxins may have been ingested.

- Consult a regional or national poisons centre for information on treatment of the poisoned patient. In the UK, specialist advice about specific poisons can be obtained by accessing TOXBASE® (www.toxbase.org).

Specific treatments

There are few specific therapies for poisons that are useful immediately. The emphasis is on intensive supportive therapy using the ABCDE approach, with correction of hypoxia, hypotension, acid/base, and electrolyte disorders.

Therapies include decontamination, limiting absorption of ingested poisons, enhancing elimination, or the use of specific antidotes. Seek advice from a poisons centre for up-to-date guidance for severe or uncommon poisonings.

- For skin exposures, initial management consists of removing clothes.

- Routine use of gastric lavage for gastrointestinal decontamination is not recommended.

- Activated charcoal adsorbs certain drugs. Its efficacy decreases over time following ingestion. There is little evidence that treatment with activated charcoal improves clinical outcome. Consider giving a single dose of activated charcoal to patients who have ingested a potentially toxic amount of a poison known to be adsorbed by activated charcoal, up to one hour previously. Give only to patients with an intact or protected airway. Multiple doses may be beneficial in life-threatening poisoning with carbemazepine, dapsone, phenobarbital, quinine and theophylline.

- Whole-bowel irrigation can reduce drug absorption by cleansing the gastro-intestinal tract using enteral administration of a polyethylene glycol solution. Consider in potentially toxic ingestion of sustained release or enteric-coated drugs, oral iron poisoning, and the removal of ingested packets of illicit drugs.

- Laxatives (cathartics) or emetics (e.g. ipecacuanha) have no role in the management of the acutely poisoned patient and are not recommended.

- Urine alkalinisation (urine pH > 7.5) by giving IV sodium bicarbonate can be useful in moderate to severe salicylate poisoning in patients who do not need haemodialysis.

- Haemodialysis removes drugs or metabolites with low molecular weight, low protein binding, small volumes of distribution and high water solubility.

- Specific antidotes should be employed in the appropriate clinical context when poisoning occurs with a known (or highly suspected) toxin'.

Specific antidotes

Opioid poisoning

Opioid poisoning causes respiratory depression, pinpoint pupils and coma followed by respiratory arrest. The opioid antagonist naloxone rapidly reverses these effects.

The route for giving naloxone depends on the skills of the rescuer: intravenous (IV), intramuscular (IM), subcutaneous (SC), and intranasal (IN) routes can be used. The non-IV routes may be quicker because time is saved in not having to establish IV access, which can be extremely difficult in an IV drug user. The initial doses of naloxone are 400 mcg IV, 800 mcg IM, 800 mcg SC or 2 mg IN. Large opioid overdoses require titration to a total naloxone dose of 10 mg. The duration of action of naloxone is 45–70 min, but respiratory depression may persist for 4–5 h after opioid overdose. Thus, the clinical effects of naloxone may not last as long as those of a significant opioid overdose.

Give increments of naloxone until the patient is breathing adequately and has protective airway reflexes. Consider the need for an ongoing infusion of naloxone if the respiratory rate is not maintained and long-acting opioid preparations have been ingested.

Acute withdrawal from opioids produces a state of sympathetic excess and can cause complications such as pulmonary oedema, ventricular arrhythmia, and severe agitation. Use naloxone reversal of opioid intoxication with caution in patients suspected of opioid dependence.

Cardiac arrest is usually secondary to a respiratory arrest and associated with severe brain hypoxia. Prognosis is poor. Once cardiac arrest has occurred, follow standard resuscitation guidelines.

Benzodiazepines

Overdose of benzodiazepines can cause loss of consciousness, respiratory depression and hypotension. Flumazenil, a competitive antagonist of benzodiazepines can be used to reverse sedation caused by benzodiazepines when there is no history or risk of seizures. Reversal of benzodiazepine intoxication with flumazenil can cause significant toxicity (seizure, arrhythmia, hypotension, and withdrawal syndrome) in patients with benzodiazepine dependence or co-ingestion of proconvulsant medications such as tricyclic antidepressants. Do not use flumazenil routinely in the comatose patient. There are no specific modifications required for cardiac arrest caused by benzodiazepines.

Figure 12.2   12-lead ECG showing features of severe tricyclic antidepressant toxicity

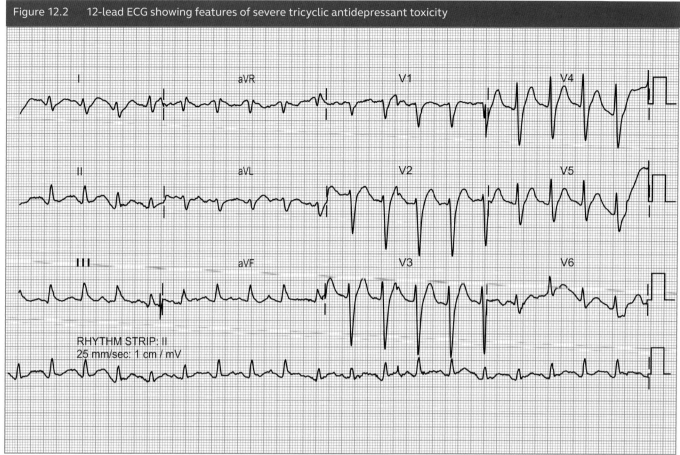

RHYTHM STRIP: II
25 mm/sec: 1 cm / mV

Tricyclic antidepressants

This includes tricyclic and related cyclic drugs (e.g. amitriptyline, desipramine, imipramine, nortriptyline, doxepin, and clomipramine). Self-poisoning with tricyclic antidepressants is common and can cause hypotension, seizures, coma and life-threatening arrhythmias. Cardiac toxicity mediated by anticholinergic and sodium channel-blocking effects can produce a broad-complex tachycardia (VT). Consider tricyclic overdose as a possible diagnosis in any adult presenting with an otherwise unexplained shockable rhythm.

Hypotension is exacerbated by alpha-1 receptor blockade. Anticholinergic effects include dilated pupils, fever, dry skin, delirium, tachycardia, ileus, and urinary retention. Most life-threatening problems occur within the first 6 h after ingestion.

A widening QRS complex and right axis deviation indicates a greater risk of arrhythmias (Figure 12.2). Consider sodium bicarbonate for the treatment of tricyclic-induced ventricular conduction abnormalities. While no study has investigated the optimal target arterial pH with bicarbonate therapy, a pH of 7.45–7.55 is commonly accepted.

Local anaesthetic toxicity

Local anaesthetic toxicity occurs typically in the setting of regional anaesthesia, when a bolus of local anaesthetic inadvertently enters an artery or vein. Systemic toxicity of local anaesthetics involves the central nervous system, and the cardiovascular system. Severe agitation, loss of consciousness, with or without tonic-clonic convulsions,

sinus bradycardia, conduction blocks, asystole and ventricular tachyarrhythmia can all occur. Toxicity can be potentiated in pregnancy, extremes of age, or hypoxaemia.

Follow standard resuscitation measures. In addition, patients with both cardiovascular collapse and cardiac arrest attributable to local anaesthetic toxicity may benefit from treatment with intravenous 20% lipid emulsion in addition to standard advanced life support. Give an initial intravenous bolus of 1.5 mL kg^{-1} 20% lipid emulsion followed by an infusion at 15 mL kg^{-1} h^{-1}. Give up to three bolus doses of lipid at 5 min intervals and continue the infusion until the patient is stable or has received up to a maximum of 12 mL kg^{-1} of lipid emulsion.

Stimulants

Stimulants include cocaine, and amphetamine (and similar drugs). Sympathetic overstimulation caused by these may cause agitation, symptomatic tachycardia, hypertensive crisis, hyperthermia and myocardial ischaemia with angina. Small doses of intravenous benzodiazepines (midazolam, diazepam, lorazepam) are effective first-line drugs. Glyceryl trinitrate and phentolamine can reverse cocaine-induced coronary vasoconstriction. Use nitrates only as second-line therapy for myocardial ischaemia. The evidence for or against the use of beta-blocker drugs, including those beta-blockers with alpha blocking properties (carvedilol and labetalol) is limited. The optimal choice of anti-arrhythmic drug for the treatment tachyarrhythmias is not known. Seek expert advice if chest pain does not settle, recurs or there is evidence suggesting an acute coronary syndrome. If cardiac arrest occurs, follow standard resuscitation guidelines.

Drug-induced severe bradycardia

Severe bradycardia from poisoning or drug overdose may be refractory to standard ALS protocols because of prolonged receptor binding or direct cellular toxicity. Atropine can be life-saving in organophosphate, carbamate or nerve agent poisoning. Give atropine for bradycardia caused by acetylcholinesterase-inhibiting substances. Large (2–4 mg IV) and repeated doses may be required to achieve a clinical effect. Isoprenaline may be useful at high doses in refractory bradycardia induced by beta-receptor blockade. Heart block and ventricular arrhythmias associated with digoxin or digitalis glycoside poisoning may be treated effectively with digoxin-specific antibody fragments.

Vasopressors, inotropes, calcium, glucagon, phosphodiesterase inhibitors and high-dose insulin-glucose-potassium infusions may all be useful in beta-blocker and calcium channel blocker overdose. Transcutaneous pacing may be effective for severe bradycardia caused by poisoning and overdose (Chapters 10 and 11).

Hypoxia

This section addresses common causes of hypoxia which place people at risk of cardiac arrest. Acting quickly, early after the onset of hypoxia is critical for ensuring the best outcomes. Once cardiac arrest has occurred as a consequence of hypoxia, outcomes are generally poor. Causes of hypoxia related cardiac arrest presented in this chapter includes, asthma and drowning. Airway obstruction and foreign body airway obstruction are covered in the airway management chapter.

The general principles for the assessment and treatment of hypoxia focuses on the ABCDE approach.

- Treat the cause of asphyxia / hypoxaemia as the highest priority because this is a potentially reversible cause of cardiac arrest.
- Establish a patent airway using the techniques described in the airways chapter (Chapter 7).
- Effective ventilation with the highest feasible inspired oxygen is a priority in patients with asphyxial cardiac arrest.

Asthma

Worldwide, approximately 340 million people of all ages and ethnic backgrounds have asthma with a high prevalence in some European countries (United Kingdom, Netherlands and Scandinavia). Annual worldwide deaths from asthma have been estimated at 420 000, with 1400 deaths reported in the UK in 2018. A national confidential enquiry in the UK in 2014 showed that most asthma-related deaths occurred before admission to hospital. Good asthma control and prevention of acute asthma is therefore important. The British Thoracic Society (BTS) and Scottish Intercollegiate Guidelines Network (SIGN) have published guidelines for the management of asthma available at www.brit-thoracic.org.uk

This guidance focuses on the treatment of patients with near-fatal asthma and cardiac arrest.

Patients at risk of asthma-related cardiac arrest

Most patients who die of asthma have chronically severe asthma. The combination of severe asthma and one or more adverse psychological factors identify patients at risk of death.

Features of severe asthma

- a history of near-fatal asthma requiring intubation and mechanical ventilation
- hospitalisation or emergency care for asthma in the past year
- requiring three or more classes of asthma medication
- increasing use and dependence of beta-2 agonists
- adverse behavioural or psychological factors such as:
  - non-adherence with treatment, monitoring, clinical attendance
  - psychiatric illnesses (e.g. depression) or deliberate self-harm
  - alcohol or drug dependence
  - learning difficulties, employment problems, social isolation.

Causes of cardiorespiratory arrest associated with asthma

Cardiac arrest in a patient with asthma is often a terminal event after a period of hypoxaemia; occasionally, it may be sudden. Cardiac arrest in patients with asthma has been linked to:

- Severe bronchospasm and mucous plugging leading to asphyxia (this condition causes the vast majority of asthma-related deaths).
- Cardiac arrhythmias caused by hypoxia, which is the commonest cause of asthma-related arrhythmia. Arrhythmias can also be caused by stimulant drugs (e.g. beta-adrenergic agonists, aminophylline) or electrolyte abnormalities.

- Dynamic hyperinflation (auto positive end-expiratory pressure (auto-PEEP)) can occur in mechanically ventilated patients with asthma. Auto-PEEP is caused by air trapping and 'breath stacking' (air entering the lungs and being unable to escape). Gradual build-up of pressure occurs and reduces venous return and blood pressure.

- Tension pneumothorax (occasionally bilateral).

The 4 Hs and 4 Ts approach to reversible causes will help identify these causes in cardiac arrest.

Initial assessment and treatment of asthma to prevent cardiorespiratory arrest

Use the ABCDE approach to assess severity and guide treatment. The severity of acute asthma is summarised in Table 12.2.

The patient with acute severe asthma requires aggressive medical management to prevent deterioration. Experienced clinicians should treat these patients in a critical care area.

- Provide controlled oxygen therapy to all hypoxaemic patients with acute severe asthma. Titrate to achieve an SpO_2 94–98%. Do not delay oxygen administration whilst waiting for a pulse oximeter.

- Salbutamol (5 mg delivered by oxygen driven nebuliser) is the main therapy for acute asthma. Repeated doses every 15–30 min, or continuous doses (5–10 mg h^{-1} – requires a special nebuliser), may be needed. Nebulised drugs will not be delivered to the lungs effectively if the patient is tired and hypoventilating. If a nebuliser is not immediately available beta-2 agonists can be temporarily administered by repeating activations of a metered dose inhaler via a large volume spacer device.

- Add nebulised ipratropium bromide (500 mcg 4–6 hourly) to beta-2 agonist treatment for patients with acute severe or life-threatening asthma or those with a poor initial response to beta-2 agonist therapy.

- Give steroids (prednisolone 40–50 mg orally or hydrocortisone 100 mg IV 6-hourly) early. Oral formulations have a longer half-life but the IV route is easier to give in near fatal asthma.

- Give a single dose of IV magnesium sulfate (2 g (8 mmol) IV over 20 min) to patients with acute severe asthma (PEF < 50% best or predicted) who have not had a good initial response to inhaled bronchodilator therapy. The most commonly reported adverse effects of IV magnesium sulfate are flushing, fatigue, nausea, headache and hypotension.

- Consider intravenous salbutamol (250 mcg IV slowly) only when inhaled therapy is not possible (e.g. a patient receiving bag-mask ventilation). If used, monitor serum lactate for evidence of toxicity.

Table 12.2   Severity of asthma exacerbations
From British Thoracic Society/Scottish Intercollegiate Guidelines Network Guideline on the Management of Asthma. www.brit-thoracic.org.uk

Asthma severity			
Near-fatal asthma	Raised $PaCO_2$ and/or mechanical ventilation with raised inflation pressures		
Life-threatening asthma	Any one of the following in a patient with severe asthma:		
	Clinical signs:		Measurements:
	Altered conscious level Exhaustion Arrhythmia Hypotension Cyanosis Silent chest Poor expiratory effect		PEF < 33% best or predicted SpO_2 < 92% PaO_2 < 8 kPa 'normal' $PaCO_2$ (4.6–6.0 kPa)
Acute severe asthma	Any one of:		
	PEF 33–50% best or predicted Respiratory rate ≥ 25 min^{-1} Heart rate ≥ 110 min^{-1} Inability to complete sentences in one breath		

- Following senior advice, consider aminophylline in severe or near-fatal asthma only. A loading dose of 5 mg kg^{-1} IV is given over 20 min (unless on maintenance therapy), followed by an infusion of 500–700 mcg kg^{-1} h^{-1}. Maintain serum theophylline concentrations below 20 mcg mL^{-1} to avoid toxicity.

- These patients are often dehydrated or hypovolaemic and will benefit from fluid replacement. Beta-2 agonists and steroids may induce hypokalaemia, which should be corrected with electrolyte supplements.

- An intensive care specialist should assess patients who fail to respond to initial treatment, or develop signs of life-threatening asthma.

- Consider tracheal intubation and controlled ventilation if, despite efforts to optimise drug therapy, the patient has:
  - deteriorating peak flow
  - a decreasing conscious level, or coma
  - persisting or worsening hypoxaemia
  - deteriorating respiratory acidosis
  - severe agitation, confusion and fighting against the oxygen mask (clinical signs of hypoxaemia)
  - progressive exhaustion, feeble respiration
  - respiratory or cardiac arrest.

- Elevation of the $PaCO_2$ alone does not indicate the need for tracheal intubation.

- The role of non-invasive ventilation (NIV) in patients with severe acute asthma is uncertain. NIV should be considered only in an ICU or equivalent clinical setting.

Cardiorespiratory arrest associated with asthma

- Follow standard BLS and ALS protocols. Ventilation will be difficult because of increased airway resistance; try to avoid gastric inflation.

- Intubate the trachea early. There is a significant risk of gastric inflation and hypoventilation of the lungs when attempting to ventilate a severe asthmatic without a tracheal tube.

- The recommended respiratory rate (10 breaths min^{-1}) and tidal volume required for a normal chest rise during CPR should not cause dynamic hyperinflation of the lungs (gas trapping).

- If dynamic hyperinflation of the lungs is suspected during CPR, compression of the chest wall and/or a period of apnoea (disconnection of tracheal tube) may relieve gas-trapping. Although this procedure is supported by limited evidence, it is unlikely to be harmful in an otherwise desperate situation.

- Dynamic hyperinflation increases transthoracic impedance, but modern impedance-compensated biphasic defibrillation waveforms are no less effective in patients with a higher impedance. As with standard ALS defibrillation protocols, consider increasing defibrillation energy if the first shock is unsuccessful and a manual defibrillator is available.

- Look for reversible causes using the 4 Hs and 4 Ts approach.

- Tension pneumothorax can be difficult to diagnose in cardiac arrest. Always consider bilateral tension pneumothoraces in asthma. See section on tension pneumothorax. Extracorporeal life support (ECLS) can provide both organ perfusion and gas exchange in cases of otherwise refractory respiratory and circulatory failure. Cases of successful treatment of asthma-related cardiac arrest in adults using ECLS have been reported.

Anaphylaxis

This guidance is based on Emergency Treatment of Anaphylaxis, Resuscitation Council UK. For more details see www.resus.org.uk.

Definition

Anaphylaxis is a serious systemic hypersensitivity reaction that is usually rapid in onset and may cause death. Severe anaphylaxis is characterised by potentially life-threatening compromise in airway, breathing and/or the circulation, and may occur without typical skin features or circulatory shock being present.

Epidemiology

Anaphylaxis is common and affects about 1 in 300 of the European population at some stage in their lives.

Anaphylaxis can be triggered by any of a very broad range of triggers with food, drugs, stinging insects, the most commonly identified triggers. The greatest risk from fatal food allergy appears to be in teenagers and adults up to age 30 years. In contrast, fatal anaphylaxis due to drugs is rare in children, and peaks in the elderly (presumably due to polypharmacy in this age group). Virtually any food or drug can be implicated, but certain foods (nuts) and drugs (muscle relaxants, antibiotics, nonsteroidal anti-inflammatory drugs) cause most reactions. A significant number of cases of anaphylaxis are idiopathic as the cause cannot be identified.

The overall prognosis of anaphylaxis is good, with a case fatality ratio of less than 1% reported in most population-based studies. The European Anaphylaxis Registry reported that only 2% of 3333 cases progressed to cardiac arrest.

Anaphylaxis and risk of death is increased in those with pre-existing asthma, particularly if the asthma is poorly controlled, severe, or if treatment with adrenaline is delayed. When anaphylaxis is fatal, death usually occurs very soon after contact with the trigger. Fatal food reactions typically cause respiratory arrest after about 30 min; insect stings cause collapse from shock after 10–15 min; and deaths caused by intravenous medication occur most commonly within five minutes. Death more than four hours after contact with the trigger is rare.

Recognition of anaphylaxis

- Anaphylaxis is likely if a patient who is exposed to a trigger (allergen) develops a sudden illness (usually within minutes of exposure) with rapidly progressing skin changes and life-threatening airway and/or breathing and/or circulation problems. The reaction is usually unexpected.

Anaphylaxis is likely when all of the following three criteria are met:

1. Sudden onset and rapid progression of symptoms
2. Life-threatening Airway and/or Breathing and/or Circulation problems
3. Skin and/or mucosal changes (flushing, urticaria, angioedema).

Exposure to a known allergen for the patient supports the diagnosis.

Remember:

- Skin or mucosal changes alone are not a sign of anaphylaxis
- Skin and mucosal changes can be subtle or absent in up to 20% of reactions (some patients can have initial bronchospasm or a decrease in blood pressure)
- There can also be gastrointestinal symptoms (e.g. vomiting, abdominal pain, incontinence). These are more common when the route of exposure is non-oral e.g. following a sting.

Sudden onset and rapid progression of symptoms

- The patient will feel and look unwell
- Most reactions occur quickly over minutes
- An intravenous trigger will cause a more rapid onset of reaction than stings which, in turn, tend to cause a more rapid onset than orally ingested triggers
- The patient is usually anxious and can experience a 'sense of impending doom'.

Life-threatening Airway, Breathing and Circulation problems

Use the ABCDE approach to recognise life-threatening Airway, Breathing and Circulation problems.

Airway problems

- Airway swelling (e.g. throat and tongue swelling (pharyngeal/laryngeal oedema)). The patient has difficulty in breathing and swallowing and feels that the throat is closing up
- Hoarse voice (new)
- Stridor – this is a high-pitched inspiratory noise caused by upper airway obstruction.

Breathing problems

- Shortness of breath – increased respiratory rate
- Wheeze
- Patient becoming tired
- Cyanosis – this is usually a late sign
- Respiratory arrest.

Circulation problems

- Pale, clammy
- Tachycardia

- Hypotension – feeling faint, collapse
- Decreased conscious level or loss of consciousness
- Anaphylaxis can cause myocardial ischaemia and ECG changes even in individuals with normal coronary arteries
- Cardiac arrest.

Circulation problems can be caused by direct myocardial depression, vasodilation and capillary leak, and loss of fluid from the circulation.

The above Airway, Breathing and Circulation problems can all alter the patient's neurological status (Disability problems) because of decreased brain perfusion. There may be confusion, agitation and loss of consciousness.

Skin and mucosal changes

These should be assessed as part of the Exposure when using the ABCDE approach.

- They are often the first feature and present in over 80% of anaphylaxis cases.
- They can be subtle or dramatic.
- There may be changes just to the skin, just to the mucosal, or both.
- There may be erythema – a patchy, or generalised, red rash.
- There may be urticaria (also called hives, nettle rash, weals or welts), which can appear anywhere on the body. The weals may be pale, pink or red, and may look like nettle stings. They can be different shapes and sizes, and are often surrounded by a red flare. They are usually itchy.
- Angioedema is similar to urticaria but involves swelling of deeper tissues, most commonly in the eyelids and lips, and sometimes in the mouth and throat.
- Although skin changes can be worrying or distressing for patients and those treating them, skin changes without airway, breathing or circulation problems do not signify anaphylaxis. Reassuringly, most patients who present with skin changes caused by an allergic reaction do not go on to develop anaphylaxis.

Differential diagnosis for anaphylaxis

Life-threatening conditions

- Sometimes anaphylaxis can present with symptoms and signs that are very similar to life-threatening asthma.
- A low blood pressure (or normal in children) with a petechial or purpuric rash can be a sign of septic shock. Seek help early if there are any doubts about the diagnosis and treatment.
- Following the ABCDE approach will help with treating the differential diagnoses.

Other conditions which can mimic anaphylaxis (but do not respond to adrenaline):

- Inducible laryngeal obstruction (ILO, formerly known as vocal cord dysfunction)
- ACE inhibitor-induced angioedema (not usually life-threatening).

Non life-threatening conditions (these usually respond to simple measures)

- Faint (vasovagal episode)
- Panic attack
- Breath-holding episode in child
- Idiopathic (non-allergic) urticaria or angioedema

There can be confusion between anaphylaxis and a panic attack. Victims of previous anaphylaxis may be particularly prone to panic attacks if they think they have been re-exposed to the allergen that caused a previous problem. The sense of impending doom and breathlessness leading to hyperventilation are symptoms that can resemble anaphylaxis. While there is no hypotension, pallor, wheeze, or urticarial rash or swelling, there may sometimes be flushing or blotchy skin associated with anxiety, adding to the diagnostic difficulty. Diagnostic difficulty may also occur with vasovagal attacks after immunisation procedures, but the absence of rash, breathing difficulties, and swelling are useful distinguishing features, as is the slow pulse of a vasovagal attack compared with a rapid pulse with anaphylaxis. Fainting will usually respond to lying the patient down and raising the legs.

Treatment of anaphylaxis to prevent cardiorespiratory arrest

As the diagnosis of anaphylaxis is not always obvious, all those who treat anaphylaxis must use the ABCDE approach to the sick patient. Treat life-threatening problems as you find them. The key steps are described in the anaphylaxis algorithm (Figure 12.3).

- Death can occur within minutes if a patient stands, walks or sits up suddenly. Patients must NOT walk or stand during acute reactions. Use caution when transferring patients who have been stabilised.
- Patients with Airway and Breathing problems may prefer to sit up as this will make breathing easier.
- Lying flat with or without leg elevation is helpful for patients with a low blood pressure.
- Patients who are breathing normally and unconscious should be placed on their side (recovery position). Monitor breathing continuously and prepare to intervene if this changes.
- Pregnant patients should lie on their left side to prevent aortocaval compression.
- Removing the trigger during anaphylaxis is not always possible. Early removal is more important than the

method of removal. Stop any drug suspected of causing anaphylaxis (e.g. stop IV infusion of a gelatin solution or antibiotic). Remove the stinger after a bee sting. Do not delay definitive treatment if removing the trigger is not feasible.

- Monitor all patients who have suspected anaphylaxis as soon as possible (e.g. by ambulance crew, in the emergency department etc.). Minimum monitoring includes pulse oximetry, non-invasive blood pressure and a 3-lead ECG.
- Initially, give the highest concentration of oxygen possible using a non-rebreather mask with resevoir. Once pulse oximetry is feasible target an SpO_2 of 94–98%.

Adrenaline is the most important drug for the treatment of anaphylaxis. As an alpha-receptor agonist, it reverses peripheral vasodilation and reduces oedema. Its beta-receptor activity dilates the bronchial airways, increases the force of myocardial contraction, and suppresses histamine and leukotriene release. Adrenaline works best when given early after the onset of the reaction. Adverse effects are extremely rare with correct doses injected intramuscularly (IM).

- The intramuscular route is the best for most individuals who have to give adrenaline to treat anaphylaxis and should be administered as early as possible.
- For adults give an initial IM adrenaline dose of 0.5 mg (0.5 mL of 1:1000 adrenaline = 0.5 mg = 500 mcg). Further doses can be given at about 5 min intervals, according to the patient's response.
- The best site for IM injection is the anterolateral aspect of the middle third of the thigh. The needle used for injection needs to be sufficiently long to ensure that the adrenaline is injected into muscle.
- If features of anaphylaxis persist despite 2 doses of IM adrenaline, follow the refractory anaphylaxis algorithm (Figure 12.4) and start an adrenaline infusion with expert support. In patients with a spontaneous circulation, intravenous adrenaline can cause life-threatening hypertension, tachycardia, arrhythmias, and myocardial ischaemia. Patients who are given IV adrenaline must be monitored closely – continuous ECG and pulse oximetry and frequent non-invasive blood pressure measurements as a minimum. It is essential that these patients receive expert help early.
- Nebulised adrenaline may be effective as an adjunct to treat upper airways obstruction caused by laryngeal oedema, but only after treatment with IM (or IV) adrenaline and not as an alternative. Recommended doses are 5 mL of 1 mg mL (1:1000) adrenaline.
- Auto-injectors are often given to patients at risk of anaphylaxis for their own use. Healthcare

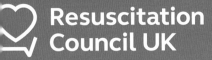
Anaphylaxis

Anaphylaxis?

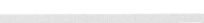 **A** = Airway  **B** = Breathing  **C** = Circulation **D** = Disability **E** = Exposure

Diagnosis – look for:
- Sudden onset of Airway and/or Breathing and/or Circulation problems[1]
- And usually skin changes (e.g. itchy rash)

Call for HELP
Call resuscitation team or ambulance

- Remove trigger if possible (e.g. stop any infusion)
- Lie patient flat (with or without legs elevated)
  - A sitting position may make breathing easier
  - If pregnant, lie on left side

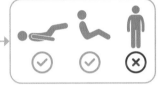

Inject at **anterolateral aspect** – middle third of the thigh

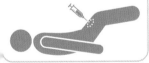

Give intramuscular (IM) adrenaline[2]

- Establish airway
- Give high flow oxygen
- Apply monitoring: pulse oximetry, ECG, blood pressure

If no response:
- Repeat IM adrenaline after 5 minutes
- IV fluid bolus[3]

If no improvement in Breathing or Circulation problems[1] despite TWO doses of IM adrenaline:
- Confirm resuscitation team or ambulance has been called
- Follow REFRACTORY ANAPHYLAXIS ALGORITHM

---

1. Life-threatening problems

Airway
Hoarse voice, stridor

Breathing
↑work of breathing, wheeze, fatigue, cyanosis, SpO$_2$ < 94%

Circulation
Low blood pressure, signs of shock, confusion, reduced consciousness

2. Intramuscular (IM) adrenaline
Use adrenaline at 1 mg/mL (1:1000) concentration

Adult and child > 12 years:	500 micrograms IM (0.5 mL)
Child 6–12 years:	300 micrograms IM (0.3 mL)
Child 6 months to 6 years:	150 micrograms IM (0.15 mL)
Child < 6 months:	100–150 micrograms IM (0.1–0.15 mL)

The above doses are for IM injection **only**.
Intravenous adrenaline for anaphylaxis to be given **only by experienced specialists** in an appropriate setting.

3. IV fluid challenge
Use crystalloid

Adults: 500–1000 mL
Children: 10 mL/kg

Figure 12.3   Anaphylaxis algorithm   159

professionals should be familiar with the use of the most commonly available auto-injector devices. If an adrenaline auto-injector is the only available adrenaline preparation when treating anaphylaxis, healthcare providers should use it.

- Give a rapid IV fluid challenge (500–1000 mL non-glucose containing crystalloid in an adult) and monitor the response; give further doses as necessary. Hartmann's solution or 0.9% saline are suitable fluids for initial resuscitation. A large volume of fluid may be needed.

- Antihistamines are not recommended for the treatment of anaphylaxis. They are of no benefit in treating life-threatening symptoms of anaphylaxis, and their use may delay more appropriate treatment (e.g. adrenaline, fluids, oxygen). Antihistamines may be helpful in alleviating cutaneous symptoms but should only be given after the patient has been stabilised. In this context, use a non-sedating oral antihistamine, such as cetirizine.

- The routine administration of corticosteroids is not advised. Consider giving steroids after initial resuscitation for refractory reactions or ongoing asthma/resistant shock. Steroids should not be given preferentially to adrenaline. The evidence that corticosteroids help shorten protracted symptoms or prevent biphasic reactions is very weak. Oral corticosteroids may be indicated where an acute asthma exacerbation may have contributed to the severity of anaphylaxis. Steroids should be given via the oral route where possible.

- Adrenaline remains the first line vasopressor for the treatment of anaphylactic reactions. Consider other vasopressors and inotropes (e.g. noradrenaline, vasopressin, metaraminol and glucagon) when initial resuscitation with adrenaline and fluids has not been successful. Only use these drugs in specialist settings (e.g. intensive care units) where there is experience in their use.

- Airway obstruction may occur rapidly in severe anaphylaxis, particularly in patients with angioedema. Warning signs are swelling of the tongue and lips, hoarseness and oropharyngeal swelling.

- Consider early tracheal intubation; delay may make intubation extremely difficult. As airway obstruction progresses, supraglottic airway devices (e.g. i-gel or LMA) are likely to be difficult to insert. Attempts at tracheal intubation may exacerbate laryngeal oedema. Early involvement of a senior anaesthetist is mandatory when managing these patients. A surgical airway may be required if tracheal intubation is not possible.

Cardiac arrest associated with anaphylaxis

Start CPR immediately and follow current guidelines. Prolonged CPR may be necessary. Rescuers should ensure that help is on its way as early ALS is essential.

Cardiac arrest with suspected anaphylaxis should be treated with the standard 1 mg dose of IV or intraosseous (IO) adrenaline for cardiac arrest.

Investigation of anaphylaxis

Undertake the usual investigations appropriate for a medical emergency (e.g. 12-lead ECG, chest X-ray, urea and electrolytes, arterial blood gases etc).

The specific test to help confirm a diagnosis of anaphylaxis is measurement of mast cell tryptase. In anaphylaxis, mast cell degranulation leads to markedly increased blood tryptase concentrations.

Mast cell tryptase sample timing

The time of onset of the anaphylactic reaction is the time when symptoms were first noticed.

a) Minimum: one sample within 2 h (but no later than 4 h) from the start of symptoms.

b) Ideally: Three timed samples:
   - Initial sample as soon as feasible after resuscitation has started – do not delay resuscitation to take sample.
   - Second sample at 1–2 h (but no later than 4 h) after the start of symptoms.
   - Third sample either at 24 h or in convalescence. This provides baseline tryptase levels – some individuals have an elevated baseline level.

c) Either serum ('liver function test' tube) or plasma samples are acceptable in most laboratories. Sample volumes as little as 0.5 mL of sample are usually sufficient, but > 2 mL is preferred.

d) Record the timing of each sample accurately on the request form and in the clinical records. Record how many minutes/hours after the onset of symptoms the sample was taken.

e) Specimens are stable for up to 2 days at room temperature, 7 days refrigerated at 2–8°C, and for longer frozen at –20°C. Samples stored beyond these times may still provide useful information and should therefore be submitted for analysis, regardless. Consult your local laboratory if you have any queries.

Discharge and follow-up after anaphylaxis

All patients should be reviewed by a senior clinician and a decision made about the need for further treatment and duration of observation. There is no reliable way of predicting who will have a biphasic reaction, so decisions about discharge must be made for each patient by an experienced clinician. NICE recommends that prior to

Refractory anaphylaxis

No improvement in respiratory or cardiovascular symptoms
despite 2 appropriate doses of intramuscular adrenaline

Seek expert[1] help early
Critical care support is essential

Start adrenaline infusion
Adrenaline is essential for treating
all aspects of anaphylaxis

&

**Establish dedicated
peripheral IV or IO access**

Give rapid IV fluid bolus
e.g. 0.9% sodium chloride

**Follow local protocol
OR**

Peripheral low-dose IV adrenaline infusion:
- 1 mg (1 mL of 1 mg/mL [1:1000]) adrenaline in
  100 mL of 0.9% sodium chloride
- Prime and connect with an infusion pump via a
  dedicated line

DO NOT 'piggy back' on to another infusion line
DO NOT infuse on the same side as a BP cuff as this will
interfere with the infusion and risk extravasation

- In both adults and children, start at 0.5–1.0 mL/kg/hour,
  and **titrate according to clinical response**
- Continuous monitoring and observation is mandatory
- ↑↑ BP is likely to indicate adrenaline overdose

**Give IM* adrenaline
every 5 minutes until adrenaline
infusion has been started**

*IV boluses of adrenaline are
not recommended, but may be
appropriate in some specialist
settings (e.g. peri-operative) while
an infusion is set up

Give high flow oxygen
Titrate to SpO₂ 94–98%

**Monitor HR, BP, pulse oximetry
and ECG for cardiac arrhythmia**
Take blood sample
for mast cell tryptase

**Continue adrenaline infusion
and treat ABC symptoms**
Titrate according to clinical response

A = Airway

Partial upper airway obstruction/stridor:
Nebulised adrenaline (5 mL of 1 mg/mL)

Total upper airway obstruction:
Expert help needed, follow difficult airway algorithm

B = Breathing

Oxygenation is more important than intubation

If apnoeic:
- Bag mask ventilation
- Consider tracheal intubation

Severe/persistent bronchospasm:
- Nebulised salbutamol and ipratropium with oxygen
- Consider IV bolus and/or infusion of salbutamol or
  aminophylline
- Inhalational anaesthesia

C = Circulation

Give further fluid boluses and titrate to response:
Child 10 mL/kg per bolus
Adult 500–1000 mL per bolus
- Use glucose-free crystalloid
  (e.g. Hartmann's Solution, Plasma-Lyte®)
Large volumes may be required (e.g. 3–5 L in adults)

Place arterial cannula for continuous BP monitoring

Establish central venous access

IF REFRACTORY TO ADRENALINE INFUSION
Consider adding a second vasopressor **in addition**
to adrenaline infusion:
- Noradrenaline, vasopressin or metaraminol
- In patients on beta-blockers, consider glucagon

Consider extracorporeal life support

Cardiac arrest – follow ALS ALGORITHM
- Start chest compressions early
- Use IV or IO adrenaline bolus (cardiac arrest protocol)
- Aggressive fluid resuscitation
- Consider prolonged resuscitation/extracorporeal CPR

[1]Intravenous adrenaline for anaphylaxis to be given only by experienced specialists in an appropriate setting.

Figure 12.4   Refractory anaphylaxis algorithm   161

discharge, a healthcare professional with the appropriate skills and competencies should offer people (or, as appropriate, their parent and/or carer) the following:

- Information about anaphylaxis, including the signs and symptoms of anaphylaxis, and the risk of a biphasic reaction (and clear instructions to return to hospital if symptoms return).
- Information on what to do if anaphylaxis occurs (use the adrenaline injector and call emergency services).
- Considered for an adrenaline auto-injector or given a replacement. If prescribed, a demonstration of the correct use of the adrenaline injector and when to use it.
- Advice about how to avoid the suspected trigger (if known).
- Information about the need for referral to a specialist allergy service and the referral process.
- Information about patient support groups (e.g. Anaphylaxis Campaign, Allergy UK).

All patients presenting with anaphylaxis should be referred to an allergy clinic to identify the cause, and thereby reduce the risk of future reactions and prepare the patient to manage future episodes themselves. Patients need to know the allergen responsible (if identified) and how to avoid it. Patients need to be able to recognise the early symptoms of anaphylaxis, so that they can summon help quickly and prepare to use their emergency medication.

Pregnancy

A maternal cardiac arrest is a cardiac arrest that occurs at any stage in pregnancy and up to 6 weeks after delivery. In a UK study the incidence of cardiac arrest was 1 in 36 000 pregnacies. Both the mother and fetus must be considered in emergencies during pregnancy. Effective resuscitation of the mother is often the best way to optimise foetal outcome. Significant physiological changes occur during pregnancy; for example, cardiac output, circulatory volume, minute ventilation, and oxygen consumption all increase. The gravid uterus can cause compression of the abdominal vessels when the mother is in the supine position, resulting in reduced venous return and cardiac output, hypotension and a reduction in uterine perfusion. Resuscitation guidelines for pregnancy are based largely on case series, extrapolation from non-pregnant cardiac arrests, manikin studies and expert opinion based on the physiology of pregnancy and changes that occur in women during labour.

Causes of cardiac arrest in pregnancy

Maternal deaths are most commonly associated with:

- cardiac disease (congenital and acquired)
- pulmonary embolism
- epilepsy and stroke
- sepsis
- mental health conditions
- bleeding
- malignancy
- hypertensive disorders of pregnancy.

Pregnant women can also have the same causes of cardiac arrest as females of the same age group (e.g. anaphylaxis, drug overdose, trauma). The risk increases with age, social deprivation and for ethnic minorities. A study of cardiac arrests in pregnancy between 2011 and 2014 identified 66 cardiac arrests of whom 28 women died (42%).

Prevention of cardiac arrest in pregnancy

In an emergency, use the ABCDE approach. Many cardiovascular problems associated with pregnancy are caused by compression of the inferior vena cava and aorta by a gravid uterus. Treat a distressed or compromised pregnant patient as follows:

- Place the patient in the left lateral position or manually displace the uterus to the left if the lateral position is not possible.
- Give high-flow oxygen, guided by pulse oximetry.
- Give a fluid bolus if there is hypotension or evidence of hypovolaemia.
- Immediately re-evaluate the need for any drugs currently being given.
- Seek expert help and involve obstetric, anaesthetic and neonatal specialists early in the resuscitation.
- Identify and treat the underlying cause.

Modifications for cardiac arrest in pregnancy

- In cardiac arrest, all the principles of basic and advanced life support apply.
- Summon help immediately. Obtain expert help, including an obstetrician, anaesthetist, and neonatologist, to facilitate effective resuscitation of both mother and fetus.
- Start CPR according to standard ALS guidelines. Ensure high-quality chest compressions with minimal interruptions. Use the standard hand position for chest compressions if feasible. Over the head CPR may be necessary in those with a morbidly raised BMI.
- After approximately 20 weeks gestation (or, if palpable outside the pelvic brim), the uterus can press down against the inferior vena cava (IVC) and the aorta, impeding venous return, cardiac output

and uterine perfusion. IVC compression limits the effectiveness of chest compressions.

- The potential for IVC compression suggests that IV or IO access should ideally be established above the diaphragm.

- Manually displace the uterus to the left to minimise IVC compression.

- Add left lateral tilt only if this is feasible. The patient's body will need to be supported on a firm surface to allow effective chest compressions (e.g. a full length tilting operating table). The optimal angle of tilt is unknown. Aim for between 15–30°. Even a small amount of tilt may be better than no tilt. The angle of tilt used needs to permit high-quality chest compressions and if needed caesarean delivery of the fetus (see below).

- If tilting on a firm surface is not possible then maintain left uterine displacement and continue effective chest compressions with the patient supine.

- The use of soft pillows and wedges for the pregnant patient requiring chest compressions is not effective.

- Start preparing for emergency caesarean section (see below) – the fetus will need to be delivered if initial resuscitation efforts fail.

- There is an increased risk of pulmonary aspiration of gastric contents in pregnancy. Early tracheal intubation decreases this risk. Tracheal intubation can be more difficult in the pregnant patient however and should only be attempted by those regularly skilled in the technique. A failed intubation drill and the use of alternative airway techniques may be needed.

- Attempt defibrillation using standard energy doses. Left lateral tilt and large breasts can make it difficult to place an apical defibrillator pad.

Reversible causes of collapse and cardiac arrest in pregnancy

Look for reversible causes using the 4 Hs and 4 Ts approach. Abdominal ultrasound by a skilled operator to detect possible causes during cardiac arrest can be useful. It can also permit an evaluation of fetal viability, multiple gestations (twins) and placental localisation. It should not however delay treatments. Specific reversible causes of collapse or cardiac arrest in pregnancy include:

Haemorrhage

This can occur both antenatally and postnatally. Causes include ectopic pregnancy, placental abruption, placenta praevia, abnormal placentation (increta/ percreta) and uterine rupture. Maternity units should have a massive haemorrhage protocol. Treatment is based on the ABCDE approach. The key step is to stop the bleeding.

Consider the following:

- fluid resuscitation including use of a rapid transfusion system and cell salvage

- tranexamic acid and correction of coagulopathy

- oxytocin, ergometrine, prostaglandins and uterine massage to correct uterine atony

- uterine compression sutures, uterine packs, and intrauterine balloon devices

- interventional radiology to identify and control bleeding

- surgical control including aortic crossclamping/ compression and hysterectomy. Placenta percreta may require extensive intra-pelvic surgery.

Drugs

Overdose can occur in women with eclampsia receiving magnesium sulfate, particularly if the patient becomes oliguric. Give calcium to treat magnesium toxicity (see electrolyte abnormalities section above). Central neural blockade for analgesia or anaesthesia can cause problems due to sympathetic blockade (hypotension, bradycardia) or local anaesthetic toxicity.

Cardiovascular disease

Myocardial infarction and aneurysm or dissection of the aorta or its branches, and peripartum cardiomyopathy cause most deaths from acquired cardiac disease. Patients with known cardiac disease need to be managed in a specialist unit. Pregnant women may develop an acute coronary syndrome, typically in association with risk factors such as obesity, older age, higher parity, smoking, diabetes, pre-existing hypertension and a family history of ischaemic heart disease. Pregnant patients can have atypical features such as epigastric pain and vomiting.

Percutaneous coronary intervention (PCI) is the reperfusion strategy of choice for ST-elevation myocardial infarction in pregnancy. Consider fibrinolysis if urgent PCI is unavailable. More women with congenital heart disease are becoming pregnant – they should be managed in specialist centres.

Pre-eclampsia and eclampsia

Eclampsia is defined as the development of convulsions and/or unexplained coma during pregnancy or postpartum in patients with signs and symptoms of pre-eclampsia.

Magnesium sulfate treatment may prevent eclampsia developing in labour or immediately postpartum in women with pre-eclampsia.

Amniotic fluid embolism

Amniotic fluid embolism usually presents around the time of delivery, often in the labouring mother, with sudden cardiovascular collapse, breathlessness, cyanosis, arrhythmias, hypotension and haemorrhage associated with disseminated intravascular coagulopathy. Patients can have warning signs preceding collapse including breathlessness, chest pain, feeling cold, light-headedness, panic, pins and needles in the fingers, nausea, and vomiting. Amniotic fluid embolism is associated with older maternal age, multiple pregnancy, placenta praevia and induction of labour, instrumental vaginal and caesarean delivery. Treatment is supportive, based on an ABCDE approach and correction of coagulopathy.

Pulmonary embolism

Pulmonary embolism causing cardiopulmonary collapse can present throughout pregnancy. CPR is started with modifications as necessary. The use of fibrinolytic therapy needs considerable thought, particularly if a peri-mortem caesarean section is being considered (see below). If the diagnosis is suspected and maternal cardiac output cannot be restored it should be given.

Peri-mortem caesarean section (resuscitative hysterotomy)

When initial resuscitation attempts fail, delivery of the fetus may improve the chances of successful resuscitation of both the mother and fetus. The best survival rate for infants over 24–25 weeks gestation occurs when delivery of the infant is achieved within 5 min after the mother's cardiac arrest. This is a difficult time to achieve in reality, but consideration of peri-mortem caesarean section should be made at an early stage after cardiac arrest has occurred, and resuscitation started. In cases of obvious fatal injury to the mother the procedure can be performed immediately. The procedure should be done at the site of cardiac arrest as moving the mother significantly impairs CPR attempts.

Delivery relieves IVC compression and may improve the likelihood of resuscitating the mother by permitting an increase in venous return during the CPR attempt. Delivery also enables access to the abdominal cavity so that aortic clamping or compression is possible. Internal cardiac massage may also be possible. Once the fetus has been delivered, resuscitation of the newborn child can also begin.

In the supine position, the gravid uterus begins to compromise blood flow in the IVC and abdominal aorta at approximately 20 weeks' gestation; however, fetal viability currently begins at approximately 24 weeks.

- **Gestational age < 20 weeks** (or the uterus is not palpable above the level of the umbilicus). Urgent caesarean delivery need not be considered, because a gravid uterus of this size is unlikely to compromise maternal cardiac output and fetal viability is not an issue.
- **Gestational age approximately 20–23 weeks.** Initiate emergency delivery of the fetus to permit successful resuscitation of the mother; survival of the delivered infant which is unlikely at this gestational age.

- **Gestational age approximately > 24 weeks.** Initiate emergency delivery to help save the life of both the mother and the infant.

Post-resuscitation care

Post-resuscitation care should follow standard guidelines. Targeted temperature management (TTM) has been used safely and effectively in early pregnancy with fetal heart monitoring and resulted in favourable maternal and fetal outcome after a term delivery. Implantable cardioverter defibrillators (ICDs) have been used in patients successfully during pregnancy.

Planning for resuscitation in pregnancy

Advanced life support in pregnancy requires co-ordination of maternal resuscitation, early caesarean delivery of the fetus if maternal cardiac output cannot be restored rapidly, and newborn resuscitation. To achieve this, units likely to deal with cardiac arrest in pregnancy should:

- have in place plans and equipment for resuscitation of both the pregnant patient and the newborn child
- ensure early involvement of obstetric, anaesthetic and neonatal teams
- ensure regular training of staff in obstetric emergencies.

Traumatic cardiorespiratory arrest

Traumatic cardiac arrest has a very high mortality, but when ROSC can be achieved, neurological outcome in survivors appears to be much better than in other causes of cardiac arrest. The response to traumatic cardiac arrest is time-critical and success depends on rapidly identifying and treating the reversible causes.

The history and a scene assessment may provide clues to the cause of cardiac arrest. Cardiac arrest from a primary medical problem (e.g. cardiac arrhythmia, hypoglycaemia, seizure) can also cause a secondary traumatic event (e.g. fall, road traffic accident). In these cases, traumatic injuries may not be the primary cause of a cardiorespiratory arrest and standard advanced life support, including chest compressions and defibrillation are appropriate.

Causes of cardiac arrest in trauma patients include: severe traumatic brain injury, hypovolaemia from massive blood loss, hypoxia from respiratory arrest or airway obstruction, direct injury to vital organs and major vessels, tension pneumothorax, and cardiac tamponade. The prevalent initial heart rhythms in traumatic cardiac arrest are generally PEA and asystole.

Commotio cordis is actual or near cardiac arrest caused by a blunt impact to the chest wall over the heart. A blow to the chest can cause VF/pVT. Commotio cordis occurs mostly during sports (most commonly baseball) and recreational activities, and patients are usually teenage males. Follow standard ALS guidelines. Early defibrillation is important for survival.

Damage control resuscitation combines permissive hypotension and haemostatic resuscitation with damage control surgery.

- Permissive hypotension (administering only enough fluid to achieve a radial pulse) may be used until surgical haemostasis is achieved.
- Caution is advised in patients with traumatic brain injury where a raised intracranial pressure may require a higher cerebral perfusion pressure.
- The duration of hypotensive resuscitation should not exceed 60 min.
- Tranexamic acid (TXA) (loading dose 1 g IV over 10 min followed by infusion of 1 g over 8 h) increases survival from traumatic haemorrhage. It is most effective within the first hour and certainly within the first three hours following trauma. Started any later than four hours after the injury may increase mortality.
- In an out-of-hospital setting, only essential life-saving interventions are undertaken on scene before rapid transfer to the nearest appropriate hospital. Do not delay for spinal immobilisation.

Treatment of traumatic cardiac arrest

- Survival from traumatic cardiac arrests is correlated with duration of CPR and pre-hospital time. Factors that are associated with survival include the presence of reactive pupils, an organised ECG rhythm and respiratory activity.
- Chest compressions are still the standard of care in patients with cardiac arrest. In cardiac arrest caused by hypovolaemia, cardiac tamponade or tension pneumothorax, chest compressions are unlikely to be as effective as in normovolaemic cardiac arrest. Thus, in these situations, chest compressions have a lower priority than the correction of reversible causes (e.g. thoracotomy, controlling haemorrhage etc) and should not delay immediate treatment of them.
- Focused ultrasound should be used by a trained operator to diagnose underlying causes of cardiac arrest and to target treatment, particularly where the causes of shock cannot be diagnosed clinically. Haemoperitoneum, haemopneumothorax, tension pneumothorax and cardiac tamponade may all be detectable on ultrasound.
- Prolonged CPR is associated with a poor outcome. If there is no response to 20 min of advanced life support, all reversible causes have been excluded, and there is no detectable cardiac activity on ultrasound, then further resuscitation efforts may be stopped.

Hypovolaemia and haemorrhage control

Uncontrolled haemorrhage is a common cause of traumatic cardiac arrest, so early haemorrhage control and restoration of circulating volume is essential.

- Treat compressible external haemorrhage with elevation and direct pressure (with or without a dressing), use tourniquets if needed and/or apply topical haemostatic agents.
- Non-compressible haemorrhage is more difficult to treat. Use splints (including a pelvic splint), and where necessary blood products, IV fluids and tranexamic acid while moving the patient to surgical/radiological haemorrhage control.
- Immediate aortic occlusion may be used in patients with exsanguinating and uncontrollable infra-diaphragmatic torso haemorrhage. This can be achieved through resuscitative thoracotomy and cross-clamping of the descending aorta or use of an intravascular occlusion device ('REBOA').
- Neurogenic shock arising after a spinal cord injury can exacerbate hypovolaemia. Indicators of spinal cord injury may include warm, vasodilated peripheries, loss of reflexes below in the injured segment, and severe hypotension with a low heart rate. In these cases, vasopressor therapy may be needed in addition to fluid replacement.
- Use IO access when IV access is not initially feasible.

Hypoxia

- Effective airway management is essential to maintain oxygenation of the severely compromised trauma patient. Early tracheal intubation by experienced rescuers can be beneficial. Use basic airway management manoeuvres and alternative airways to maintain oxygenation if tracheal intubation cannot be accomplished immediately. If these measures fail, a surgical airway is indicated.
- In low cardiac output conditions, positive pressure ventilation causes further circulatory depression, and can even cause cardiac arrest, by impeding venous return to the heart. Monitor ventilation with continuous waveform capnography. Setting the lowest minute volume consistent with normocapnia will minimise rises in transpulmonary pressure and reduces the negative effect on cardiac output.
- During CPR, use 100% oxygen. In peri-arrest or post-ROSC patients, titrate oxygen levels to achieve an SpO$_2$ of 94–98%.

Tension pneumothorax

See section on tension pneumothorax.

Cardiac tamponade

- Cardiac tamponade occurs when the pericardial sac is filled with fluid under pressure, which leads to compromise of cardiac function and ultimately cardiac arrest.

- It most commonly occurs after penetrating trauma and cardiac surgery. Mortality is high and immediate decompression of the pericardium is required to give any chance of survival.

- In traumatic cardiac arrest with penetrating trauma to the chest or epigastrium, immediate resuscitative thoracotomy with a clamshell incision, and opening of the pericardium to relieve tamponade can be life-saving.

- Needle aspiration of tamponade, with or without ultrasound guidance, is unreliable because the pericardium is commonly full of clotted blood.

Resuscitative thoracotomy

- Immediate resuscitative thoracotomy is indicated in patients with penetrating chest trauma in whom less than 15 min have elapsed since loss of vital signs. Teams must be trained in the procedure, have adequate equipment to deal with intrathoracic findings, and have sufficient access to the patient. Ideally the procedure should be performed in an operating theatre.

- Patients with no pulse after penetrating chest or cardiac injuries, who arrive at hospital after a short on-scene and transport time with witnessed signs of life or ECG activity, are candidates for emergency department resuscitative thoracotomy.

Tension pneumothorax

In tension pneumothorax, the entry and trapping of air in the pleural cavity causes mediastinal shift, thereby obstructing venous return. It may be caused by trauma, asthma, other respiratory disease, or clinical procedures (e.g. central venous catheter insertion). Tension pneumothorax may be the cause of the cardiac arrest, or develop during the cardiac arrest as positive pressure ventilation may convert a non-tension pneumothorax in to a tension pneumothorax. In traumatic cardiac arrest, 13% of patients have a tension pneumothorax.

Recognition of tension pneumothorax

Tension pneumothorax should be considered in all patients with cardiac arrest. Diagnosis is based on clinical assessment or point-of-care ultrasound (POCUS). Clinical signs of a tension pneumothorax include:

- Respiratory distress or hypoxia (prior to cardiac arrest)

- Haemodynamic compromise (prior to cardiac arrest)

- Absent breath sounds on auscultation

- Chest crepitations

- Subcutaneous emphysema

- Tracheal deviation

- Jugular venous distention.

Presentation of tension pneumothorax in cardiac arrest may be atypical. In some cases, patients may develop bilateral tension pneumothoraces.

Treatment of tension pneumothorax

In patients with a suspected tension pneumothorax, the chest cavity should be immediately decompressed. The method of decompression will depend on the skillset of the clinicians present. Strategies for decompression include:

- Needle decompression – this is the most rapid method for decompressing the chest. A needle is inserted perpendicular to the chest wall in either the 2nd intercostal space (just above the 3rd rib) or the 4th/5th intercostal space in the mid-axilliary line. Due to the risk of failure with a 14-gauge intravenous cannula, it is recommended that, where available, specific long, non-kinking needles are used and that an open thoracostomy is performed as soon as appropriately trained clinicians are present. A chest drain should be sited following return of spontaneous circulation.

- Open thoracostomy – an incision is made in the chest wall (5th intercostal space mid-axillary line) followed by dissection into the pleural space. Where appropriately trained clinicians are available, open thoracostomy should be the initial strategy for chest decompression. A chest drain should be sited following return of spontaneous circulation.

- Clamshell thoracotomy – this may be required in the context of a traumatic cardiac arrest. This should only be undertaken by appropriately trained clinicians.

Perioperative cardiac arrest

Perioperative cardiac arrest can be caused by the underlying condition being treated, physiological effects of the surgery, anaesthetic drugs and fluids, complications relating to existing co-morbidities, or adverse events.

- Overall survival from perioperative cardiac arrest is high, compared to cardiac arrest in other settings.

- The incidence of perioperative cardiac arrest during general anaesthesia (GA) is higher than that of regional anaesthesia (RA).

- Causes of perioperative cardiac arrest include hypovolaemia (e.g. bleeding), cardiac problems, and anaesthesia related problems.

- The commonest cause of anaesthesia-related cardiac arrest involves airway management. Failure of ventilation, medication-related events, complications associated with central venous access, and perioperative myocardial infarction are also common.

- The primary arrest rhythms during perioperative cardiac arrest recorded in a large single centre (Mayo Clinic) series were asystole in 41.7%, VF in 35.4%, PEA in 14.4% and unknown in 8.5%. In contrast to cardiac arrest in other circumstances, the rhythm associated with the best chance of survival to hospital discharge was asystole (43% survival).

Management of perioperative cardiac arrest

The incidence of intra-operative cardiac arrest is about 5 per 10 000. Patients are normally fully monitored and, as such, there should be little or no delay in diagnosing cardiac arrest. High-risk patients will often also have invasive blood pressure monitoring, which is invaluable in the event of cardiac arrest. If cardiac arrest is a strong possibility, apply self-adhesive defibrillation electrodes before induction of anaesthesia, ensure adequate venous access and prepare resuscitation drugs and fluids. Use fluid warmers and forced air warmers to limit perioperative hypothermia and monitor the patient's temperature.

- Asystole and VF will be detected immediately, but the onset of PEA might not be so obvious – loss of the pulse oximeter signal and very low end-tidal CO_2 values will be good clues and should provoke a pulse check. Do not waste time attempting to measure non-invasive blood pressure.

- In the event of cardiac arrest, follow the ALS algorithm, but with appropriate modifications. Adjust the position and height of the operating table or trolley to optimise delivery of chest compressions.

- CPR is optimal in the supine position, but is possible in patients who are prone and where immediate turning to a supine position is not possible. Risk factors for cardiac arrest in prone patients include cardiac abnormalities in patients undergoing major spinal surgery, hypovolaemia, air embolism, wound irrigation with hydrogen peroxide, and occluded venous return. Resuscitation Council UK has produced specific guidance on the Management of cardiac arrest during neurosurgery in adults: https://www.resus.org.uk/library/publications/publication-management-cardiac-arrest-during

In many cases of perioperative cardiac arrest, physiological deterioration is gradual and the cause of the cardiac arrest is known and hence the arrest anticipated. In those where this is not the case, follow the standard ABCDE approach to identify and treat reversible causes.

- Catastrophic haemorrhage is usually obvious, but may be occult if it involves bleeding into body compartments (abdomen, chest) or into soft tissues in patients with multiple limb fractures. Pelvic and retroperitoneal haemorrhage can also cause rapid hypovolaemia and should be excluded (e.g. by ultrasound if pre-operative haemodynamic instability). In cases where direct surgical intervention

is unable to control haemorrhage, consider early interventional radiography.

- Loss of the airway is a common cause of perioperative cardiac arrest. Always use waveform capnography to ensure the lungs are ventilated.

- Undiagnosed tension pneumothorax is a readily treatable cause of cardiac arrest (see the management of tension pneumothorax above).

- Cardiovascular collapse has several causes, but in the context of perioperative cardiac arrest, common causes include hypovolaemia, anaphylaxis (most commonly with neuromuscular blockers), and vagal stimulation. Focused transthoracic echocardiography is a useful tool to exclude cardiac tamponade (if suspected) and to assess myocardial contractility and filling.

Specific modifications for perioperative cardiac arrest

- Chest compression in the prone position can be achieved with or without sternal counter-pressure. Consider open cardiac compressions in patients where the thorax is open or the heart can be easily accessed.

- In the case of VF/pVT, call for a defibrillator. If one is not immediately available, give a precordial thump. If that is unsuccessful, give chest compressions and ventilation until the defibrillator arrives. Look for reversible causes immediately – hypoxaemia and hypovolaemia will be the most common in this setting.

- If there is asystole or extreme bradycardia stop any surgical activity likely to be causing excessive vagal activity – if this is the likely cause, give 0.5 mg atropine IV and further doses as required. Start CPR and immediately look for other reversible causes.

- If adrenaline is required according to the ALS algorithm, give the initial dose in increments (e.g. 50–100 mcg IV), rather than a 1 mg bolus. If 1 mg in total has been given with no response, consider further adrenaline doses of 1 mg IV.

- Waveform capnography and invasive arterial monitoring (when available) will help guide resuscitation (Chapter 6).

- See section on Anaphylaxis (above) for the treatment of cardiac arrest associated with anaphylaxis. Titrate IV adrenaline using 50 mcg boluses according to response. If repeated adrenaline doses are needed, start an IV adrenaline infusion. The pre-filled 10 mL syringe of 1:10 000 adrenaline contains 100 mcg mL^{-1}.

- See section on Toxins (above) for the treatment of systemic toxicity of local anaesthetics with IV lipid.

- Stop operative surgery unless it is addressing a reversible cause of the cardiac arrest.

Cardiac arrest following cardiac surgery

Cardiac arrest following major cardiac surgery is relatively common in the immediate post-operative phase. There are usually specific causes of cardiac arrest, such as tamponade, hypovolaemia, myocardial ischaemia, tension pneumothorax, or pacing failure. These are all potentially reversible and if treated promptly cardiac arrest after cardiac surgery has a relatively high survival rate.

- The key to successful resuscitation is recognition of the need to perform emergency resternotomy early, especially in the context of tamponade or haemorrhage, where externa,l chest compressions may be ineffective.

- If VF or asystole, attempt external defibrillation or emergency temporary pacing at maximum amplitude.

- Start external chest compressions immediately in patients who arrest with monitoring indicating no output. Verify the effectiveness of compressions by looking at the arterial trace, aiming to achieve a systolic blood pressure > 60 mmHg and a diastolic blood pressure > 25 mmHg at a rate of 100–120 min^{-1}. Inability to obtain these targets with external chest compressions indicates the need for emergency resternotomy because ineffective chest compressions may indicate cardiac tamponade and/or hypovolaemia.

- There is concern that external chest compressions can cause sternal disruption or cardiac damage.

- Consider other reversible causes:
  - Hypoxia – check tracheal tube position, use waveform capnography, and ventilate with 100% oxygen during resuscitation
  - Tension pneumothorax
  - Pacing failure – check pacing box output and pacing wire integrity. In asystole, secondary to a loss of cardiac pacing, chest compressions may be delayed momentarily as long as the surgically inserted temporary pacing wires can be connected rapidly and pacing re-established (DDD mode at 100 min^{-1} at maximum amplitude).

- Treat a witnessed and monitored VF/pVT cardiac arrest immediately with up to three quick successive (stacked) defibrillation attempts. Three failed shocks in the post-cardiac surgery setting should trigger the need for emergency resternotomy. Further defibrillation is attempted as indicated in the ALS algorithm and is performed with internal paddles at 20 J if resternotomy has been performed.

- Use adrenaline very cautiously and titrate to effect (IV doses of up to 100 mcg in adults). Consider amiodarone 300 mg in patients with refractory shockable rhythms (VF/pVT), but do not delay resternotomy. Atropine is not recommended for asystole and temporary or external pacing should be employed.

- Emergency resternotomy is an integral part of resuscitation after cardiac surgery, once all other reversible causes have been excluded. Once adequate airway and ventilation has been established, and if three attempts at defibrillation have failed in VF/pVT, undertake resternotomy without delay. Emergency resternotomy is also indicated in asystole or PEA, when other treatments have failed, and should be performed within 5 min of the cardiac arrest by anyone with appropriate training.

Drowning

Drowning is a common cause of accidental death. The World Health Organization (WHO) reports that every hour of every day, more than 40 people die from drowning. In general, males are much more likely to drown than females. In the UK, there are approximately 350 accidental deaths from drowning each year. Drowning is commonest in males aged 20–30, and occurs mostly in inland waters (e.g. lakes, rivers) and during summer months.

Definition of drowning

Drowning is defined as a process resulting in primary respiratory impairment from submersion/immersion in a liquid medium. Implicit in this definition is that a liquid/air interface is present at the entrance of the person's airway, preventing the person from breathing air. The person may live or die after this process, but whatever the outcome, they have been involved in a drowning incident.

Submersion occurs when the face is underwater or covered in water. Asphyxia and cardiac arrest occurs within a matter of minutes of submersion. Immersion, by contrast, is when the head remains above water, in most cases by means of the support of a lifejacket. In most situations of immersion, the person remains immersed with an open airway and becomes hypothermic, although aspiration of water may occur if water splashes over the face or if the person becomes unconscious with their face in the water. The difference between submersion and immersion is important in understanding the difference in epidemiology, pathophysiology, clinical course and prognosis.

Pathophysiology of drowning

Following submersion, the person initially breath holds by reflex, and frequently swallows water. As breath holding continues, hypoxia and hypercapnia develop. A reflex laryngospasm may temporarily prevent the entrance of water into the lungs. Eventually these reflexes abate and the person aspirates water. The key is that bradycardia as a consequence of hypoxia occurs before sustaining a cardiac arrest. Correction of hypoxaemia by ventilation-only resuscitation is critical and in itself may lead to ROSC in some cases, probably because the presence of a circulation had not been detected.

Water rescue

- Whenever possible, bystanders should attempt to save the drowning person without entry into the water. Talking to the person, reaching with a rescue aid (e.g. stick or clothing), or throwing a rope or buoyant rescue aid may be effective if the person is close to dry land.

- Rescue can present significant risk to the rescuer, but a sensible risk assessment is necessary to ensure that potentially survivable persons are rescued promptly.

- If entry into the water is essential, take a buoyant rescue aid, flotation device or boat. It is safer to enter the water with two rescuers than alone.

- Trained rescuers are often professionals with specialist equipment to assist with search and rescue and will base rescue efforts on the likelihood of survival. Submersion durations of less than 5–10 min are associated with a very high chance of a good outcome, and submersion durations of more than 25 min are associated with a low chance of good outcome.

- In the UK, combined emergency services guidance recommends review of search and rescue efforts at 30 and 60 min for submersion. Extended rescue efforts up to 90 min may be appropriate for children or those submerged in icy cold water, although the protective effects of extreme hypothermia are unlikely to be sufficient in the UK where water is insufficiently cold to cool rapidly and provide neuroprotection.

- Trained individuals should consider in-water ventilation (with the support of a buoyant rescue aid) only if there is likely to be a delay in reaching land or a rescue craft.

- Remove the person from the water promptly. The chances of a drowning person sustaining a spinal injury are very low. Spinal precautions are unnecessary unless there is a history of diving in shallow water, or signs of severe injury after water-slide use, water-skiing, kite-surfing, or watercraft racing. If the person is pulseless and apnoeic, remove them from the water as quickly as possible while attempting to limit neck flexion and extension.

- Hypovolaemia after prolonged immersion can cause cardiovascular collapse/arrest on removal from water, especially if the person is upright. Keep the person in a horizontal position during and after retrieval from the water.

Initial resuscitation once retrieved from water

- Check for response by opening the airway and check for signs of life. The drowning person rescued from the water within a few minutes of submersion is likely to exhibit abnormal (agonal) breathing. Do not confuse this with normal breathing.

- Give 5 initial ventilations, supplemented with oxygen if available.

- If the person has not responded to initial ventilations, place them on a firm surface before starting chest compressions. Provide CPR in a ratio of 30 compressions to 2 ventilations. Most drowning people will have sustained cardiac arrest secondary to hypoxia. In these patients, compression-only CPR is likely to be ineffective and should be avoided.

- Massive amounts of foam caused by mixing air with water and surfactant can sometimes come out of the mouth of people. If this occurs, continue rescue breaths/ventilation until an ALS provider arrives and is able to intubate the person's trachea.

- Regurgitation of stomach contents and swallowed water is common. If this prevents ventilation, turn the person on their side and remove the regurgitated material using directed suction if possible.

Modifications to advanced life support after drowning

Airway and breathing

- Give high-flow oxygen (10–15 L min^{-1}), ideally through a non-rebreather mask with reservoir to the spontaneously breathing person.

- For people who fail to respond to initial basic airway measures, who have a reduced level of consciousness or are in cardiac arrest, consider early tracheal intubation and controlled ventilation by skilled personnel. Reduced pulmonary compliance requiring high inflation pressures may limit the use of a supraglottic airway device.

- In the drowning person who has not arrested or who has achieved ROSC, titrate the inspired oxygen concentration to achieve an SpO$_2$ of 94–98%. Confirm adequate oxygenation and ventilation with arterial blood gases once available. Set positive end expiratory pressure (PEEP) to at least 5–10 cm H$_2$O. However, PEEP values of 15–20 cm H$_2$O may be required if the patient is severely hypoxaemic. Decompress the stomach with a gastric tube.

Circulation and defibrillation

- Palpation of the pulse as the sole indicator of the presence or absence of cardiac output is not always reliable, particularly in the wet and cold drowning patient. As soon as possible, check the ECG and end-tidal CO$_2$ and consider echocardiography to confirm the presence or not of a cardiac output.

- If the person is in cardiac arrest, follow standard ALS protocols. If the person is hypothermic, modify the approach in accordance with the guidance for treatment of hypothermia (see below).

- Assess the rhythm and attempt defibrillation if indicated according to standard guidelines. Dry the person's chest before applying defibrillator pads.
- After prolonged immersion, most people will have become hypovolaemic as the hydrostatic pressure of water on the body is removed. Give rapid IV fluid to correct hypovolaemia. This should commence out-of-hospital, if transfer time is prolonged.

Discontinuing resuscitation efforts

- Making a decision to discontinue resuscitation efforts on a person of drowning is difficult. No single factor accurately predicts good or poor survival. Frequently, decisions may later prove to have been incorrect.
- Continue resuscitation unless there is clear evidence that such attempts are futile (e.g. massive traumatic injuries, rigor mortis, putrefaction etc.), or timely evacuation to a medical facility is not possible.
- Neurologically favourable outcomes have been reported in several people submerged for longer than 25 min, however these rare case reports almost invariably occur in children submerged in ice-cold water, when immersion hypothermia has preceded hypoxia or in submersion of car occupants. A retrospective study of 160 children who drowned in the Netherlands found that outcomes were extremely poor if ALS took longer than 30 min to achieve ROSC even if hypothermia was present.

Post-resuscitation care after drowning

- Follow standard post-resuscitation guidelines (Chapter 13).
- Many people of drowning are at risk of developing acute respiratory distress syndrome (ARDS) and standard protective ventilation strategies for ARDS should be followed.
- Extracorporeal membrane oxygenation (ECMO) has been used for those in refractory cardiac arrest, those with refractory hypoxaemia and in selected cases of submersion in ice cold water, although success rates remain low.
- Pneumonia is common after drowning. Prophylactic antibiotics have not been shown to be of benefit but they may be considered after submersion in grossly contaminated water such as sewage.
- Neurological outcome, notably severe permanent neurological damage, is primarily determined by the duration of hypoxia.

Accidental hypothermia

Hypothermia exists when the body core temperature is below 35°C and is classified arbitrarily as mild (32–35°C), moderate (28–32°C), or severe (< 28°C). The Swiss staging system based on clinical signs can be used by rescuers at the scene to describe people:

Stage I: mild hypothermia (conscious, shivering, core temperature 35–32°C).

Stage II: moderate hypothermia (impaired consciousness without shivering, core temperature 32–28°C).

Stage III: severe hypothermia (unconscious, vital signs present, core temperature 28–24°C).

Stage IV: cardiac arrest or low flow state (no or minimal vital signs, core temperature < 24°C).

Stage V: death due to irreversible hypothermia (core temperature < 11.8°C).

Diagnosis of hypothermia

- Accidental hypothermia may be under-diagnosed in warmer weather. When thermoregulation is impaired, for example, in the elderly and very young, hypothermia may follow a mild insult. The risk of hypothermia is increased by alcohol or drug ingestion, exhaustion, illness, injury or neglect. Risk increases when there is a decrease in the level of consciousness.
- Hypothermia may be suspected from the clinical history or a brief external examination of a collapsed patient.
- A low-reading thermometer is needed to measure core temperature and confirm the diagnosis.
  - The core temperature in the lower third of the oesophagus correlates well with heart temperature, but measurement can only be performed in patients with an advanced airway.
  - Tympanic measurement with a thermocouple-based device is a reliable alternative, but may be considerably lower than core temperature if the environment is very cold, the probe is not well insulated, or the external auditory canal is filled with snow or water.
  - Commonly used tympanic thermometers based on infrared technique do not seal the ear canal and are not designed for low core temperature readings.
- Once in hospital, use a consistent core temperature measurement site throughout resuscitation and rewarming. Bladder and rectal temperatures lag behind core temperature and are not recommended in patients with severe hypothermia.

Decision to resuscitate the hypothermic patient

- Cooling of the human body decreases cellular oxygen consumption by about 6% per 1°C decrease in core temperature. In some cases, hypothermia can exert a protective effect on the brain and vital organs and intact neurological recovery is possible, even after prolonged cardiac arrest if deep hypothermia develops before asphyxia.

- Beware of diagnosing death in a hypothermic patient, because hypothermia can produce a very slow, small-volume, irregular pulse and unrecordable blood pressure. In a hypothermic patient, no signs of life (Swiss hypothermia stage IV) alone are unreliable for declaring death. At 18°C the brain can tolerate periods of circulatory arrest for ten times longer than at 37°C. Dilated pupils can be caused by a variety of insults and must not be regarded as a sign of death. Survival has been reported after cardiac arrest and a core temperature of 11.7°C.

- Intermittent CPR during rescue can be of benefit if continuous CPR cannot be delivered. In these circumstances, in a patient with hypothermic cardiac arrest and a core temperature < 28°C (or unknown), give 5 min of CPR, alternating with periods ≤ 5 min without CPR. Patients with a core temperature < 20°C, should receive 5 min of CPR, alternating with periods of up to 10 min without CPR.

- In the pre-hospital setting, resuscitation should be withheld only if the cause of a cardiac arrest is clearly attributable to a lethal injury, fatal illness, prolonged asphyxia, or if the chest is incompressible. In all other patients the traditional guiding principle that 'no one is dead until warm and dead' should be considered. In remote wilderness areas, the impracticalities of achieving rewarming have to be considered. In the hospital setting, involve senior doctors and use clinical judgment to determine when to stop resuscitating a hypothermic arrest patient.

Modifications to advanced life support in the hypothermic patient

- Check for signs of life for up to 1 min. Palpate a central artery and assess the cardiac rhythm (if ECG monitor available). Capnography, echocardiography, near-infrared spectroscopy or ultrasound with Doppler can be used to establish whether there is an adequate cardiac output or peripheral blood flow. If there is any doubt, start CPR immediately.

- Hypothermia can cause stiffness of the chest wall, making ventilations and chest compressions difficult. Consider the use of mechanical chest compression devices.

- Do not delay careful tracheal intubation when it is indicated. The advantages of adequate oxygenation and protection from aspiration outweigh the minimal risk of triggering VF by performing tracheal intubation.

- Once CPR is under way, confirm hypothermia with a low-reading thermometer.

- The hypothermic heart may be unresponsive to cardioactive drugs, attempted electrical pacing and defibrillation. Drug metabolism is slowed, leading to potentially toxic plasma concentrations of any drug given. The evidence for the efficacy of drugs in severe hypothermia is limited.

  - Withhold adrenaline, and other CPR drugs until the patient has been warmed to a core temperature ≥ 30°C.

  - Once 30°C has been reached, the intervals between drug doses should be doubled when compared to normothermia (i.e. adrenaline every 6–10 min).

  - As normothermia is approached (≥ 35°C), use standard drug protocols.

  - If VF is detected, defibrillate according to standard protocols. If VF persists after three shocks, delay further attempts until core temperature is ≥ 30°C. CPR and rewarming may have to be continued for several hours to facilitate successful defibrillation.

  - If prolonged transport required, or terrain difficult, a mechanical CPR device is recommended.

  - Perform continuous CPR during transfer if possible; delayed CPR may be used in arrested patients < 28°C when CPR on-site is not possible or too dangerous.

  - In-hospital prognostication of successful rewarming should be based on the HOPE or ICE scores.

Rewarming after accidental hypothermia

General Principles

- General measures for all people include removal from the cold environment, prevention of further heat loss and rapid transfer to hospital.

- In the field, a patient with moderate or severe hypothermia (hypothermia stage ≥ II) should be immobilised and handled carefully, oxygenated adequately, monitored (including ECG and core temperature), and the whole body dried and insulated.

- Remove wet clothes, while minimising excessive movement of the person.

- Conscious people (hypothermia stage I) can mobilise as exercise rewarms a person more rapidly than shivering.

- Patients will continue cooling after removal from a cold environment (i.e. after drop). This can result in a life-threatening decrease in core temperature triggering a cardiac arrest during transport (i.e. 'rescue death').

Patients who stop shivering (e.g. hypothermia stage II– IV, and those sedated or anaesthetised patients) will cool faster.

Pre-hospital rewarming and transfer

- Rewarming may be passive, active external, or active internal.

- In mild hypothermia, passive rewarming is appropriate as patients are still able to shiver. This is best achieved by full body insulation with wool blankets, aluminium foil, cap and a warm environment.

- In hypothermia stages II–IV, the application of chemical heat packs to the trunk has been recommended. In conscious patients who are able to shiver, this improves comfort but does not speed rewarming. If the patient is unconscious and the airway is not secured, arrange the insulation around the patient lying in a recovery (lateral decubitus) position.

- Rewarming in the field with heated intravenous fluids and warm humidified gases is not feasible.

- Intensive active rewarming must not delay transport to a hospital where advanced rewarming techniques, continuous monitoring and observation are available.

- Patients with signs of imminent cardiac arrest (temperature < 30°C, ventricular arrythmia, or systolic blood pressure < 90mmHg) should be transferred directly to an 'ECMO centre' in settings where this is feasible.

In-hospital rewarming and post-resuscitation care

- Pre-arrest rewarm using active external methods (i.e. with forced warm air) and minimally invasively methods (i.e. with warm IV infusions).

- In deteriorating hypothermic patients, or those in hypothermic cardiac arrest, rewarming should be performed with extra-corporeal life support (ECLS), preferably using ECMO in preference to cardiopulmonary bypass.

  - Non-ECLS rewarming should be initiated in a peripheral hospital if an ECLS centre cannot be reached within 6 h.

  - Where an ECLS centre is not available, rewarming can be attempted using a combination of external and internal rewarming techniques (e.g. forced warm air, warm infusions, forced peritoneal lavage).

  - Continuous haemodynamic monitoring and warm IV fluids are essential. Patients will require large volumes of IV fluids during rewarming, as vasodilation causes expansion of the intravascular space. Avoid hyperthermia during and after rewarming.

  - Once ROSC has been achieved, use standard post-resuscitation care.

Hyperthermia

Hyperthermia occurs when the body's ability to thermoregulate fails and core temperature exceeds that normally maintained by homeostatic mechanisms.

Hyperthermia may be exogenous, caused by environmental conditions or secondary to endogenous heat production.

Environment-related hyperthermia occurs where heat, usually in the form of radiant energy, is absorbed by the body at a rate faster than can be lost by thermoregulatory mechanisms. Hyperthermia occurs along a continuum of heat-related conditions starting with heat stress, progressing to heat exhaustion, heat stroke and culminating in multi-organ dysfunction and cardiac arrest in some instances.

Malignant hyperthermia (MH) is a rare disorder of skeletal muscle calcium homeostasis characterised by muscle contracture and life-threatening hypermetabolic crisis following exposure of genetically predisposed individuals to halogenated anaesthetics and depolarising muscle relaxants.

Hyperthermia and malignant hyperthemia

Hyperthermia occurs due to failed thermoregulation, leading to the body temperature increasing above normothermia (36.5–37.5°C). Due to increasing global temperatures, the incidence of hyperthermia is rising. Malignant hyperthermia is a form of hyperthermia, caused by administration of anaesthetic drugs to individuals with a genetic predisposition to malignant hyperthermia.

Hyperthermia is a continuum of heat-related illness ranging from milder illness (heat syncope) to severe illness (heat stroke). In heat stroke, a systemic inflammatory response causes changes in mental state and organ dysfunction. This may lead to cardiac arrest.

Mortality from heat stroke ranges between 10–33%. There are two forms of heat stroke:

1. Classic non-exertional heat stroke occurs during high environmental temperatures.

2. Exertional heat stroke occurs during strenuous physical exercise in high environmental temperatures and/or high humidity and usually effects healthy young adults.

Predisposing factors for hyperthermia

The key risk associated factor associated with heat stroke is an impaired ability to sweat. The elderly are at increased risk for heat-related illness because of underlying illness, medication use, declining thermoregulatory mechanisms, and limited social support. There are several other risk factors, including: lack of acclimatisation, dehydration, obesity, alcohol, cardiovascular disease, skin conditions (e.g. psoriasis, eczema) hyperthyroidism, phaeochromocytoma, and medication use (e.g. anticholinergics, diamorphine, cocaine, amphetamine, phenothiazines, sympathomimetics, calcium channel blockers, beta-blockers).

Clinical presentation of hyperthermia

The clinical presentation of hyperthermia depends both on the severity of illness, which is associated with core body temperature.

Patients with milder forms of hyperthermia (e.g. heat syncope, heat exhaustion) may present with intense thirst, weakness, syncope, dizziness.

The diagnosis of heat stroke is based on a triad of clinical symptoms:

- Severe hyperthermia with core body temperature > 40°C
- Neurological symptoms (including confusion, seizure, coma)
- Exposure to high environmental temperatures (classic heat stroke) or recent strenuous physical exertion (exertional heat stroke).

Other symptoms include tachycardia, tachypnoea, hypotension, organ failure, and hot, dry skin.

Heat stroke can resemble septic shock and may be caused by similar mechanisms.

Patients with milder forms of heat-related illness may present with normal or increased body temperature, syncope, dizziness, thirst, anxiety and weakness.

Other clinical conditions presenting with increased core temperature need to be considered, including drug toxicity, drug withdrawal syndrome, serotonin syndrome, neuroleptic malignant syndrome, sepsis, central nervous system infection, endocrine disorders (e.g. thyroid storm, phaeochromocytoma).

Treatment of hyperthermia

Treatment for heat stroke is time-critical and comprises supportive therapy to optimise airway, breathing, circulation, and disability. Key treatments include:

- The patient should be transferred to a cool environment and laid flat.
- Immediately start cooling and begin transfer to hospital.
- Patients should be cooled to < 39°C (ideally 38.0–38.5°C). Rapid cooling is safe (cooling rates of 0.2–0.35°C min^{-1} are achievable).
- Measurement of core body temperature should be used to guide treatment.
- The most rapid cooling is achieved with cold-water immersion or full-body conductive cooling systems.

If these systems are not available or not practical, then use any available system to achieve the most rapid rate of cooling (e.g. misting/ fanning/ cool IV fluids/ extracorporeal circuits/ intravascular cooling).

- Administer intravenous isotonic or hypertonic fluids. Hypertonic fluid is recommended when blood sodium is ≤ 130 mmol L (up to 3 x 100 mL NaCl 3% may be administered).
- Large volumes of intravenous fluid may be required to support blood pressure.
- Correct electrolytes abnormalities.
- Patients with severe heat stroke need to be managed in a critical care setting.
- No specific drugs are recommended to support cooling.
- Seizures should be treated in accordance with local protocols.
- If cardiac arrest occurs, continue active cooling and follow standard advanced life support and cool the patient. Animal studies suggest the prognosis is poor compared with normothermic cardiac arrest. The risk of unfavourable neurological outcome increases for each degree of body temperature > 37°C.

Patients with milder forms of heat-related illness should be removed to a cool environment and laid flat. The patient should be given isotonic or hypertonic fluid via the oral or intravenous route (depending on severity of their condition). If intravenous fluid is required, then 1–2 litres crystalloid at 500 mL h^{-1} is typically adequate. Correction of electrolyte abnormalities should be considered. If cooling is required, then simple strategies (e.g. fanning/ misting) are likely to be sufficient.

Malignant hyperthermia

Malignant hyperthermia is a rare, life-threatening genetic sensitivity of skeletal muscles to volatile anaesthetics and depolarising neuromuscular blocking drugs occurring during or after anaesthesia. In the event of malignant hyperthermia:

- stop triggering agents immediately
- give oxygen
- correct acidosis and electrolyte abnormalities
- start active cooling
- give dantrolene.

If the patient sustains a cardiac arrest, continue active cooling and follow the standard ALS algorithm. Patients should be carefully monitored following treatment as relapse occurs in 25% patients within 72 h. Other drugs such as 3,4-methylenedioxymethamphetamine (MDMA, 'ecstasy') and amphetamines also cause a condition similar to malignant hyperthermia and the use of dantrolene may be beneficial.

Obesity

Effective CPR in obese patients can be challenging due to difficulties with:

- access and transportation
- airway management
- vascular access
- high-quality chest compressions
- defibrillation.

It may not be possible to move obese patients so they are supine and on a firm surface. In morbidly obese patients access to the chest may be physically limited. A step or platform may be required. Chest compressions can be performed from the head end of the patient if necessary. Provide standard chest compressions up to a maximum of 6 cm.

Intravenous access may be extremely challenging and the intraosseous route should be considered early. Standard doses of drugs should be used.

Manual ventilation with a bag-mask should be minimised and be performed by experienced staff using a two-person technique in order to avoid gastric inflation. If a supraglottic airway (SGA) is inserted then leaks may occur necessitating a standard 30:2 compression-ventilation ratio. An experienced provider should intubate the trachea early so that the period of bag-mask ventilation is minimised. Tracheal intubation may be particularly difficult and higher airway pressures should also be anticipated.

Placement of defibrillator pads may be technically demanding. Consider escalating defibrillation energy to maximum for repeated shocks.

12: Summary learning

The conditions described in this chapter account for a large proportion of cardiac arrests in younger patients.

Use the ABCDE approach for early recognition and treatment to prevent cardiac arrest.

High-quality CPR and treatment of reversible causes is the mainstay of treatment of cardiac arrest from any cause.

Call for expert help early when specialist procedures are needed (e.g. delivery of the fetus for cardiac arrest in pregnancy).

My key take-home messages from this chapter are:

Further reading

Alfonzo AV, Harrison A, Baines R, et al. Clinical Practice Guidelines Treatment of Acute Hyperkalaemia in Adults. The Renal Association. 2020 https://renal.org/sites/renal.org/files/RENAL%20ASSOCIATION%20HYPERKALAEMIA%20GUIDELINE%202020.pdf

Aseni P, Rizzetto F, Grande AM, et al. Emergency Department Resuscitative Thoracotomy: Indications, surgical procedure and outcome. A narrative review. Am J Surg. 2020 Oct 2;S0002-9610(20)30607-3. doi: 10.1016/j.amjsurg.2020.09.038.

Brown DJ, Brugger H, Boyd J, Paal P. Accidental hypothermia. N Engl J Med 2012;367:1930-8.

Chu J, Johnston TA, Geoghegan J, on behalf of the Royal College of Obstetricians and Gynaecologists. Maternal Collapse in Pregnancy and the Puerperium. BJOG 2020;127:e14–e52.

Dunning J, Fabbri A, Kolh PH, et al. Guideline for resuscitation in cardiac arrest after cardiac surgery. Eur J Cardiothorac Surg 2009;36:3-28.

Epstein Y, Yanovich R. Heatstroke. N Engl J Med. 2019 Jun 20;380(25):2449-2459.

Global Asthma Network. Global asthma report 2018. http://www.globalasthmareport.org/resources/global_asthma_report_2018.pdf

Hopkins PM, Girard T, Dalay S, Jenkins B, Thacker A, Patteril M, McGrady E. Malignant hyperthermia 2020: Guideline from the Association of Anaesthetists. Anaesthesia. 2021 Jan 5. doi: 10.1111/anae.15317.

Ildris AH, Bierens JJLM, Perkins GD, Wenzel V, et al. 2015 Revised Utstein-Style Recommended Guidelines for Uniform Reporting of Data From Drowning-Related Resuscitation: An ILCOR Advisory Statement. Circ Cardiovasc Qual Outcomes. 2017 Jul;10(7):e000024.

Lipman S, Cohen S, Einav S, et al. The Society for Obstetric Anesthesia and Perinatology consensus statement on the management of cardiac arrest in pregnancy. Anesthesia and analgesia 2014;118:1003-16.

Lockey DJ, Lyon RM, Davies GE. Development of a simple algorithm to guide the effective management of traumatic cardiac arrest. Resuscitation 2013;84:738-42.

Lott C, Truhlár A, Alfonzo A, Barelli A, González-Salvado V, Hinkelbein J, Nolan JP, Paal P, Perkins GD, Thies K-C, Yeung J, Zideman DA, Soar J. European Resuscitation Council Guidelines 2021: Cardiac arrest in special circumstances. Resuscitation. 2021;161.

Management of Severe Local Anaesthetic Toxicity. Association of Anaesthetists of Great Britain and Ireland, 2010. www.aagbi.org

Muraro A, Roberts G, Worm M, et al. Anaphylaxis: guidelines from the European Academy of Allergy and Clinical Immunology. Allergy 2014;69:1026-45.

National Institute for Clinical Excellence. Pre-hospital initiation of fluid replacement therapy for trauma. London: National Institute for Clinical Excellence; 2004.

National Institute for Health and Care Excellence. [CG134] Anaphylaxis: assessment to confirm an anaphylactic episode and the decision to refer after emergency treatment for a suspected anaphylactic episode.2011. https://www.nice.org.uk/guidance/cg134

Nolan JP, Böttiger BW, Cariou A, Cronberg T, Friberg H, Gengrugge C, Haywood K, Lilja G, Moulaert VRM, Nikolaou N, Olasveengen TM, Skrifvars MB, Taccone FS, Soar J. European Resuscitation Council and European Society of Intensive Care Medicine Guidelines 2021: Post-resuscitation Care. Resuscitation. 2021;161.

Olasveengen TM, Mancini ME, Perkins GD, et al. Adult Basic Life Support: International Consensus on Cardiopulmonary Resuscitation and Emergency Cardiovascular Care Science With Treatment Recommendations. Adult Basic Life Support Collaborators. Resuscitation. 2020 Nov;156:A35-A79.

Resuscitation Council (UK). Management of cardiac arrest during neurosurgery in adults. 2014. www.resus.org.uk/library/publications/publication-management-cardiac-arrest-during

Royal College of Physicians. Why asthma still kills: the national review of asthma deaths (NRAD). Confidential Enquiry Report 2014. http://www.rcplondon.ac.uk/sites/default/files/why-asthma-still-kills-full- report.pdf.)

BTS/SIGN British guideline on the management of asthma. 2019. https://www.brit-thoracic.org.uk/quality-improvement/guidelines/asthma

Soar J, Berg KM, Andersen LW, et al. Adult Advanced Life Support: 2020 International Consensus on Cardiopulmonary Resuscitation and Emergency Cardiovascular Care Science with Treatment Recommendations. Resuscitation. 2020 Nov;156:A80-A119.

Soar J, Pumphrey R, Cant A, et al. Emergency treatment of anaphylactic reactions–guidelines for healthcare providers. Resuscitation 2008;77:157-69.

Soar J, Böttiger BW, Carli P, Couper K, Deakin CD, Djärv T, Lott C, Olasveengen TM, Paal P, Pellis T, Perkins GD, Sandroni C, Nolan JP. European Resuscitation Council Guidelines 2021: Advanced Life Support. Resuscitation. 2021;161.

Surviving Sepsis Campaign http://www.survivingsepsis.org/

Szpilman D, Bierens JJ, Handley AJ, Orlowski JP. Drowning. New Eng J Med 2012;366:2102-10.

Zafren K, Durrer B, Herry JP, Brugger H. Lightning injuries: prevention and on- site treatment in mountains and remote areas. Official guidelines of the International Commission for Mountain Emergency Medicine and the Medical Commission of the International Mountaineering and Climbing Federation (ICAR and UIAA MEDCOM). Resuscitation 2005;65:369-72.

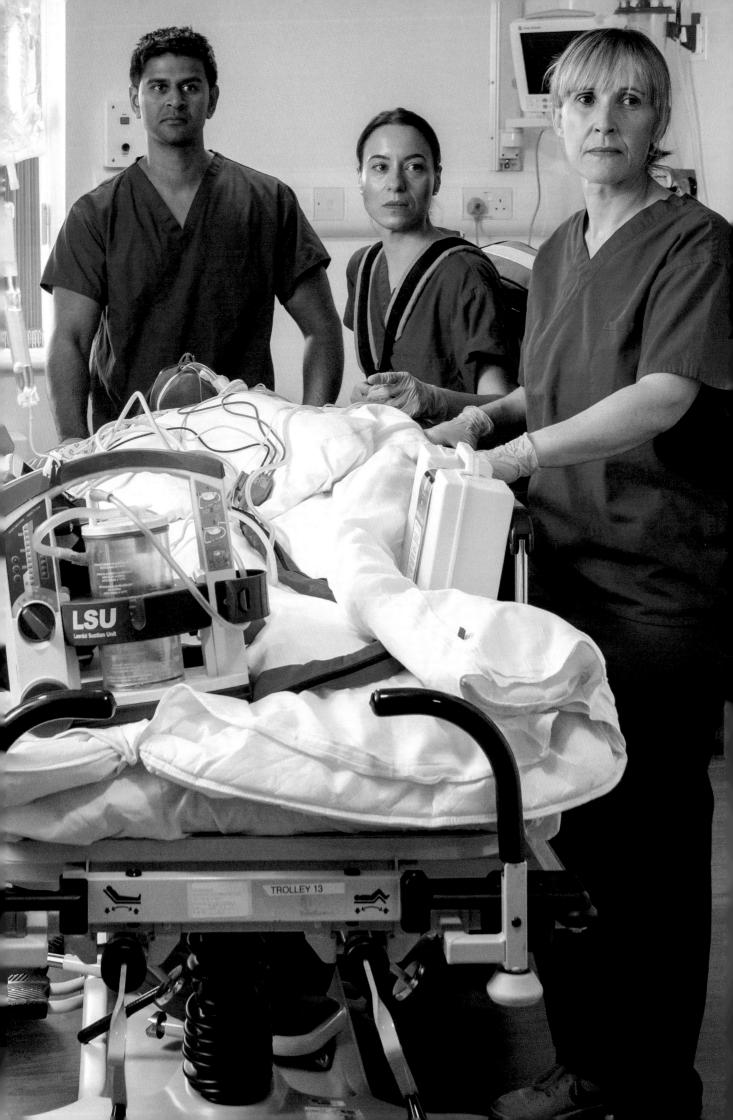

Post-resuscitation care

In this chapter

The post-cardiac arrest syndrome

Optimising organ function

The post-resuscitation care algorithm

Prognostication

The learning outcomes will enable you to:

Understand the need for continued resuscitation after return of spontaneous circulation

Understand the post-cardiac arrest syndrome

Facilitate safe transfer of the patient

Consider the role and limitations of assessing prognosis after cardiac arrest

Introduction

Return of a spontaneous circulation (ROSC) is an important step in the continuum of resuscitation. However, the next goal is to return the patient to a state of normal cerebral function, and to establish and maintain a stable cardiac rhythm and normal haemodynamic function. This requires further treatment, tailored to each patient's individual needs.

The quality of treatment provided in this post-resuscitation phase – the final ring in the Chain of Survival – significantly influences the patient's ultimate outcome. The post-resuscitation phase starts at the location where ROSC is achieved but, once stabilised, the patient needs transfer to the most appropriate high-care area (e.g. intensive care unit (ICU), coronary care unit (CCU)) for continued monitoring and treatment.

The post-cardiac arrest syndrome

The post-cardiac arrest syndrome comprises:

- post-cardiac arrest brain injury
- post-cardiac arrest myocardial dysfunction
- systemic ischaemia/reperfusion response
- persistent precipitating pathology.

The severity of this syndrome will vary with the duration and cause of cardiac arrest. It may not occur at all if the cardiac arrest is brief. Post-cardiac arrest brain injury manifests as coma, seizures, myoclonus, varying degrees of neurocognitive dysfunction and brain death. Post-cardiac arrest brain injury may be exacerbated by microcirculatory failure, impaired autoregulation, hypotension, hypercarbia, hypoxaemia, hyperoxaemia, pyrexia, hypoglycaemia, hyperglycaemia and seizures. Significant myocardial dysfunction is common after cardiac arrest but typically starts to recover by 2–3 days, although full recovery may take significantly longer. The whole body ischaemia/reperfusion of cardiac arrest activates immune and coagulation pathways contributing to multiple organ failure and increasing the risk of infection. Thus, the post-cardiac arrest syndrome has many features in common with sepsis, including intravascular volume depletion, vasodilation, endothelial injury and abnormalities of the microcirculation.

> The quality of treatment provided in the post-resuscitation phase significantly influences the patient's ultimate outcome

Continued resuscitation

In the immediate post-resuscitation phase, pending transfer to an appropriate high-care area, treat the patient by following the ABCDE approach described in the post-resuscitation care algorithm (Figure 13.1).

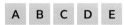

Airway and breathing

Following most cardiac arrests tracheal intubation will occur during CPR or if the patient remains comatose after ROSC. Tracheal intubation following ROSC in comatose patients will facilitate post-resuscitation care that includes controlled oxygenation and ventilation, protection of the lungs from aspiration of stomach contents, control of seizures, and temperature control. Consider tracheal intubation, sedation and controlled ventilation in any patient with obtunded cerebral function.

Patients who have had a brief period of cardiac arrest and have responded immediately to appropriate treatment (e.g. witnessed ventricular fibrillation (VF) reverting to sinus rhythm after early defibrillation) may achieve an immediate return of normal cerebral function. These patients do not require tracheal intubation and ventilation, but should be given oxygen by face mask to maintain a normal arterial oxygen saturation.

Hypoxaemia and hypercarbia both increase the likelihood of a further cardiac arrest and may contribute to secondary brain injury. Several animal studies indicate that hyperoxaemia (excessively high arterial blood oxygen concentration) causes oxidative stress and harms post-ischaemic neurones. Observational studies in humans have produced conflicting results: most, but not all, have shown an association between hyperoxaemia and a poor outcome. Based on this evidence, as soon as arterial blood oxygen saturation can be monitored reliably (by blood gas analysis and/or pulse oximetry (SpO_2)), adjust the inspired oxygen concentration to maintain the arterial blood oxygen saturation in the range of 94–98%.

After ROSC, blood carbon dioxide values ($PaCO_2$) are commonly increased because of intra-arrest hypoventilation and poor tissue perfusion, causing a mixed respiratory acidosis and metabolic acidosis. Increased $PaCO_2$ (hypercapnia) increases cerebral blood flow, cerebral blood volume and intracerebral pressure. Hypocapnia causes vasoconstriction that may decrease blood flow and cause cerebral ischaemia. Observational studies using cardiac arrest registries document an association between hypocapnia and poor neurological outcome; therefore, adjust ventilation to achieve normocarbia and monitor this using the end-tidal CO_2 and arterial blood gas values.

Examine the patient's chest and look for symmetrical chest movement. Listen to ensure that the breath sounds are equal on both sides. A tracheal tube that has been inserted too far will tend to go down the right main bronchus and fail to ventilate the left lung. If ribs have been fractured during chest compression (documented in up to 70% of out-of-hospital cardiac arrests receiving CPR) there may be a pneumothorax (reduced or absent breath sounds) or a flail chest wall segment. Listen for evidence of pulmonary oedema or pulmonary aspiration of gastric contents. Insert a gastric tube – this will decompress the stomach following mouth-to-mouth or bag-mask ventilation, prevent splinting of the diaphragm, and enable drainage of gastric contents.

Circulation

Cardiac rhythm and haemodynamic function are likely to be unstable following a cardiac arrest. Continuous monitoring of the ECG is essential. Seek evidence of poor cardiac function. Record the pulse and blood pressure and assess peripheral perfusion: warm, pink digits with a rapid capillary refill usually imply adequate perfusion. Grossly distended neck veins when the patient is semi-upright may indicate right ventricular failure, but in rare cases could indicate pericardial tamponade. Left ventricular failure may be indicated by fine inspiratory crackles heard on auscultation of the lungs, and the production of pink frothy sputum. If the facility for direct continuous arterial blood pressure monitoring is available (e.g. in the emergency department) insert an arterial cannula to enable reliable monitoring during transfer. Once in a high-care area, insert a central venous catheter to enable infusion of multiple drugs and consider use of non-invasive cardiac output monitoring device. Infusion of fluids may be required to increase right heart filling pressures or conversely, diuretics and vasodilators may be needed to treat left ventricular failure.

Record a 12-lead ECG as soon as possible. Acute ST-segment elevation or new left bundle branch block in a patient with a typical history of acute myocardial infarction is an indication for treatment to try to re-open an occluded coronary artery (reperfusion therapy) – this is usually achieved by emergency percutaneous coronary intervention (PCI) (Chapter 4). Services should aim to achieve a 'call-to-balloon' time (i.e. time from call for help to attempted re-opening of the culprit artery) of < 120 min whenever possible. If this is not feasible consider fibrinolytic therapy. Cardiopulmonary resuscitation, even if prolonged, is not a contraindication to fibrinolytic therapy.

In OHCA patients without ST-segment elevation, several large observational series showed that absence of ST-segment elevation does not completely exclude the presence of a recent coronary occlusion. For this reason, primary PCI should be considered and discussed with an interventional cardiologist in all post-cardiac-arrest patients who are suspected of having coronary

Adult post-resuscitation care

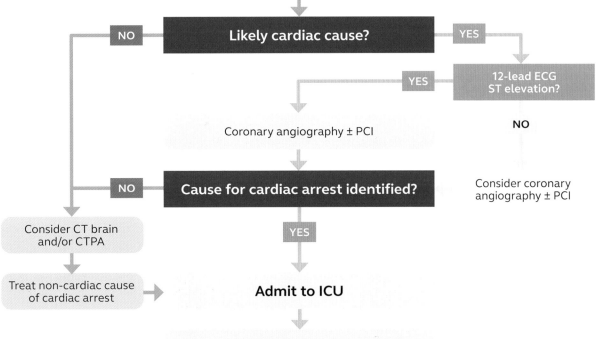

IMMEDIATE TREATMENT

Airway and breathing
- Maintain SpO$_2$ 94–98%
- Insert advanced airway
- Waveform capnography
- Ventilate lungs to normocapnia

Circulation
- 12-lead ECG
- Obtain reliable intravenous access
- Aim for SBP >100 mmHg
- Fluid (crystalloid) – restore normovolaemia
- Intra-arterial blood pressure monitoring
- Consider vasopressor/inotrope to maintain SBP

Control temperature
- Constant temperature 32–36°C
- Sedation; control shivering

DIAGNOSIS

Likely cardiac cause? NO / YES

YES — **12-lead ECG ST elevation?**

NO — Consider coronary angiography ± PCI

Coronary angiography ± PCI

Cause for cardiac arrest identified? NO / YES

NO — Consider CT brain and/or CTPA → Treat non-cardiac cause of cardiac arrest

YES — **Admit to ICU**

OPTIMISING RECOVERY

ICU management
- Temperature control: constant temperature 32–36°C for ≥ 24 h; prevent fever for at least 72 h
- Maintain normoxia and normocapnia; protective ventilation
- Avoid hypotension
- Echocardiography
- Maintain normoglycaemia
- Diagnose/treat seizures (EEG, sedation, anti-epileptic drugs)
- Delay prognostication for at least 72 h

Functional assessments before hospital discharge

Structured follow-up after hospital discharge

Rehabilitation

Secondary prevention
e.g. ICD, screen for inherited disorders, risk factor management

Figure 13.1 Post-resuscitation care algorithm – **SBP** systolic blood pressure, **PCI** percutaneous coronary intervention, **CTPA** computed tomography pulmonary angiogram, **ICU** Intensive care unit, **MAP** mean arterial pressure, **CO/CI** cardiac output/cardiac index, **EEG** electroencephalography, **ICD** implanted cardioverter defibrillator

artery disease as the cause of their arrest, even if they are sedated and mechanically ventilated. The decision for early coronary angiography is based on the presence of haemodynamic or electrical instability and ongoing myocardial ischaemia, while taking into account comorbidities, symptoms before arrest, initial cardiac rhythm for cardiac arrest, ECG pattern post ROSC, and echocardiography. In patients with a low probability of an ischaemic cause of cardiac arrest, delaying coronary angiography for few hours or days may buy time for initial management in ICU, enabling early initiation of post-resuscitation care (haemodynamic optimisation, protective ventilation, TTM) and prognostication. This 'wait and see' strategy will avoid coronary angiography altogether in patients with the lowest probability of an acute coronary lesion. These two strategies (early versus delayed coronary angiography) were evaluated in patients with VF OHCA and without evidence of shock in a randomised controlled trial that showed no difference in 90 day survival.

Disability and exposure

Although cardiac arrest is frequently caused by primary cardiac disease, other precipitating conditions must be excluded, particularly in-hospital patients (e.g. massive blood loss, respiratory failure, pulmonary embolism). Assess the other body systems rapidly so that further resuscitation can be targeted at the patient's needs. To examine the patient properly full exposure of the body may be necessary.

Although it may not be of immediate significance to the patient's management, assess neurological function rapidly and record the Glasgow Coma Scale score (Table 13.1). The maximum score possible is 15; the minimum score possible is 3.

Consider the need for targeted temperature management (TTM) in any patient who remains comatose after initial resuscitation from cardiac arrest (see below). When TTM is considered an appropriate treatment, it should started as soon as possible – do not wait until the patient is in the ICU before starting to cool.

Further assessment

History

Obtain a comprehensive history as quickly as possible. Those involved in caring for the patient immediately before the cardiac arrest may be able to help (e.g. emergency medical personnel, primary/community care physician, and relatives). Consider other causes of cardiac arrest if there is little to suggest primary cardiac disease (e.g. drug overdose, subarachnoid haemorrhage). Make a note of any delay before the start of resuscitation (no-flow time), and the duration of the resuscitation (low-flow time); this may have prognostic significance, although is generally unreliable and certainly should not

Table 13.1   The Glasgow Coma Scale score

Eye opening	Spontaneously	4
	To speech	3
	To pain	2
	Nil	1
Verbal	Oriented	5
	Confused	4
	Inappropriate words	3
	Incomprehensible sounds	2
	Nil	1
Best motor response	Obeys commands	6
	Localises	5
	Normal flexion	4
	Abnormal flexion	3
	Extension	2
	Nil	1

be used alone to predict outcome. The patient's baseline physiological reserve (before the cardiac arrest) is one of the most important factors taken into consideration by the ICU team when determining whether prolonged multiple organ support is appropriate.

Monitoring

Continuous monitoring of ECG, arterial blood pressure, respiratory rate, pulse oximetry, capnography, core temperature and urinary output is essential to detect changes during the period of instability that follows resuscitation from cardiac arrest.

Investigations

Several physiological variables may be abnormal immediately after a cardiac arrest and urgent biochemical and cardiological investigations should be undertaken (Table 13.2).

Arterial blood gases

Guidance on the interpretation of arterial blood gas values is given in Chapter 15.

Hypoperfusion during the period of cardiac arrest will usually cause a metabolic acidosis. This will cause a low pH (acidaemia), low standard bicarbonate, a base deficit, and a high lactate value. The rate at which the acidaemia and lactataemia resolves in the post-resuscitation period is an important guide to the adequacy of tissue perfusion. The most effective way of correcting any acidaemia is by addressing the underlying cause. For example, poor peripheral perfusion is treated best by giving fluid and inotropic drugs and not by giving sodium bicarbonate.

Giving bicarbonate may, paradoxically, increase intracellular acidosis, as it is converted to carbon dioxide with the release of hydrogen ions within the cell.

Table 13.2 Investigations after restoration of circulation

Full blood count	To exclude anaemia as a contributor to myocardial ischaemia and provide baseline values	
Biochemistry	To assess renal function	
	To assess electrolyte concentrations (K$^+$, Mg^{2+}, and Ca^{2+})	
	To ensure normoglycaemia	
	To commence serial cardiac troponin measurements	
	To provide baseline values	
12-lead ECG	To record cardiac rhythm	
	To look for evidence of acute coronary syndrome	
	To look for evidence of abnormalities that could cause primary arrhythmogenic cardiac arrest, e.g. Brugada syndrome, long QT syndromes	
	To provide a baseline record	
Chest radiograph	To establish the position of tracheal tube, a gastric tube, and/or a central venous catheter	
	To check for evidence of pulmonary oedema	
	To check for evidence of pulmonary aspiration	
	To exclude pneumothorax	
	To assess cardiac contour	
Arterial blood gases	To ensure adequacy of ventilation and oxygenation	
	To ensure correction of acid/base imbalance	
Echocardiography	To identify contributing causes to cardiac arrest	
	To assess LV and RV structure and function	
CT scan	To exclude intracranial bleed or stroke as a primary cause of cardiac arrest particularly if there were neurological symptoms before cardiac arrest	
	To exclude pulmonary embolism or other respiratory causes of cardiac arrest	

Indications for bicarbonate include cardiac arrest associated with hyperkalaemia or tricyclic overdose. Do not give bicarbonate routinely to correct acidaemia after cardiac arrest.

Indications and timing of computed tomography (CT) scanning

Early identification of a respiratory or neurological cause for out-of-hospital cardiac arrest (OHCA) can be achieved by performing a brain and chest CT-scan (usually CT pulmonary angiography to exclude pulmonary embolism) at hospital admission, before or after coronary angiography. In the absence of signs or symptoms suggesting a neurological or respiratory cause (e.g. headache, seizures or neurological deficits for neurological causes, shortness of breath or documented hypoxia or if there is clinical or ECG evidence of myocardial ischaemia, coronary angiography is undertaken first, followed by CT scan in the absence of causative lesions.

Patient transfer

Following the period of initial post-resuscitation care and stabilisation, the patient will need to be transferred to an appropriate critical care environment (e.g. ICU or CCU). The decision to transfer a patient from the place where stabilisation has been achieved should be made only after discussion with senior members of the admitting team.

Continue all established monitoring during the transfer and secure all cannulae, catheters, tubes and drains. Make a full reassessment immediately before the patient is transferred. Ensure that portable suction apparatus, an oxygen supply and a defibrillator/monitor accompany the patient and transfer team.

The transfer team should comprise individuals capable of monitoring the patient and responding appropriately to any change in patient condition, including a further cardiac arrest. The Faculty of Intensive Care Medicine and the Intensive Care Society (UK) have published guidelines for the transfer of the critically ill adult (www.ficm. ac.uk). These outline the requirements for equipment and personnel when transferring critically ill patients.

Optimising organ function

The extent of secondary organ injury after ROSC depends on the ability to minimise the harmful consequences of post-cardiac-arrest syndrome. There are opportunities to limit the insult to organs following cardiac arrest.

Heart and cardiovascular system

Post-resuscitation myocardial dysfunction causes haemodynamic instability, which manifests as hypotension, low cardiac output and arrhythmias. Perform early echocardiography in all patients in order to detect and quantify the degree of myocardial dysfunction. Post-resuscitation myocardial dysfunction often requires inotropic support, at least transiently.

Although dobutamine is the most established treatment in the setting of myocardial dysfunction, the systematic inflammatory response that occurs frequently in post-cardiac arrest patients causes vasoplegia and severe vasodilation. Thus, noradrenaline, with or without dobutamine, and fluid is usually the most effective treatment. Infusion of relatively large volumes of fluid is tolerated remarkably well by patients with post-cardiac arrest syndrome. If treatment with fluid resuscitation, inotropes and vasoactive drugs is insufficient to support the circulation, consider insertion of an intra-aortic balloon pump (IABP). Treatment may be guided by blood pressure, heart rate, urine output, rate of plasma lactate clearance, and central venous oxygen saturation.

There is insufficient evidence to recommend specific haemodynamic goals; such goals should be considered on an individual patient basis and are likely to be influenced by post–cardiac arrest status and pre-existing comorbidities. In the absence of definitive data, target the mean arterial blood pressure to achieve an adequate urine output (≥ 0.5 mL kg^{-1} h^{-1}) and normal or decreasing plasma lactate values, taking into consideration the patient's normal blood pressure, the cause of the arrest and the severity of any myocardial dysfunction. These targets may vary depending on individual physiology and co-morbid status but a systolic blood pressure of at least 100 mmHg (or mean blood pressure ≥ 65 mmHg) is usually required.

Immediately after a cardiac arrest there is typically a period of hyperkalaemia. Subsequent endogenous catecholamine release and correction of metabolic and respiratory acidosis promotes intracellular transportation of potassium, causing hypokalaemia. Hypokalaemia may predispose to ventricular arrhythmias. Give potassium to maintain the serum potassium concentration between 4.0–4.5 mmol L^{-1}.

Referral for implantable cardioverter defibrillator

Consider the possible requirement for an implantable cardioverter defibrillator (ICD) in any patient who has been resuscitated from cardiac arrest in a shockable rhythm outside the context of proven acute ST-segment elevation myocardial infarction. All such patients should be referred before discharge from hospital for assessment by a cardiologist with expertise in heart rhythm disorders (Chapter 4).

Brain: optimising neurological recovery

Cerebral perfusion

Immediately after ROSC there is a period of cerebral hyperaemia. In many post-cardiac arrest patients, cerebral blood flow autoregulation is impaired or the lower limit is right-shifted. This means that at lower mean arterial pressure (MAP) values, in some patients, cerebral blood flow may be MAP-dependent with an increased risk of cerebral hypoperfusion (if MAP too low) or hyperaemia and intracranial hypertension (if MAP too high). As discussed above, following ROSC, maintain mean arterial pressure near the patient's normal level.

Sedation

Although it has been common practice to sedate and ventilate patients for at least 24 h after ROSC, there are no data to support a defined period of ventilation, sedation and neuromuscular blockade after cardiac arrest. Patients need to be well sedated during treatment with targeted temperature management, and the duration of sedation and ventilation is therefore influenced by this treatment. There are no data to indicate whether or not the choice of sedation influences outcome, but a combination of opioids and hypnotics is usually used. Short-acting drugs (e.g. propofol, alfentanil, remifentanil) will enable earlier reliable neurological assessment. Adequate sedation will reduce oxygen consumption. During hypothermia, optimal sedation can reduce or prevent shivering, which enables the target temperature to be achieved more rapidly.

Control of seizures

Seizures are reported in 20–30% of cardiac arrest patients in the ICU and are usually a sign of a severe hypoxic-ischaemic brain injury. Seizures may be observed as clinical convulsions (clinical seizure) and/or as typical activity in the EEG (electrographic seizure). Myoclonus is sudden, brief, shock-like involuntary muscle contractions and is by far the most common type of clinical seizure in post-arrest patients. It is often generalised but may be focal (periodic eye-opening, swallowing, diaphragmic contractions) or multi-focal. It typically develops during the first 1–2 days after the arrest and is often transient during the first week. It is associated with a poor prognosis but some patients survive with a good outcome. Focal and generalised tonic-clonic seizures also occur after cardiac arrest, and it is not uncommon that an individual patient has several seizure sub-types.

Use intermittent or continuous electroencephalography (EEG) to detect epileptic activity in patients with clinical seizure manifestations. Patients with electrographic status epilepticus may or may not have clinically detectable seizure manifestations that may be masked by sedation. Whether systematic detection and treatment of electrographic epileptic activity improves patient outcome is not known.

Seizures may increase the cerebral metabolic rate and have the potential to exacerbate brain injury caused by cardiac arrest: treat seizures with levetiracetam and/or sodium valproate. After the first event, start maintenance therapy. Additional treatment options include perampanel, zonisamide or topiramate. Consider increased doses of propofol or benzodiazepines to suppress myoclonus and electrographic seizures. Thiopental may be considered in selected patients.

There is currently no evidence supporting prophylactic treatment with anti-epileptic drugs in the post-arrest setting. Routine seizure prophylaxis in post-cardiac arrest patients is not recommended because of the risk of adverse effects and the poor response to anti-epileptic drugs among patients with clinical and electrographic seizures.

Myoclonus and electrographic seizure activity, including status epilepticus, are related to a poor prognosis but individual patients may survive with good outcome.

Prolonged observation may be necessary after treatment of seizures with sedatives, which will decrease the reliability of a clinical examination.

Glucose control

There is a strong association between high blood glucose after resuscitation from cardiac arrest and poor neurological outcome. However, severe hypoglycaemia is associated with increased mortality in critically ill patients, and comatose patients are at particular risk from unrecognised hypoglycaemia. Based on the available data and expert consensus, following ROSC, maintain blood glucose at $\leq$ 10 mmol L^{-1} and avoid hypoglycaemia (< 4.0 mmol L^{-1}).

Temperature control

Treatment of hyperpyrexia

A period of hyperthermia (hyperpyrexia) is common in the first 2–3 days after cardiac arrest. Several studies document an association between post-cardiac arrest pyrexia and poor outcome. Although the effect of elevated temperature on outcome is not proved, treat any hyperthermia occurring after cardiac arrest with antipyretics or active cooling.

Targeted temperature management

Animal and human data indicate that mild induced hypothermia is neuroprotective and improves outcome after a period of global cerebral hypoxia-ischaemia.

Cooling suppresses many of the pathways leading to delayed cell death, including apoptosis (programmed cell death). Hypothermia decreases the cerebral metabolic rate for oxygen (CMRO$_2$) by about 6% for each 1°C reduction in core temperature and this may reduce the release of excitatory amino acids and free radicals. Hypothermia blocks the intracellular consequences of excitotoxin exposure (high calcium and glutamate concentrations) and reduces the inflammatory response associated with the post-cardiac arrest syndrome.

All studies of post-cardiac arrest mild induced hypothermia have included only patients in coma. One randomised trial and a pseudo-randomised trial demonstrated improved neurological outcome at hospital discharge or at six months in comatose patients after out-of-hospital VF cardiac arrest. Cooling was initiated within minutes to hours after ROSC and a temperature range of 32–34°C was maintained for 12–24 h. In the Targeted Temperature Management (TTM) trial, 950 all-rhythm OHCA patients were randomised to 36 h of temperature control (comprising 28 h at the target temperature followed by slow rewarm) at either 33°C or 36°C. There was no difference in mortality and detailed neurological outcome at six months was also similar. Importantly, patients in both arms of this trial had their temperature well controlled so that fever was prevented in both groups.

The term 'targeted temperature management' or temperature control is now preferred over the previous term therapeutic hypothermia. The Advanced Life Support Task Force of the International Liaison Committee on Resuscitation (ILCOR) made several treatment recommendations on TTM:

- Maintain a constant, target temperature between 32–36°C for those patients in whom temperature control is used. Whether certain subpopulations of cardiac arrest patients may benefit from lower (32–34°C) or higher (36°C) temperatures remains unknown.

- TTM is recommended for adults after out-of-hospital cardiac arrest with an initial shockable rhythm who remain unresponsive after ROSC.

- TTM is suggested for adults after out-of-hospital cardiac arrest with an initial nonshockable rhythm who remain unresponsive after ROSC.

- TTM is suggested for adults after in-hospital cardiac arrest with any initial rhythm who remain unresponsive after ROSC.

- If TTM is used, it is suggested that the duration is at least 24 h.

- Prevent and treat fever in persistently comatose adults after completion of TTM between 32°C and 36°C.

How to control temperature

A target temperature of 36°C is not the same as normothermia and in most cases will still require cooling and active temperature management to achieve and maintain this target.

The practical application of TTM is divided into three phases: induction, maintenance and rewarming. External and/or internal cooling techniques can be used to initiate and maintain TTM.

Animal data indicate that earlier cooling after ROSC produces better outcome but this has yet to be demonstrated in humans. If a lower target temperature (e.g. 33°C) is chosen, an infusion of 30 mL kg^{-1} of 4°C saline or Hartmann's solution will decrease core temperature by approximately 1.0–1.5°C and is probably safe in a well monitored environment. Pre-hospital cooling using this technique is not recommended because there is some evidence of increased risk of pulmonary oedema and re-arrest during transport to hospital.

Methods of inducing and/or maintaining TTM include:

- Simple ice packs and/or wet towels are inexpensive; however, these methods may be more time consuming for nursing staff, may result in greater temperature fluctuations, and do not enable controlled rewarming. Ice cold fluids alone cannot be used to maintain hypothermia, but even the addition of simple ice packs may control the temperature adequately.

- Cooling blankets or pads.

- Water or air circulating blankets.

- Water circulating gel-coated pads.

- Transnasal evaporative cooling – this technique enables cooling before ROSC but the two trials undertaken using this technique have shown no significant benefits on patient outcomes.

- Intravascular heat exchanger, placed usually in the femoral or subclavian veins.

- Extracorporeal circulation (e.g. cardiopulmonary bypass, extracorporeal membrane oxygenation (ECMO)).

In most cases, it is easy to cool patients initially after ROSC because the temperature normally decreases within this first hour. Admission temperature after OHCA is usually between 35–36°C. If a target temperature of 36°C is chosen, allow a slow passive rewarm to 36°C. If a target temperature of 33°C is chosen, initial cooling is facilitated by neuromuscular blockade and sedation, which will prevent shivering. Magnesium sulfate, a naturally occurring NMDA receptor antagonist, that reduces the shivering threshold slightly, can also be given to reduce the shivering threshold.

In the maintenance phase, a cooling method with effective temperature monitoring that avoids temperature fluctuations is preferred. This is best achieved with external or internal cooling devices that include continuous temperature feedback to achieve a set target temperature. The temperature is typically monitored from a thermistor placed in the bladder and/or oesophagus. There are no data indicating that any specific cooling technique increases survival when compared with any other cooling technique; however, internal devices enable more precise temperature control compared with external techniques.

Plasma electrolyte concentrations, effective intravascular volume and metabolic rate can change rapidly during rewarming, as they do during cooling. Rebound hyperthermia is associated with worse neurological outcome. Thus, rewarming should be achieved slowly: the optimal rate is not known, but the consensus is currently about 0.25–0.5°C of rewarming per hour.

Physiological effects and complications of hypothermia

The well-recognised physiological effects of hypothermia need to be managed carefully.

- Shivering will increase metabolic and heat production, thus reducing cooling rates.

- Mild hypothermia increases systemic vascular resistance and can cause arrhythmias (usually bradycardia). However, several studies have documented an association between bradycardia and better outcome.

- Hypothermia causes a diuresis and electrolyte abnormalities such as hypophosphataemia, hypokalaemia, hypomagnesaemia and hypocalcaemia.

- Hypothermia decreases insulin sensitivity and insulin secretion, causing hyperglycaemia, which will need treatment with insulin.

- Mild hypothermia impairs coagulation and increases bleeding although this has not been confirmed in many clinical studies.

- Hypothermia can impair the immune system and increase infection rates.

- The clearance of sedative drugs and neuromuscular blockers is reduced by up to 30% at a core temperature of 34°C.

Contraindications to hypothermia

Within the recommended TTM range of 32–36°C there are few, if any, recognised contraindications. Previously suggested contraindications to TTM at 33°C included severe systemic infection and pre-existing medical coagulopathy, but not fibrinolytic therapy. Results from a post hoc analysis of the TTM-trial suggest that if there is severe cardiovascular impairment at 33°C a higher temperature might be targeted.

Prognostication

The prognostication of comatose post-cardiac arrest patients is very complex, should be undertaken only by experienced clinicians and is outside the scope of the Advanced Life Support course. This brief summary covers only the broad concepts of prognostication; detailed guidance is provided in the European Resuscitation Council and European Society of Intensive Care Medicine (ESICM) Guidelines for Post-resuscitation care 2021.

Hypoxic-ischaemic brain injury is common after resuscitation from cardiac arrest. Among patients surviving to ICU admission but subsequently dying in-hospital, neurological withdrawal of treatment (following prognostication of poor neurological outcome) is the cause of death in approximately two-thirds after OHCA and approximately 25% after in-hospital cardiac arrest. For this reason, when dealing with patients who are comatose after resuscitation from cardiac arrest minimising the risk of a falsely pessimistic prediction is essential.

Ideally, when predicting a poor outcome, these tests should have 100% specificity or zero false positive rate (FPR) (i.e. no individuals should have a 'good' long-term outcome if predicted to have a poor outcome). However, most prognostication studies include so few patients that it is very difficult to be completely confident in the results. Moreover, many studies are confounded by self-fulfilling prophecy, which is a bias occurring when the treating physicians are not blinded to the results of the outcome predictor and use it to make a decision on withdrawal of life sustaining treatment (WLST). Finally, both TTM itself and sedatives or neuromuscular blocking drugs used to maintain it may potentially interfere with prognostication tests, especially those based on clinical examination.

Prognostication of the comatose post-cardiac arrest patient should be multimodal, in other words involve multiple types of tests of brain injury, and should be delayed sufficiently to enable full clearance of sedatives and any neurological recovery to occur – in most cases, prognostication is not reliable until after 72 h from cardiac arrest. The tests are categorised:

- **clinical examination** – GCS score, pupillary response to light, corneal reflex, presence of seizures
- **neurophysiological studies** – somatosensory evoked potentials (SSEPs) and electroencephalography (EEG)
- **biochemical markers** – neuron-specific enolase (NSE) is the most commonly used
- **imaging studies** – brain CT and magnetic resonance imaging (MRI).

Rehabilitation

Although neurological outcome is considered to be good for the majority of cardiac arrest survivors, cognitive and emotional problems and fatigue are common. Long-term cognitive impairments are present in half of survivors.

Memory is most frequently affected, followed by problems in attention and executive functioning (planning and organisation). The cognitive impairments can be severe, but are mostly mild. These patients may benefit from a formal programme of rehabilitation but such an approach is currently rare in the UK.

Organ donation

Post-cardiac arrest patients who do not survive represent an opportunity to increase the number of potential organ donors, either after brain death or as non-heart-beating donors. Non-randomised studies have shown that graft survival at one year is similar from donors who have had CPR compared with donors who have not had CPR.

Cardiac arrest centres

There is wide variation in patient survival rates among hospitals caring for patients after resuscitation from cardiac arrest. There is indirect evidence that regional cardiac systems of care improve outcome after ST-elevation myocardial infarction (STEMI). Many studies have reported an association between survival to hospital discharge and transport to a recognised centre of care (e.g. cardiac arrest centre), but there is inconsistency in the hospital factors that are most related to patient outcome. There is also inconsistency in the services that together define a cardiac arrest centre. Most experts agree that such a centre must have a cardiac catheterisation laboratory that is immediately accessible 24/7 and the facilities to provide intensive care with TTM. The availability of a neurology service that can provide neuroelectrophysiological monitoring (electroencephalography (EEG)) and investigations (e.g. EEG and somatosensory evoked potentials (SSEPs)) is also essential. Despite the lack of high-quality data to support implementation of cardiac arrest centres, post-cardiac arrest care is being increasingly regionalised.

13: Summary learning

After cardiac arrest, return of spontaneous circulation is just the first stage in a continuum of resuscitation.

The quality of post-resuscitation care will influence significantly the patient's final outcome.

These patients require appropriate monitoring, safe transfer to a critical care environment, and continued organ support.

The post-cardiac arrest syndrome comprises post-cardiac arrest brain injury, post-cardiac arrest myocardial dysfunction, the systemic ischaemia/reperfusion response, and persistence of precipitating pathology.

Prognosticating the final neurological outcome for those patients remaining comatose after cardiopulmonary resuscitation is complex.

My key take-home messages from this chapter are:

Further reading

Nolan JP, Neumar RW, Adrie C, et al. Post-cardiac arrest syndrome: epidemiology, pathophysiology, treatment, and prognostication. A Scientific Statement from the International Liaison Committee on Resuscitation; the American Heart Association Emergency Cardiovascular Care Committee; the Council on Cardiovascular Surgery and Anesthesia; the Council on Cardiopulmonary, Perioperative, and Critical Care; the Council on Clinical Cardiology; the Council on Stroke. Resuscitation 2008;79:350-79.

Nolan JP, Böttiger BW, Cariou A, Cronberg T, Friberg H, Gengrugge C, Haywood K, Lilja G, Moulaert VRM, Nikolaou N, Olasveengen TM, Skrifvars MB, Taccone FS, Soar J. European Resuscitation Council and European Society of Intensive Care Medicine Guidelines 2021: Post-resuscitation Care. Resuscitation. 2021;161.

Sandroni C, D'Arrigo S, Cacciola S, et al Prediction of poor neurological outcome in comatose survivors of cardiac arrest: a systematic review. Intensive Care Med 2020;46:1803–1851.

Soar J, Berg KM, Andersen LW, et al. Advanced life support: 2020 International Consensus on Cardiopulmonary Resuscitation and Emergency Cardiovascular Care Science With Treatment Recommendations. Resuscitation 2020;156:A80–A119.

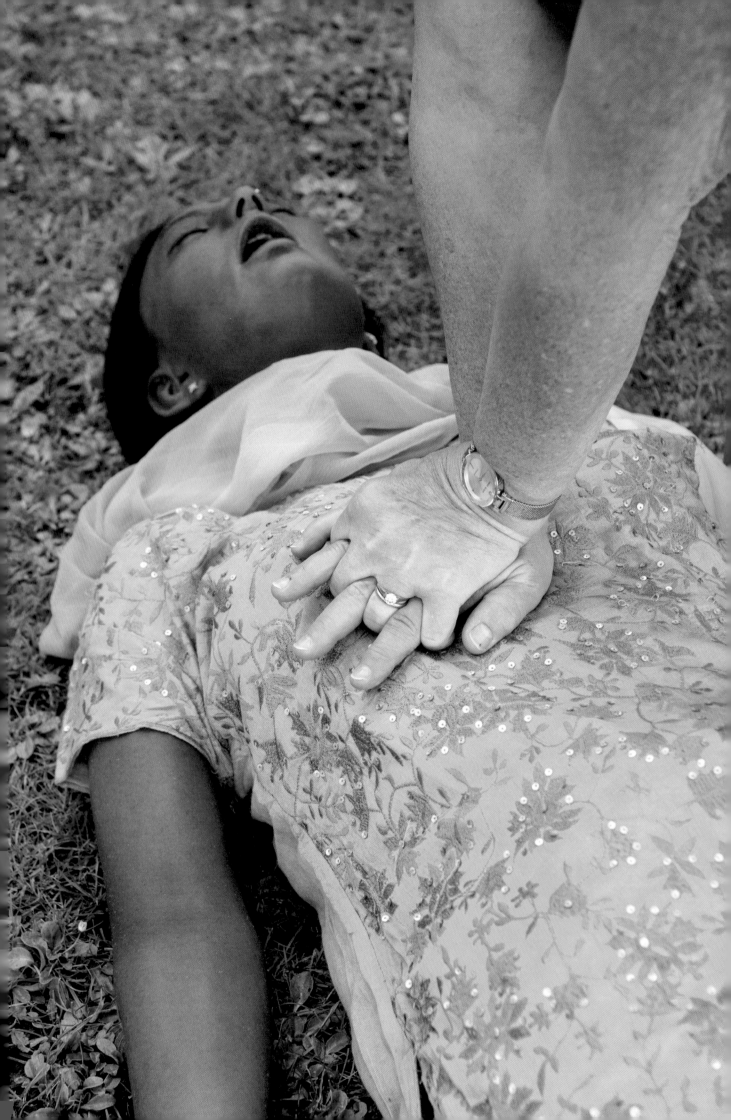

Pre-hospital cardiac arrest

In this chapter

Resuscitation at the scene versus transfer to hospital

Team approach to pre-hospital cardiac arrest

Pre-hospital airway management

Circulatory support

Recognition of life extinct

Pre-hospital post-resuscitation care

Team handover and crew debriefing

Audit

The learning outcomes will enable you to:

Apply the team approach to pre-hospital resuscitation

Understand the optimal approach to managing the airway, breathing and circulation in the pre-hospital setting

Consider the principles of recognition of life extinct (ROLE)

Consider the main features of a team handover and crew debriefing

Introduction

The principles of basic and advanced life support are the same for the pre-hospital setting as they are for in-hospital cardiac arrest, but out-of-hospital can be constrained by a combination of factors including a lack of trained staff, the environment (both on scene or during transport), equipment and drugs and physical access to the patient.

The actions described in the Advanced Life Support (ALS) algorithm can also be applied to the pre-hospital setting (Chapter 6). Resuscitation in special circumstances (e.g. drowning, trauma) is addressed in Chapter 12. Most pre-hospital services will have standard operating procedures (SOPs) that cover many of the topics discussed below.

Survival after out-of-hospital cardiac arrest (OHCA) relies on early recognition and CPR from bystanders. When an ambulance is called, ambulance service telephone dispatchers will provide assistance to bystanders to help identify cardiac arrest and start CPR before the ambulance arrives. Automated external defibrillators (AEDs) are available in many public places (e.g. train stations, shopping centres). An AED should be used as soon as possible. In many areas the ambulance dispatcher will be able to tell bystanders the location of the nearest AED. Resuscitation by bystanders with CPR and an AED before the ambulance arrives offers the best chance of survival after OHCA.

Resuscitation at scene versus transfer to hospital

Treatment on scene aims to identify and treat immediate life-threatening problems and achieve return of spontaneous circulation (ROSC) in those who have had a cardiac arrest. Remain on scene to achieve ROSC unless reversible causes that cannot be dealt with on scene are identified and can potentially be dealt with in-hospital (e.g. emergency department, cardiac catheterisation laboratory, operating theatre). Ideally the decision to transport a patient to hospital should be reached as soon as the need for skills/interventions not available on scene becomes apparent. The deteriorating patient who cannot be stabilised on scene requires early recognition and transport to a suitable hospital (e.g. patient with penetrating trauma and haemodynamic compromise).

Survival after out-of-hospital cardiac arrest (OHCA) relies on early recognition and CPR from bystanders

Resuscitation by bystanders with CPR and an AED before the ambulance arrives offers the best chance of survival after OHCA

Team approach

Pre-hospital cardiac arrest requires a system to be in place to achieve the best possible chance of survival. The system not only requires technical skills, but also requires non-technical skills:

- teamwork
- situational awareness
- leadership
- decision-making.

Appoint an experienced team leader who should assign each member of the team a specific role. Ensure that there is 360° access to the patient (Figure 14.1).

Position 1
Airway (at head of patient) – the person must be trained and equipped to provide the full range of airway skills.

Position 2
High-quality chest compressions and defibrillation if needed – at patient's left side. Be prepared to alternate with operator at position 3 to avoid fatigue.

Position 3
High-quality chest compressions and access to the circulation (intravenous (IV), intraosseous (IO)) – at patient's right side.

Position 4
Team leader – stand back and oversee the resuscitation attempt, only becoming involved if required. The team leader should have an awareness of the whole incident and ensure high-quality resuscitation is maintained and appropriate decisions made.

A Pre-hospital airway management

The aim is to maintain a patent airway enabling adequate oxygenation and ventilation of the lungs. Although tracheal intubation has been considered the gold standard in airway management, lack of supportive outcome data, the practical challenges of implementing its use in the pre-hospital setting and the risks of very serious harm and death (e.g. prolonged desaturation, unrecognised oesophageal intubation or bronchial intubation) have questioned the role of intubation. In particular, do not attempt tracheal intubation in children unless you are an expert in the procedure in this age group, as simpler and safer techniques (e.g. bag-mask ventilation) may be just as effective at maintaining adequate oxygenation and ventilation.

Stepwise approach to airway care

In practice, several airway interventions (e.g. no airway interventions, mouth-to-mouth, bag-mask, supraglottic airway, tracheal intubation) and devices are used in a stepwise manner during CPR and after ROSC. Rescuers should use the skills in which they are proficient. Stepwise airway care provides a progressive approach to obtaining and maintaining an open airway. During a cardiac arrest, it is very important to maintain high-quality chest compressions with minimal interruption for airway interventions. Start with a head tilt/chin lift or jaw thrust, using the latter in patients at risk of cervical spine injury. Simple airway adjuncts (e.g. oropharyngeal airway or nasopharyngeal airway (Chapter 7)) can assist with opening the airway at this stage. In unresponsive

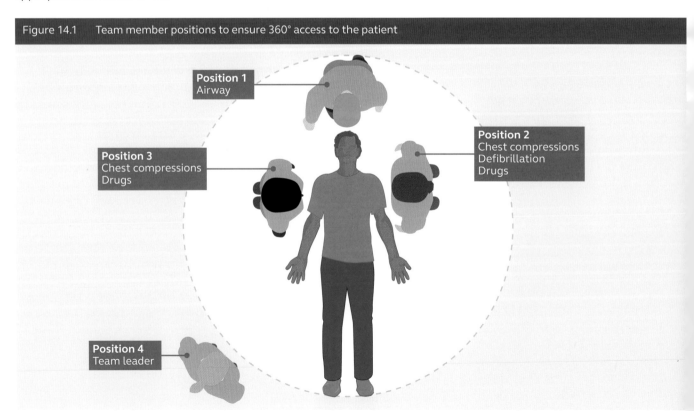

Figure 14.1   Team member positions to ensure 360° access to the patient

Position 1
Airway

Position 2
Chest compressions
Defibrillation
Drugs

Position 3
Chest compressions
Drugs

Position 4
Team leader

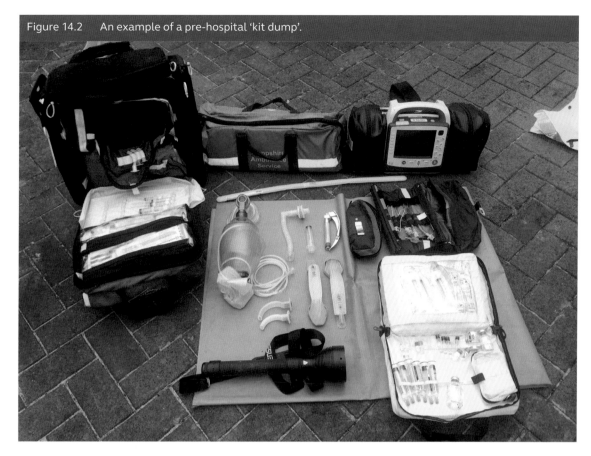

Figure 14.2 An example of a pre-hospital 'kit dump'.

patients, particularly those in respiratory arrest or where ventilation is required, a supraglottic airway (SGA) insertion may be most appropriate.

Tracheal intubation

The tracheal tube is the most challenging of all airway devices to insert successfully and requires adequate initial training and ongoing practice. There is no evidence that outcome from out-of-hospital cardiac arrest is improved by tracheal intubation and several studies have suggested that simpler airway techniques during CPR (i.e. bag-mask, SGA) result in at least as good, if not better, patient outcomes.

Pre-hospital tracheal intubation – practical considerations

Views of the larynx are often suboptimal because of restricted neck movement/jaw opening, poor lighting, vomit and other airway secretions, poor patient positioning, and difficult access to the patient. The following can help achieve safe and successful pre-hospital tracheal intubation.

- Ensure 360° access around the patient where possible.
- Ensure all the necessary equipment is placed by the patient as a 'kit dump' (Figure 14.2).
- Use a checklist to check all equipment is available, allocate roles and make a rescue plan if initial attempts at intubation or ventilation fail.
- Patient positioning: whenever possible, place the patient supine on an ambulance trolley (preferably one that tips head-down in case of vomiting). Intubation is easier when the trolley is at knee level of the airway person.

- Do not routinely use cricoid pressure for tracheal intubation during CPR. Many patients have already aspirated and cricoid pressure can make tracheal intubation more difficult.
- Use a bougie, if necessary, over which a tracheal tube can be rail-roaded. A bougie should always be available.
- Choose the correct-sized laryngoscope blade; generally a size 4 MAC blade can be used for most adults. Videolaryngoscopy can help with difficult intubation – a variety of devices are available but require specific training in their use. A good view of the cords on the video screen does not mean tube placement will be easy.
- Secure the tracheal tube immediately after insertion (adult males 22–23 cm, adult females 21–22 cm), using a tie, commercial clamp or tape. A tie around the patient's head or neck can decrease venous drainage of blood from the head and brain and increase the intracranial pressure – do not over tighten the tie and consider using tape in patients where intracranial pressure may be raised (e.g. head injury). The same is true for securing SGAs. When moving the patient, hold the tracheal tube, even when it is secured. Regularly check the tracheal tube length during transit to ensure that it has not dislodged.
- During CPR aim to minimise the interruption to chest compressions for tube placement to less than 5 s – this means doing the initial laryngoscopy whilst compressions are ongoing, a brief pause to optimise the view and pass the tube and then restarting compressions. Plan actions and pauses whilst compressions are ongoing.

Tracheal intubation – complications

Complications associated with tracheal intubation include:

1. **Hypoxaemia** – do not allow desaturation while attempting intubation; oxygenate the lungs between intubation attempts.

2. **Unrecognised oesophageal intubation** – use waveform capnography to exclude oesophageal intubation (Chapter 7).

3. **Endobronchial intubation** – insert the tracheal tube to no more than the appropriate length, listen to breath sounds in both axillae, and ensure both lungs are ventilated. Monitor the position of the tube during transit.

B Breathing

Initial management

Having opened the airway, the first priority is to rapidly assess, identify and treat reversible causes of impaired breathing. Assessment of breathing follows the look, listen and feel approach. In sick patients, expose the chest sufficiently to look for signs of injury, chest wall expansion and asymmetry between each side. Listening with a stethoscope is particularly difficult in the noisy pre-hospital setting. Feeling for equal chest wall expansion, bony injury or surgical emphysema is useful; the latter in most cases indicates a pneumothorax or rupture of a large airway is likely. It can be difficult to measure oxygen saturation reliably with a pulse oximeter when patients are cold, or have a low blood pressure. If a pulse oximeter placed on the finger fails to read adequately, other sites that may work include the toes, nose, ear lobes, tongue or lip (although care must be taken in their interpretation as SaO_2 values from these sites may be less reliable).

Gastric distention

Positive pressure ventilation using a bag-mask can lead to gastric insufflation, respiratory compromise, regurgitation of stomach contents and aspiration. Gentle ventilation with a bag-mask (sufficient to just enable the chest wall to rise) minimises airway pressure and reduces the fraction of air forced down the oesophagus and into the stomach. Low tidal volumes also minimise adverse haemodynamic effects on the circulation. SGAs minimise the risk of gastric distention and should be considered in preference to a bag-mask.

Tension pneumothorax

A tension pneumothorax requires immediate treatment by decompression (Chapter 12). The aim of pre-hospital management is to relieve the tension and convert a tension pneumothorax to a simple pneumothorax; the latter is generally not life-threatening and will enable transfer to hospital for definitive care. In patients very close to a destination hospital, needle decompression can be sufficient to transport the patient before the tension pneumothorax recurs. In patients with longer transit times or requiring air transfer, who are breathing spontaneously, a chest drain with a one-way valve will need to be inserted, usually in the 5th intercostal space in the midaxillary line. In patients receiving positive pressure ventilation, a thoracostomy (5th intercostal space in the midaxillary line) is preferable to a chest drain as it is less invasive, a quicker procedure and avoids complications associated with the chest drain itself.

Oxygenation and ventilation

Give high-flow oxygen to correct and avoid hypoxia. As soon as the oxygen saturation can be reliably measured, adjust the inspired oxygen concentration to achieve a target oxygen saturation (e.g. 94–98% after ROSC from cardiac arrest – Chapter 13).

Hyperventilation (from excessive tidal volumes, respiratory rate, or both) is common and can cause haemodynamic instability. Hypocarbia induced by hyperventilation can cause excessive cerebral vasoconstriction and ischaemia. The use of mechanical ventilators may prevent hyperventilation and minimise peak airway pressures, as well as freeing a rescuer for other tasks.

C Circulation

Defibrillation

Defibrillation is one of the few interventions that improves outcome from sudden cardiac arrest, but its application is time critical, with mortality increasing 10% for every minute's delay in defibrillation. Attach the defibrillation electrodes and deliver the first shock as soon as possible. When attending as a solo responder, immediate assessment of the rhythm and defibrillation when indicated, should take precedence over airway or breathing interventions (Chapter 9). Attempt defibrillation in patients with VF of any magnitude.

A few patients who present in VF are difficult to cardiovert (i.e. they remain in VF). In such cases, ensure correct defibrillation electrode placement particularly of the apical electrode, consider a change in electrode position, (e.g. move from the standard anterior-lateral to an anterior-posterior or bi-axillary position) and increase the defibrillation energy level output if initial lower energy shocks fail to defibrillate. Dual (double) sequential defibrillation has not been proven to be of benefit and should only be used in the context of a controlled trial. Ventricular fibrillation recurs in 50% of patients within 2 min of successful termination and in 75% of patients during the entire cardiac arrest. Give amiodarone (300 mg IV) after three defibrillation attempts, irrespective of whether those episodes are concurrent or separate.

Defibrillating and performing effective chest compressions whilst moving these patients to the ambulance and transporting to hospital is difficult. If necessary, put the patient down or stop the ambulance while further therapy is given.

Vascular access

Obtain IV access if this has not been done already. Peripheral venous cannulation is quick and relatively easy and is preferable to IO access as the initial cannulation choice.

If IV access is considered too difficult or cannot be established, consider gaining IO access (Chapter 6). Some pre-hospital services recommend a maximum of two attempts at IV access or a maximum of 2 min for attempts before considering IO access. During CPR, effective chest compressions and early defibrillation is the first priority and the role of drugs is uncertain, so do not delay other more useful interventions for vascular access. Tibial and humeral sites are readily accessible. Follow any drug injection (IV or IO) by a flush of at least 20 mL of fluid to facilitate drug delivery to the central circulation.

Chest compressions

Start chest compressions as soon as cardiac arrest is confirmed. Whenever possible, perform CPR on a firm surface because soft surfaces (e.g. mattresses make it difficult to estimate how deep the chest is being compressed and can lead to under-compression.

CPR monitoring, feedback and prompt devices

Some defibrillators and specific feedback/prompt devices monitor CPR quality (e.g. compression rate, depth, leaning, ventilation rate) during CPR. These devices give the rescuer real-time objective feedback on the quality of CPR. If these devices are used they should be part of an overall quality improvement programme that monitors CPR quality and provides rescuers with post-event feedback on performance.

Mechanical chest compression devices

The routine use of automated mechanical chest compression devices is not superior to manual chest compressions. However, automated mechanical chest compression devices can give high-quality manual chest compressions in situations where sustained high-quality manual chest compressions are impractical or compromise rescuer safety (e.g. during transport, enclosed spaces).

Mechanical devices should only be used within a structured, monitored programme, which includes comprehensive competency-based training and regular opportunities to refresh skills. Improper use of mechanical compression devices can delay life-saving interventions such as defibrillation, and cause harmful pauses in chest compressions when switching from manual to mechanical compressions.

Examples of scenarios where mechanical chest compressions are suitable include transport of patients to hospital for correction of a potentially reversible cause:

- Patients with acute myocardial infarction and VF or pVT refractory to 5 shocks (i.e. persistence or recurrence of VF or pVT), for whom a decision is made to transport during persistent arrhythmia to access coronary angiography and percutaneous coronary intervention.
- The patient with hypothermia in whom prolonged resuscitation is considered.

Continuous waveform capnography as a guide to circulatory status

Continuous waveform capnography is a useful guide for managing the circulation and must be used for all patients immediately following tracheal intubation, during the resuscitation attempt and following ROSC. It has several roles in addition to monitoring tracheal tube placement and ventilation rate (Chapter 6):

- early indication of ROSC
- monitoring the quality of CPR
- helping with prognostication.

Recognition of life extinct

The Association of Ambulance Services Chief Executives (through the Joint Royal Colleges Ambulance Liaison Committee, UK Ambulance Service – Clinical Practice Guidelines), and Resuscitation Council UK have both provided clinical guidelines around both the futility of starting resuscitation in certain circumstances and when it may be appropriate to stop a resuscitation attempt. In the presence of cardiorespiratory arrest, and in the absence of a documented do not attempt cardiopulmonary resuscitation (DNACPR) decision or refusal of CPR in an Advance Decision to Refuse Treatment (ADRT) ('living will'), ambulance clinicians should start CPR unless the patient has a condition unequivocally associated with death.

When not to start resuscitation

The UK Ambulance Service Clinical Practice Guidelines (2019) list the following situations as unequivocally associated with death:

- decapitation
- massive cranial and cerebral destruction
- hemicorporectomy (or similar massive injury)
- incineration (> 95% full thickness burns)
- decomposition/putrefaction
- rigor mortis and hypostasis.

Resuscitation should also not be started in patients where a valid DNACPR decision has been made (Chapter 16).

These decisions are difficult to confirm in an out-of-hospital setting and it may be appropriate to start and continue resuscitation whilst the facts are clarified. If a patient is inaccessible and assessment is difficult, an ECG must be taken before any decision to withhold resuscitation is taken. There are situations where an experienced practitioner clearly identifies that the patient is in the final stages of a terminal illness and resuscitation is unlikely to be appropriate or successful. In these circumstances the practitioner must be able to explain the grounds for the decision not to start resuscitation, and these must be documented. Discussion with a senior clinician is recommended in these situations.

When to stop resuscitation

In patients where ROSC is not achieved on scene, despite appropriate ALS and treatment of potentially reversible causes, little is to be gained from transporting adult patients to hospital.

The asystolic patient

As with UK Ambulance Service Clinical Practice Guidelines (2019), if, following ALS interventions, the patient has been persistently and continuously asystolic for 20 min and all reversible causes have been identified and corrected, resuscitation may be discontinued.

In cases of cardiac arrest < 18 years old, drowning, hypothermia, poisoning or overdose and pregnancy these patients should be transported to the nearest facility with ongoing resuscitation, while minimising delays on scene.

Pulseless electrical activity

The decision about when to stop resuscitation if pulseless electrical activity (PEA) persists is less clear and there is limited evidence to support when one should stop resuscitation in a PEA cardiac arrest. Although there is ongoing electrical activity, the outcome is usually poor. The use of cardiac ultrasound may assist in decision-making. UK Ambulance Service Clinical Practice Guidelines (2019) recommend involving senior clinicians in decision support where the patient remains in PEA after 20 min of ALS and where paramedics on scene believe continuing resuscitation is futile.

When making this decision, take into consideration the length of time in cardiac arrest before CPR was started, the absence of treatable reversible causes, patient co-morbidities, the rate/width of the QRS complexes and the trend and absolute value of end-tidal CO_2.

Young age, myocardial infarction and potentially reversible causes of cardiac arrest (e.g. pulmonary embolus, hypothermia) are associated with a better outcome, particularly from witnessed cardiac arrests with bystander CPR.

Ventricular fibrillation

Where practical, patients with persistent VF or pulseless VT should be taken to a cardiac arrest centre with ongoing CPR, minimising time on scene, because further treatment (e.g. coronary angiography and primary percutaneous intervention (PCI)) may be successful.

Communication with relatives

Although priorities during the management of a cardiac arrest are focused on the patient, it is important to consider the relatives who are often present. Relatives are also patients and treating them sensitively can help with the mourning process if resuscitation is unsuccessful (Chapter 17). Allow relatives to be present during the resuscitation attempt, providing they do not interfere with clinical care.

Pre-hospital post-resuscitation care

General principles

The focus of post-resuscitation care is directed at optimising perfusion of the brain and heart (Chapter 13). Use the ABCDE approach (Chapter 3).

Monitor the patient with:
- pulse oximetry
- continuous waveform capnography to monitor end-tidal CO_2
- blood pressure
- ECG
- 12-lead ECG where appropriate
- blood glucose measurement
- temperature.

Haemodynamic management

Following ROSC, hypotension and arrhythmias are common. Treat hypotension with a 250 mL IV/IO bolus of 0.9% saline, repeated as necessary. Treat arrhythmias according to the peri-arrest guidelines (Chapter 11). For more details about post-resuscitation care and optimising the circulation see Chapter 13. In the event of severe hemodynamic instability unresponsive to atropine and/or fluids and/or pacing, consider using inotropic support. Boluses of adrenaline 0.05–0.1 mg IV/IO can be titrated against blood pressure and repeated as necessary. When titrating adrenaline aim for an initial systolic BP above 100 mmHg. The use of intravenous adrenaline is undertaken only in the setting of robust clinical governance with medical support (e.g. by telephone). If the 12-lead ECG shows an acute STEMI, transport the patient to a hospital capable of delivering primary PCI, regardless of the patient's conscious level.

Ventilation

Change from hand ventilation to mechanical ventilation of the patient's lungs, ensuring that there is adequate rise and fall of the chest. Waveform capnography is mandatory for intubated patients.

Aim to maintain the SpO_2 at 94–98% and the end-tidal CO_2 at 4.6–6 kPa (35–45 mmHg). End-tidal CO_2 values may be lower in patients with a poor cardiac output.

Targeted temperature management

The benefits of therapeutic hypothermia for post-arrest patients are unclear, but immediate temperature management aims to achieve a core temperature no higher than 36.0°C. Passive cooling is appropriate for these patients. Do not cover the patient in blankets and maintain ambulance temperature no higher than ambient. Do not use rapid high-volume (2 L) cold intravenous fluid infusion immediately after ROSC for rapid cooling – it is associated with an increased incidence of re-arrest and pulmonary oedema. Cooling with cold IV fluids must only be done with close monitoring.

The combative patient

Following ROSC, patients may be cerebrally irritated and combative. Exclude hypoglycaemia. These patients can benefit from formal anaesthetic management, but incremental doses of IV diazepam or midazolam may be indicated with appropriate online medical support if advanced medical care is not available on scene. If sedation is used ensure that oxygenation and ventilation are adequate.

Transporting the patient to hospital

Attempts to provide resuscitation whilst moving the patient to the ambulance and transporting to hospital are likely to be sub-optimal. Aim to achieve ROSC on scene. In patients who achieve ROSC, and in those who have not achieved ROSC within 20 min but in whom resuscitation is being continued, aim to leave the scene as soon as possible.

When the decision is made to transport the patient with ROSC, maintain the patient in a position most likely to optimise cerebral perfusion:

- supine
- feet-first if coming down stairs
- slightly head-up (30°) once in the vehicle.

| A | B | C | D | E |

Assess using the ABCDE approach before leaving the scene and transport the patient to the nearest appropriate hospital.

Patient destination

Cardiac arrest centres

Ambulance services should transfer patients following cardiac arrest with ST-elevation on their ECG to a regional cardiac arrest centre so they can undergo urgent coronary angiography and PCI if indicated. This should be the case irrespective of the patient's conscious level. Other patients who are likely to have a primary cardiac cause for their cardiac arrest should also be considered for direct transfer to a regional cardiac arrest centre.

Pre-alerting

Alert the receiving hospital as soon as possible whenever transporting a patient in cardiac arrest or once ROSC has been achieved. When pre-alerting, ensure that you identify the hospital, department and name of the person receiving your message.

Use a structured method to give the key information. Typically, this is done using 'ATMIST' (Table 14.1).

Table 14.1   A structured approach to providing key information – the ATMIST mnemonic

	Medical	Trauma
A	Age	Age
T	Time of onset	Time of incident
M	Medical complaint/history	Mechanism of injury
I	Investigations (brief examination of findings)	Injuries (top to toe)
S	Vital Signs (first set and significant changes)	Vital Signs (first set and significant changes)
T	Treatment, including ETA and any specialist resources needed on arrival	Treatment, including ETA and any specialist resources needed on arrival

ETA – expected time of arrival

Most patients will be transported to an emergency department resuscitation room where a handover from the ambulance to hospital clinician will take place. Ensure that the receiving hospital is aware of the patient's conscious level – cardiac arrest centres often do not have anaesthetic support as part of their receiving team and will need to summon such personnel if the patient is unconscious.

Team handover and debriefing

Handover

Use a handover template to transfer information rapidly during resuscitation. A commonly used EMS handover template is ATMIST (Age, Name, Time of onset, Medical history, Investigations, vital Signs, Treatment – see above). Speak loudly and clearly using the template headings; pauses will enable important points to be understood and assimilated. Be concise and try and limit the handover.

Adjuncts to handover such as pictures from the scene can be extremely useful. If you have taken them show them to the hospital team leader.

Debriefing

Following an out-of-hospital resuscitation attempt, an immediate debrief with the attending EMS team is valuable. This 'Hot' debrief can provide a valuable learning opportunity and also ensure the welfare of the pre-hospital resuscitation team. Debriefing in a structured manner is particularly useful to explore non-technical elements of resuscitation such as communication, leadership and team working. Ideally, the debrief is led by a person trained and capable of leading the session in a non-threatening, constructive manner, and should include review of records and data from the resuscitation attempt.

Audit

Quality of CPR/defibrillator downloads

Modern defibrillators include the ability to obtain downloads of data related to the quality of CPR. The systematic analysis of such data and provision of feedback to ambulance clinicians is recommended and has been shown to improve the quality of CPR.

Out-of-Hospital Cardiac Arrest Outcomes (OHCAO) database

Ongoing, systematic collection and analysis of data about out-of-hospital cardiac arrest and bystander CPR is essential to the planning, implementation, and evaluation of effective CPR programs. The British Heart Foundation and Resuscitation Council UK established a national OHCAO registry in partnership with the National Association of Ambulance Medical Directors and University of Warwick. The OHCAO registry (https://warwick.ac.uk/fac/sci/med/research/ctu/trials/ohcao/) collects process and outcome information about patients who are treated by ambulance services for cardiac arrest and which is based on the international Utstein template. The registry will provide a tool to support local quality improvement initiatives and will facilitate measuring the impact of resuscitation interventions.

14: Summary learning

Most of the interventions used in hospital for resuscitation can be also be applied to patients with out-of-hospital cardiac arrest by highly skilled pre-hospital teams.

Allocate roles and tasks and ensure the appropriate kit is available during resuscitation.

Pre-hospital tracheal intubation is difficult and should be undertaken only by experts. If not skilled in tracheal intubation, use a bag-mask or a supraglottic airway.

Follow standard operating procedures (SOPs) for decisions about starting or stopping resuscitation at the scene, and for identifying patients for transport to hospital with ongoing CPR.

My key take-home messages from this chapter are:

Further reading

Deakin CD, Clarke T, Nolan J, et al. A critical reassessment of ambulance service airway management in pre-hospital care: Joint Royal Colleges Ambulance Liaison Committee Airway Working Group. EMJ 2010;27:226-33.

Lott C, Truhlár A, Alfonzo A, Barelli A, González-Salvado V, Hinkelbein J, Nolan JP, Paal P, Perkins GD, Thies K-C, Yeung J, Zideman DA, Soar J. European Resuscitation Council Guidelines 2021: Cardiac arrest in special circumstances. Resuscitation. 2021;161.

National Institute for Health and Care Excellence. Clinical Guideline 185. Acute Coronary Syndromes. 2020. https://www.nice.org.uk/guidance/ng185

Olasveengen TM, Semeraro F, Ristagno G, Castren M, Handley A, Kuzovlev A, Monsieurs KG, Raffay V, Smyth M, Soar J, Svavarsdottir H and Perkins GD. European Resuscitation Council Guidelines 2021: Basic Life Support. Resuscitation. 2021;161.

Nolan JP, Böttiger BW, Cariou A, Cronberg T, Friberg H, Gengrugge C, Haywood K, Lilja G, Moulaert VRM, Nikolaou N, Olasveengen TM, Skrifvars MB, Taccone FS, Soar J. European Resuscitation Council and European Society of Intensive Care Medicine Guidelines 2021: Post-resuscitation Care. Resuscitation. 2021;161.

Soar J, Berg KM, Andersen LW, et al. Adult Advanced Life Support: 2020 International Consensus on Cardiopulmonary Resuscitation and Emergency Cardiovascular Care Science with Treatment Recommendations. Resuscitation. 2020 Nov;156:A80-A119.

Soar J, Böttiger BW, Carli P, Couper K, Deakin CD, Djärv T, Lott C, Olasveengen TM, Paal P, Pellis T, Perkins GD, Sandroni C, Nolan JP. European Resuscitation Council Guidelines 2021: Advanced Life Support. Resuscitation. 2021;161.

The UK Out-of-Hospital Cardiac Arrest Outcomes (OHCAO) Project: https://warwick.ac.uk/fac/sci/med/research/ctu/trials/ohcao/

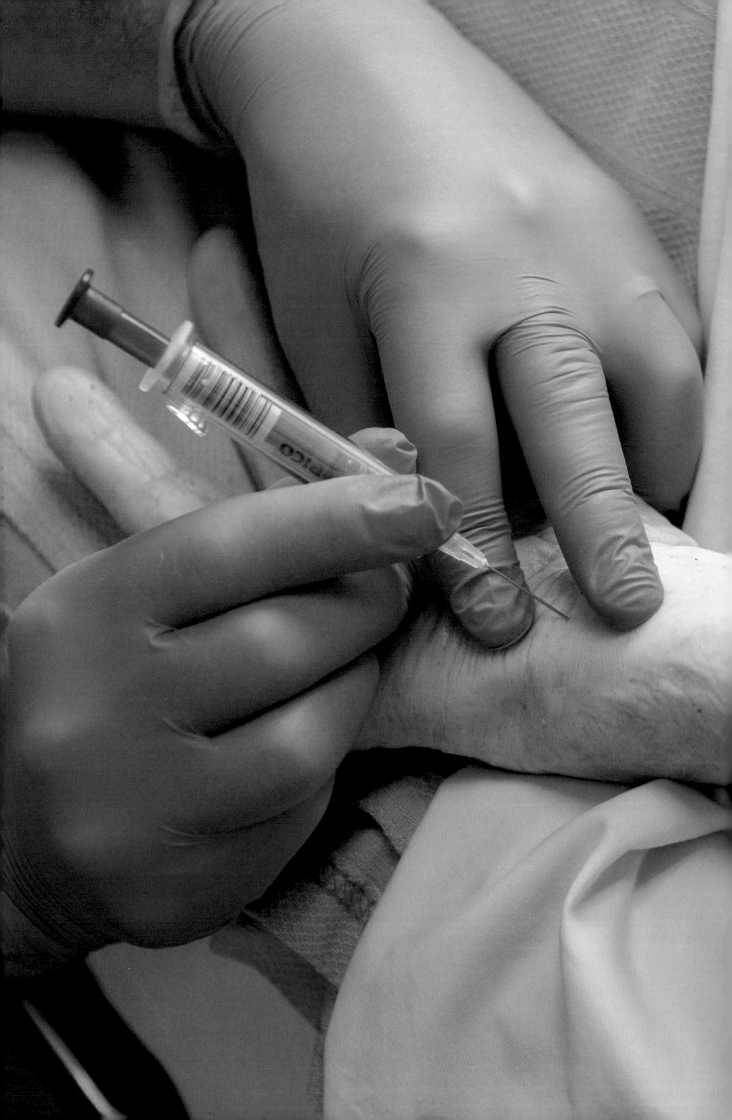

Blood gas analysis and pulse oximetry

In this chapter

Introduction to blood gas analysis

Interpreting blood gas values using the 6-step approach

Example case studies

Practical aspects of blood gas analysis during resuscitation

Pulse oximetry

Targeted oxygen therapy

The learning outcomes will enable you to:

List the range of values produced by a blood gas analysis

Describe the link between respiration and metabolism in terms of pH regulation

Use the 6-step approach to blood gas interpretation

Describe the principles of pulse oximetry

Describe the principles of using oxygen therapy safely and effectively

Introduction

Blood gas analysers produce a range of results, including pH, partial pressure of oxygen (PaO_2), partial pressure of carbon dioxide ($PaCO_2$), blood bicarbonate concentration, and base excess. Most will also produce a range of supplementary values, including haemoglobin, many electrolytes, and blood glucose.

Interpreting the results of an arterial blood sample to determine a patient's acid-base status and respiratory gas exchange is a key component in the management of any unwell patient. It is essential to have a system to ensure that nothing is overlooked or misinterpreted. The body needs the pH of the blood to be within a normal range (7.35 to 7.45) to function optimally. In order to achieve this, an intricate system of balance involving the lungs and kidneys is used to compensate for any abnormalities. If the pH of the blood is not within this normal range, then body systems start to fail.

There is a higher risk of this situation if there is failure of one or both of the compensatory organs, or if there is an overwhelming stress on the system (e.g. cardiac arrest or sepsis). It is therefore important to analyse blood gas results as they will provide information about the efficiency of the compensatory mechanisms as well as guide the clinician to providing the correct treatment to address the situation.

Interpreting blood gas values using the 6-step approach

There are six important questions to ask when interpreting a blood gas result:

1. How is the patient?

2. Is the patient hypoxaemic?

3. What is the pH?

4. What has happened to the $PaCO_2$?

5. What has happened to the bicarbonate?

6. Are there any other important values to consider?

Step 1: How is the patient?

Without the clinical history it is difficult to interpret blood gas values. Understanding the events preceding a review of a patient will enable the team to make predictions about what they might expect to find. For example, one might predict that analysis of arterial blood shortly after successful resuscitation would show signs of a respiratory acidosis caused by a period of inadequate ventilation, and a metabolic acidosis due to the period of cardiac arrest. We would therefore expect the patient to have a low pH and a high $PaCO_2$. The blood gas will help to quantify how ill the patient is, and serial measurements can show how a patient is responding to treatment. If the measured values do not match the team's predictions, it can be a prompt to review the diagnosis or plan. Knowing how the patient is will also help determine how quickly a team must respond to their needs.

Gas measurements: partial pressure

Blood gas machines measure the partial pressure of oxygen and carbon dioxide.

Partial pressure measurements are usually given in kiloPascals (kPa), but occasionally may be in millimetres of mercury (mmHg).

The partial pressure of a gas is the contribution it makes towards the total pressure of the mixture.

Since atmospheric pressure is close to 100 kPa, then it's easy to estimate the partial pressure of each gas in the atmosphere: since oxygen is 21% of the mixture, its pressure is close to 21 kPa.

This is important because increasing the partial pressure of oxygen can help a damaged lung take in more of the gas.

For example when you give a patient 40% oxygen, you are giving them oxygen at a partial pressure of 40 kPa, almost twice what they were breathing in air. This creates a bigger pressure gradient between the gas in the lung and the blood, which often helps its uptake.

At atmospheric pressure, the partial pressure of a gas in a mixture in kPa is numerically the same as the percentage (%) of the gas by volume.

Step 2: Is the patient hypoxaemic?

It is important to always think about PaO_2 in terms of how much oxygen the patient is breathing. Room air contains 21% oxygen, and atmospheric pressure is very close to 100 kPa, so normally people breathe in about 21 kPa of oxygen. When the lungs functional normally, this gives an arterial PaO_2 of 10–13 kPa.

The PaO_2 is always lower than the atmospheric partial pressure because air is humidified as it is breathed in, then it mixes with expired CO_2 in the alveoli, both of which dilute the oxygen a little.

If you give a patient extra oxygen then more oxygen will be present in the alveoli, so you would predict that their PaO_2 should also rise. If it doesn't, then this would mean there is something wrong with the lungs, preventing normal oxygen uptake into the blood.

As a rough 'rule of thumb' the PaO_2 should be about 10 less than the inspired concentration (%) in a healthy patient. If this patient started breathing 40% oxygen, we would therefore expect their PaO_2 to rise to 30 kPa. If it is lower than this prediction, there is probably something wrong with the lungs. That means that although a PaO_2 of 12 kPa when breathing air would be completely normal, if you measured that same value in someone when they are breathing additional oxygen it could actually be a very abnormal result.

If the blood gases indicate that the patient is hypoxaemic, this may require immediate action before evaluating the rest of the blood gases.

Step 3: What is the pH?

The acidity or alkalinity of the blood (or any solution) is determined by the concentration of hydrogen ions [H^+]. The greater the concentration, the more acid the solution. In the body, the concentration of hydrogen ions is extremely low, normally around 40 nanomoles per litre (nmol L^{-1}). To make it easier to deal with such small concentrations of hydrogen ions, we use the pH scale; this is a logarithmic scale expressing the hydrogen ion concentration between 1 and 14.

The pH of normal arterial blood lies between 7.35–7.45, or [H^+] 44–36 nmol L^{-1}.

There are two key points to remember about the pH scale:

1. The numerical value of pH changes inversely with hydrogen ion concentration; a decrease in blood pH below 7.35 indicates an increase in [H^+] above normal, a condition referred to as an acidaemia. Conversely, an increase in blood pH above 7.45 indicates a reduction in [H^+] below normal, a condition referred to as an alkalaemia.

2. Small changes in pH represent big changes in hydrogen ion [H^+] concentration; a pH change from 7.4 to 7.1 means that the [H^+] has increased from 40 nmol L^{-1} to 80 nmol L^{-1} (i.e. it has doubled for a pH change of 0.3).

Many of the complex reactions within cells are controlled by enzymes that function only within a very narrow pH range; hence, normal pH is controlled tightly between 7.35–7.45.

Step 4: What has happened to the PaCO$_2$?

In other words, is any abnormality in pH wholly or partially due to a defect in the respiratory system?

If the PaCO$_2$ is abnormal, check whether the PaCO$_2$ has risen or fallen, and compare it with the pH:

4a. If the pH is < 7.35 (acidaemia): is the PaCO$_2$ increased (> 6.0 kPa)?
If so, there is a respiratory acidosis that may be accounting for all or part of the derangement. There could also be a metabolic component, see Step 5a.

4b. If the pH is > 7.45 (alkalaemia): is the PaCO$_2$ reduced (< 4.7 kPa)?
If so, there is a respiratory alkalosis, but this is an unusual isolated finding in a patient breathing spontaneously with a normal respiratory rate. It is seen more often in patients who are being mechanically ventilated with excessively high rates and/or tidal volumes. It may occasionally be seen when patients are hyperventilating because of severe pain or an acute anxiety attack.

Carbon dioxide (CO_2) is an important waste product of metabolism. Too much CO_2, for example if the patient is hypoventilating (or indeed has stopped breathing entirely), will make patients more acidaemic. This happens because CO_2 combines with water to generate hydrogen ions and bicarbonate:

$$CO_2 + H_2O \rightleftharpoons H^+ + HCO_3^-$$

This is termed a **respiratory acidosis**, because it is a ventilatory change that is triggering the rise in hydrogen ion concentration, and therefore the fall in pH.

The reaction can go the other way too; hyperventilation causes CO_2 to fall, making the bicarbonate and hydrogen recombine to restore the equilibrium of the reaction. Hydrogen concentration falls, so patients become alkalaemic. This would be termed a respiratory alkalosis, again because the first change was in ventilation.

The lungs are therefore very important in the regulation of pH, particularly since the respiratory system can respond very rapidly. The normal PaCO$_2$ is between 4.7–6.0 kPa.

Under normal circumstances, the respiratory centre in the brain stem is very sensitive to blood [H^+]. Within a few minutes of sensing a rise in hydrogen concentration it stimulates the person to breathe more. This increases CO_2 excretion, making blood PaCO$_2$ fall, and therefore decreases [H^+]. This is called respiratory compensation – the respiratory centre has sensed a change in pH, so triggers a response that should return pH towards normal.

The lungs are the primary mechanism by which [H^+] is adjusted by regulating PaCO$_2$.

Step 5: What has happened to the base excess or bicarbonate?

In other words, is any abnormality in pH wholly or partially due to a defect in the metabolic system?

5a. If the pH is < 7.35 (acidaemia): Is there a base deficit (< –2 mmol L⁻¹) (i.e. more negative), and/or the bicarbonate reduced (< 22 mmol L⁻¹)?
If so, there is a metabolic acidosis accounting for all or part of the derangement. There could be a respiratory component if the $PaCO_2$ is also increased – see Step 4a; this is a situation commonly seen after a cardiac arrest.

5b. If the pH is > 7.45 (alkalaemia): Is there a base excess (> +2 mmol L⁻¹) and/or the bicarbonate increased (> 26 mmol L⁻¹)?
If so, there is a metabolic alkalosis accounting for all or part of the derangement. There could be a respiratory component if the $PaCO_2$ is also decreased – see Step 4b, but this would be unusual.

Buffering hydrogen ions in the body

Bicarbonate (HCO_3^-) is the most important buffer and is generated by the kidneys. Acids not immediately eliminated by the respiratory system can be buffered by HCO, adding more bicarbonate essentially 'mops up' some of the excess hydrogen ions in the reverse of the reaction described above in relation to CO_2:

$$H^+ + HCO_3^- \rightleftharpoons H_2CO_3^-$$

Under normal circumstances, the concentration of bicarbonate is 22–26 mmol L⁻¹.

The kidneys are largely responsible for maintaining HCO_3^- values, and they do this by either re-absorbing bicarbonate ions filtered into the urine, or by generating new bicarbonate. These systems have a large capacity, but unlike respiratory compensation the response of the kidneys is slow, taking several days. Metabolic compensation for respiratory acidosis is often seen in COPD patients with a chronically raised $PaCO_2$; the long-term rise in $PaCO_2$ causes an acidaemia, which the kidneys respond to by raising bicarbonate values.

If the kidneys fail to produce sufficient bicarbonate, the resultant **metabolic acidosis** will lead to a decrease in pH below 7.35 (acidaemia).

Occasionally, the situation arises where there is an excess of bicarbonate. This is most commonly caused by loss of acid, such as from persistent vomiting. This will have the effect of excessive buffering of hydrogen ions and will produce a **metabolic alkalosis** and increase the pH above 7.45 (alkalaemia).

An alternative method of measuring metabolic acid-base status is **base excess**. This is a measure of the amount of excess acid or base in the blood as a result of a metabolic derangement. The normal values of base excess are +2 to -2 mmol L⁻¹, and it is calculated as the amount of strong acid or base that would have to be added to a blood sample with an abnormal pH to restore it to normal (pH 7.4).

A patient with a **base excess of +8 mmol L⁻¹** would require 8 mmol L⁻¹ of **strong acid** to be added to return their pH to normal (in other words they have too many alkaline substances in their blood, so need more acid to neutralize it). This patient therefore has a metabolic alkalosis.

Conversely, a patient with a **base excess of -8 mmol L⁻¹** would require the addition of 8 mmol L⁻¹ of **strong base** to normalise their pH, because they lack sufficient alkaline substances to neutralize their acid load.

> **A base excess more negative than -2 mmol L⁻¹ indicates a metabolic acidosis.**

> **A base excess greater than +2 mmol L⁻¹ indicates a metabolic alkalosis.**

Step 6: Are there any other important values?

Blood gas analysers are particularly valuable because they give results very quickly. Most blood gas machines will produce a range of results in addition to the partial pressure and pH-related values mentioned above.

Generally it will be possible to get electrolytes such as sodium, potassium, chloride, and calcium; haemoglobin, glucose, and lactate are also widely available. At least one blood gas sample will be needed in most cardiac arrests to look for reversible causes.

The values available on a blood gas result are also highly relevant when deciding how to treat a critically ill patient. Not all the values will necessarily be equally important in every situation and it is reasonable to prioritise the results you think are most relevant, but you should be systematic when looking through the results. It is not uncommon to encounter an abnormal value that you were not expecting, and need to treat this too.

Finally, remember that there are many important tests which can only be done by a laboratory, so blood gas analysis is only one of the investigations you will need to perform. It does not replace the need to send samples for formal testing.

Summary

By using this stepwise approach to analysis of arterial blood gases, you will be able to identify if there is a problem, what the source of the problem is, and how to treat the problem. There now follows a series of examples, based on clinical cases, to highlight key points.

Case study 1

21 year-old woman, thrown from her horse at a local event. On the way to hospital, she has become increasingly drowsy and the paramedics have inserted an oropharyngeal airway and given high-flow oxygen via a face mask with a reservoir.

1. **How is the patient?**
    From the history we would predict the reduction in level of consciousness to reduce ventilation, increasing $PaCO_2$, causing a respiratory acidosis. It may also impair oxygenation. There is unlikely to be much compensation because the situation is acute. On arrival at hospital, following a rapid ABCDE assessment, an arterial blood sample is taken and shows:

Blood gas results		
PaO_2	18.8 kPa	10–13 kPa
pH	7.26	7.35–7.45
$PaCO_2$	8.2 kPa	4.7–6.0 kPa
Bicarbonate	26.0 mmol L^{-1}	22–26 mmol L^{-1}
Base excess	-1.4 mmol L^{-1}	-2 – +2 mmol L^{-1}

2. **Is the patient hypoxaemic?**
    Although the PaO_2 is just above the 'normal' range, breathing high-flow oxygen we would expect a PaO_2 around 75 kPa. Therefore there is a significant impairment in oxygenation.

3. **What is the pH?**
    The patient clearly has an acidaemia with a pH well below normal.

4. **What has happened to the $PaCO_2$?**
    The $PaCO_2$ is increased, consistent with the low pH, so the patient has a respiratory acidosis.

5. **What has happened to the bicarbonate?**
    The base excess within normal limits, as is the bicarbonate. This confirms that there is no significant metabolic contribution or compensation.

6. **Are there any other important values to consider?**
    In any unconscious patient it is useful to consider the blood glucose. Even here in a case of trauma it may be a contributor; depending on the patient's history, it is possible that a hypoglycaemic episode triggered the fall. Crush injuries can cause hyperkalaemia, so potassium should be checked. Haemoglobin can usefully be checked early in the resuscitation, although remember that it may appear normal until fluid resuscitation has started. A normal haemoglobin does not necessarily mean the patient is normovolaemic.

In summary, the patient has an acute respiratory acidosis with impaired oxygenation.

Case study 2

A 19 year-old man with asthma is bought to the emergency department (ED) by his parents. Over the past 4 hours, he has become increasingly wheezy with no response to his inhalers. He is now very distressed, tachypnoeic and has audible wheeze. He is receiving oxygen at 15 L min^{-1} via a face mask with reservoir.

1. **How is the patient?**
   From the history we would predict the bronchospasm will impair oxygenation and the hyperventilation should reduce his PaCO$_2$ causing a respiratory alkalosis. There is unlikely to be much compensation because the situation is acute. Following a rapid ABCDE assessment, an analysis of an arterial blood sample shows:

Blood gas results		
PaO$_2$	23.6 kPa (FiO$_2$ ≈ 85%)	10–13 kPa
pH	7.57	7.35–7.45
PaCO$_2$	3.4 kPa	4.7–6.0 kPa
Bicarbonate	23.1 mmol L^{-1}	22–26 mmol L^{-1}
Base excess	-1.8 mmol L^{-1}	-2 – +2 mmol L^{-1}

2. **Is the patient hypoxaemic?**
   Although the PaO$_2$ is above the normal range, breathing 85% oxygen we would expect a PaO$_2$ around 75 kPa. Therefore there is a significant impairment in oxygenation.

3. **What is the pH?**
   The patient clearly has a pH above the normal range, an alkalaemia.

4. **What has happened to the PaCO$_2$?**
   The PaCO$_2$ is decreased, consistent with a raised pH; the patient has a respiratory alkalosis. The PaCO$_2$ measurement is crucial in patients with acute severe asthma; a 'normal' PaCO$_2$ may even be a critical sign that the patient is tiring, and can no longer maintain the hyperventilation that was sustaining them.

5. **What has happened to the bicarbonate?**
   The base excess and bicarbonate are within normal limits. This confirms that there is no significant metabolic contribution or compensation.

6. **Are there any other important values to consider?**
   Repeated salbutamol nebulisers can reduce serum potassium values, and may cause lactate to rise, so these would be the most important values to consider for this patient.

In summary, the patient has an acute respiratory alkalosis with impaired oxygenation (Type I respiratory failure) and requires continued medical therapy for acute severe asthma.

Case study 3

A 52 year-old man, complaining of crushing central chest pain, is bought to the emergency department by his wife. He is attached to an ECG monitor, given oxygen 40% via a facemask, sublingual GTN and aspirin to chew. An intravenous cannula is inserted and he is given intravenous morphine. During an ABCDE assessment, he suddenly has a cardiac arrest. After 4 minutes of resuscitation he has a palpable pulse and starts to breathe spontaneously.

1. **How is the patient?**
   From the history we would predict the impaired ventilation to result in hypoxaemia, an increased PaCO$_2$, and respiratory acidosis. The impaired circulation will cause an increase in anaerobic respiration, production of lactate, and a metabolic acidosis. This will also decrease bicarbonate as it is used to buffer the excess acid. The acute presentation and failure of circulation is likely to prevent any degree of compensation. Analysis of an arterial blood sample shows:

Blood gas results		
PaO$_2$	8.9 kPa (FiO$_2$ ≈ 40%)	10–13 kPa
pH	7.11	7.35–7.45
PaCO$_2$	7.2 kPa	4.7–6.0 kPa
Bicarbonate	14 mmol L^{-1}	22–26 mmol L^{-1}
Base excess	-10.6 mmol L^{-1}	-2 – +2 mmol L^{-1}

2. **Is the patient hypoxaemic?**
   The patient is hypoxaemic despite breathing 40% oxygen; we would expect a PaO$_2$ around 30 kPa. Therefore there is a significant impairment in oxygenation.

3. **What is the pH?**
   The patient clearly has a very low pH; a severe acidaemia.

4. **What has happened to the PaCO$_2$?**
   The PaCO$_2$ is increased, consistent with the low pH, so the patient has a respiratory acidosis.

5. **What has happened to the bicarbonate?**
   The base excess and bicarbonate are both reduced. This is consistent with a metabolic acidosis.

6. **Are there any other important values to consider?**
   Anaemia can exacerbate acute coronary syndromes, so haemoglobin should be checked. Electrolyte disturbances can be a cause of sudden cardiac arrest, so would also be particularly relevant to this case.

In summary, the patient has a mixed respiratory and metabolic acidosis with impaired oxygenation following the cardiac arrest. He will still require assisted ventilation and treatment of the underlying cause of the arrest.

Derangements of both PaCO$_2$ and base excess or bicarbonate – compensation

Case study 3 demonstrates that sometimes the respiratory and metabolic changes occur in the same direction. That post-arrest patient had a high PaCO$_2$ and a low bicarbonate, both of which contribute to decreasing pH.

Other conditions may show changes where the respiratory and metabolic components go in 'opposite directions', and often show minimal disturbance of the pH. In these situations one of the derangements is a result of the original illness, which provokes a compensatory reaction in the other system. Both the respiratory and metabolic systems are capable of reacting to changes in the other, the aim being to minimise long term changes in pH.

The simplest way to determine which is the primary change and which is the compensatory change is to look at the direction of change in the pH, then examine the PaCO$_2$ and bicarbonate. Ask yourself first if the change in pH can be explained by the change in PaCO$_2$? A high PaCO$_2$ should cause a low pH, so if you see these together then there is a respiratory acidosis, and if there is metabolic compensation then the bicarbonate will be higher than normal. If the pH is low but the CO$_2$ is also low, then carbon dioxide can't explain the pH change; this means the primary problem is metabolic and the respiratory system is trying to compensate. You would expect the bicarbonate to be low in this case.

Case study 4

A 68 year-old man with a long history of COPD is reviewed on the medical ward before discharge.

1. **How is the patient?**
   From the history we would predict the patient to have a chronically raised PaCO$_2$ causing a respiratory acidosis. However, there is likely to be significant compensation in the form of a metabolic alkalosis. Oxygenation is also likely to be impaired, but given the patient is ready for discharge, this may be normal for him. Analysis of an arterial blood sample shows:

Blood gas results		
PaO$_2$	8.9 kPa	10–13 kPa
pH	7.34	7.35–7.45
PaCO$_2$	7.3 kPa	4.7 6.0 kPa
Bicarbonate	30.2 mmol L^{-1}	22–26 mmol L^{-1}
Base excess	+5.3 mmol L^{-1}	-2 – +2 mmol L^{-1}

2. **Is the patient hypoxaemic?**
   The PaO$_2$ is significantly reduced. Breathing air we would expect a PaO$_2$ around 11 kPa. Therefore there is impairment in oxygenation, although given the history this is likely to be chronic.

3. **What is the pH?**
   The patient has a borderline acidaemia with a pH just below the normal range.

4. **What has happened to the PaCO$_2$?**
   The PaCO$_2$ is increased. This should cause a low pH, so we can say there is a respiratory acidosis. The pH is not as low as one might expect, so we may predict there is a degree of compensation happening.

5. **What has happened to the bicarbonate?**
   The base excess and bicarbonate are both increased, confirming that there is metabolic compensation. This compensation has helped minimise or compensate for the pH disturbance caused by the respiratory acidosis. Since metabolic compensation takes some time, we can be confident that the respiratory problem is probably chronic.

6. **Are there any other important values to consider?**
   Since this blood gas has been taken in a routine situation, there aren't likely to be acute changes to be concerned about, but it is sensible to check each value carefully in case of surprises. Given the patient is chronically hypoxaemic you would predict their haemoglobin may be higher than normal, but this is a normal response to hypoxaemia, and not something that would ordinarily need to be corrected.

In summary, the patient has a chronic respiratory acidosis with a compensatory metabolic alkalosis, with significantly impaired oxygenation (Type II respiratory failure). He will require optimisation of medical management of his COPD prior to discharge.

Case study 5

A 22 year-old male, recently diagnosed with insulin dependent diabetes mellitus (IDDM) presents to the emergency department, having been unwell for 48 hours, with a gradually increasing blood glucose concentration, despite taking his insulin. He is tachypnoeic, tachycardic and a point-of-care measurement of his blood glucose is 23 mmol L^{-1}.

1. **How is the patient?**
    From the history the most likely problem is that the patient has diabetic ketoacidosis (DKA) (i.e. a metabolic acidosis). However, the fact that he is tachypnoeic suggests that he is trying to compensate by reducing his $PaCO_2$ that effectively reduces the [H+] causing a respiratory alkalosis. Following a rapid ABCDE assessment, analysis of an arterial blood sample while breathing oxygen, 6 L min^{-1} via a facemask shows:

Blood gas results		
PaO_2	22.2 kPa	10–13 kPa
pH	7.14	7.35–7.45
$PaCO_2$	33.8 kPa	4.7–6.0 kPa
Bicarbonate	19.1 mmol L^{-1}	22–26 mmol L^{-1}
Base excess	-7.9 mmol L^{-1}	-2 – +2 mmol L^{-1}

2. **Is the patient hypoxaemic?**
    The PaO_2 is slightly lower than might be predicted for someone breathing 40% oxygen, which may indicate the possibility of an underlying chest infection.

3. **What is the pH?**
    The pH is well below the lower limit of normality, he has a significant acidaemia.

4. **What has happened to the $PaCO_2$?**
    The $PaCO_2$ is decreased. This should cause a respiratory alkalosis, so doesn't explain the change in pH. This must be the compensatory response.

5. **What has happened to the bicarbonate?**
    The base excess and bicarbonate are both decreased. This confirms that there is a metabolic acidosis. The change in pH would have been greater without the concurrent respiratory changes to compensate.

6. **Are there any other important values to consider?**
    The blood glucose value will be the most important value to check in this patient, but electrolyte abnormalities are also very common in DKA. Potassium and sodium should also be checked, and your hospital will have protocols about the safe way to manage any abnormalities you see.

In summary, the patient has a metabolic acidosis (as a result of impaired glucose metabolism and the development of ketoacids) with a compensatory respiratory alkalosis. He will require careful IV fluid and electrolyte replacement along with a fixed rate insulin infusion according to local DKA protocols.

Practical aspects of blood gas analysis during resuscitation

During cardiac arrest, arterial blood gas values should be interpreted with caution because they correlate poorly with the severity of hypoxaemia, hypercapnia and acidosis in the tissues. They can also be quite difficult to obtain when the patient is pulseless. During cardiac arrest, venous blood gases (VBGs) may reflect more accurately the acid-base state of the tissues. These are interpreted using the same 6-step approach, but remember that venous blood will have a much lower PaO_2 (and higher $PaCO_2$) than arterial blood, so you cannot use the same reference ranges for the gases measured on a venous blood gas sample.

Once return of spontaneous circulation is achieved, arterial blood gas analysis will provide a useful guide to post-resuscitation care, such as appropriately setting a ventilator to achieve optimal oxygenation and CO_2 levels. Arterial lactate concentration can also be used to indicate the adequacy of tissue oxygenation. Immediately after cardiac arrest lactate concentration will be raised, reflecting the lactic acidosis caused by a period of inadequate cardiac output. After ROSC a progressively decreasing lactate is a valuable indicator of improving tissue perfusion, and can show the patient is responding to treatment.

In the peri-arrest setting, it may be easiest to obtain a sample of arterial blood (in a heparinised syringe) from the femoral artery because the pulse is likely to be stronger than at the radial artery. The radial artery may be preferable once the patient has an adequate cardiac output and blood pressure. The radial artery is also the best site for arterial cannulation; this enables continuous beat-to-beat blood pressure monitoring and frequent arterial blood sampling during post-resuscitation care.

Venous blood gas samples (VBG) are often used in the assessment of acutely unwell patients instead of ABGs. They are particularly useful for monitoring metabolic disturbances when there is no clinical indication of any respiratory compromise. They are generally more comfortable for an awake patient, so can be useful when multiple measurements in a short space of time are required. A specific example is in DKA, where serial samples enable the clinician to monitor for resolution of the metabolic abnormalities whilst also providing a point of care test for essential electrolytes (specifically potassium in DKA). When interpreting electrolyte values a degree of caution should be exercised if results are unexpectedly or disproportionately abnormal. Prolonged tourniquets application, repeated aspiration of the syringe, or transferring blood between syringes can cause red blood cells in the sample to haemolyse. This may make tests inaccurate, so results that do not fit the clinical picture should always be confirmed.

Table 15.1   Haemoglobin oxygen dissociation curve

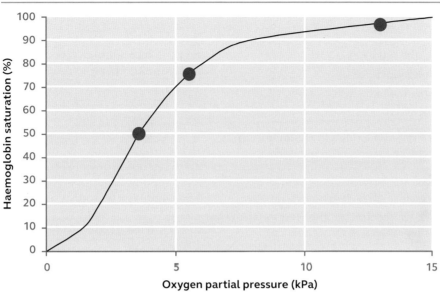

VBGs from a central venous line (if one is present) may provide a better indication of acid-base status because the blood is being sampled after it has passed through the tissues. This is particularly useful in the cardiac arrest setting, where the lack of effective circulation means that ABGs do not accurately reflect tissue metabolism. Central lines are time-consuming and potentially difficult to insert, so although useful if already present it would be very uncommon to put a new line in during a cardiac arrest.

Pulse oximetry

Role of pulse oximetry

Pulse oximetry is a vital adjunct to the assessment of hypoxaemia. Clinical recognition of decreased arterial oxygen saturation of haemoglobin (SaO$_2$) is subjective and unreliable: a person may not appear to be cyanosed until their arterial oxygen saturations are as low as 80–85%; objective measurements by pulse oximetry is therefore much more reliable. Pulse oximeters work by detecting changes in oxygenated haemoglobin in the blood. They do this by shining light through the tissue, but they depend on having a reasonable circulation to the area of the body where the probe is attached.

Pulse oximeters often provide an audible tone related to the SpO$_2$ value, with a decreasing tone reflecting increasing hypoxaemia. This can be helpful, since you can detect changes in SpO$_2$ just by listening, even if you aren't looking at the screen. Some pulse oximeters, particularly those in areas like the emergency department (ED), intensive care unit (ICU), or operating room, also display a waveform. This gives useful information about the quality of the signal the system is measuring. A poor signal may indicate a low blood pressure or poor tissue perfusion, and may also mean the measured arterial blood saturations are inaccurate.

Limitations of pulse oximetry

The relationship between oxygen saturation and PaO$_2$ is demonstrated by the oxyhaemoglobin dissociation curve (Figure 15.1). The sinusoid shape of the curve means that an initial decrease from a normal PaO$_2$ is not accompanied by a drop of similar magnitude in the oxygen saturation of the blood, and early hypoxaemia may be masked. For example, at the point where the SpO$_2$ reaches 94% the PaO$_2$ will have decreased from about 13.0 kPa to about 10 kPa. In other words, the partial pressure of oxygen will have decreased by more than a fifth for a decrease of only 6–8% in SpO$_2$. Below 94% the graph becomes very steep, so relatively small decreases in saturation cause disproportionately large decreases in PaO$_2$. At 75% saturation (the saturation of normal venous blood), PaO$_2$ is only 5.3 kPa.

There are several potential sources of error with pulse oximetry:

- Presence of other haemoglobins: carboxyhaemoglobin (carbon monoxide poisoning), methaemoglobin (congenital or acquired), fetal haemoglobins and sickling red cells (sickle cell disease).

- Surgical and imaging dyes (e.g. methylene blue) can cause falsely low saturation readings.

- Nail varnish (especially blue, black and green).

- High-ambient light levels (fluorescent and xenon lamps).

- Motion artefact.

- Reduced pulse volume:
  - hypotension
  - low cardiac output
  - vasoconstriction
  - hypothermia.

Pulse oximeters are not affected by:

- anaemia (reduced haemoglobin)
- jaundice (hyperbilirubinaemia)
- skin pigmentation.

Pulse oximetry does not provide a reliable signal during CPR. It may also be difficult to record if the patient is hypovolaemic or hypothermic. Remember that the pulse oximeter will only measure blood oxygen saturations where the system can detect a pulse. If blood oxygen saturations are completely unrecordable, this is more likely to reflect a 'C' problem than a 'B' problem.

Targeted oxygen therapy

Give high-concentration oxygen immediately to critically ill patients with acute hypoxaemia (initial SpO_2 < 85%) or in the peri-arrest situation. Give this initially with a non-rebreather mask with reservoir and an oxygen flow of 15 L min^{-1}. During cardiac arrest use 100% inspired oxygen concentration to maximise arterial oxygen content and delivery to the tissues. After an initial assessment you can then reduce the amount of oxygen given to the patient as appropriate.

Patients with respiratory failure can be divided into two groups:

Respiratory failure

Type I:

Low PaO_2 (< 8 kPa), normal $PaCO_2$ (< 7 kPa). In these patients it is safe to give a high concentration of oxygen initially with the aim of returning their PaO_2 to normal. Once clinically stable, you can adjust the inspired oxygen concentration to maintain the patient's SpO_2 at 94–98%.

Type II:

Low PaO_2 (< 8 kPa), increased $PaCO_2$ (> 7 kPa). This is often described as hypercapnic respiratory failure and is often caused by COPD. If given excessive oxygen, these patients may develop worsening respiratory failure with further increases in $PaCO_2$ and the development of a respiratory acidosis. If unchecked, this will eventually lead to unconsciousness, and respiratory or cardiac arrest. The target oxygen saturation in this at-risk population is 88–92%. However, when critically ill and their arterial blood oxygen saturation is unknown, give these patients high-flow oxygen initially, then analyse the arterial blood gases and use the results to adjust the inspired oxygen concentration. When clinically stable and a reliable pulse oximetry reading is obtained, adjust the inspired oxygen concentration to maintain an SpO_2 of 88–92%.

Giving these patients oxygen is not intrinsically dangerous, but failing to monitor them carefully and regularly is. If you are concerned a patient may have Type-II respiratory failure and is receiving oxygen therapy make sure you do frequent observations, and initially you may need to take serial ABG samples. If their CO_2 is rising then they may be receiving too much oxygen, and it might need to be turned down. You may need assistance from respiratory physicians or intensive care as the patient may require ventilatory support.

Patients with acute coronary syndromes

In patients with an acute coronary syndrome, and who are not critically or seriously ill, aim to maintain an SpO_2 of 94–98% (or 88–92% if the patient is also at risk of hypercapnic respiratory failure). This may be achievable without supplementary oxygen.

15: Summary learning

Arterial blood gas analysis results are interpreted systematically using the 6-step approach.

Pulse oximetry enables arterial blood oxygen saturation to be monitored continuously.

Use an inspired oxygen concentration of 100% until return of spontaneous circulation (ROSC) is achieved.

After ROSC is achieved, and once the SpO_2 can be monitored reliably, titrate the inspired oxygen concentration to keep the SpO_2 in the range 94–98%.

My key take-home messages from this chapter are:

Further reading

Al-Sheikh B, Stacey S Essentials of equipment in anaesthesia, critical care, and perioperative medicine 5th Edition 2018, Elsevier, London, UK.

West JB, Luks, AM West's respiratory physiology: the essentials 10th Edition, 2016 Wolters Kluwer, Philadelphia, USA.

WHO Guidelines on Drawing Blood: Best practices in phlebotomy (Chapter 5: arterial blood sampling): https://www.ncbi.nlm.nih.gov/books/NBK138661/

BTS Guideline for oxygen use in healthcare and emergency settings: https://www.brit-thoracic.org.uk/quality-improvement/guidelines/emergency-oxygen/

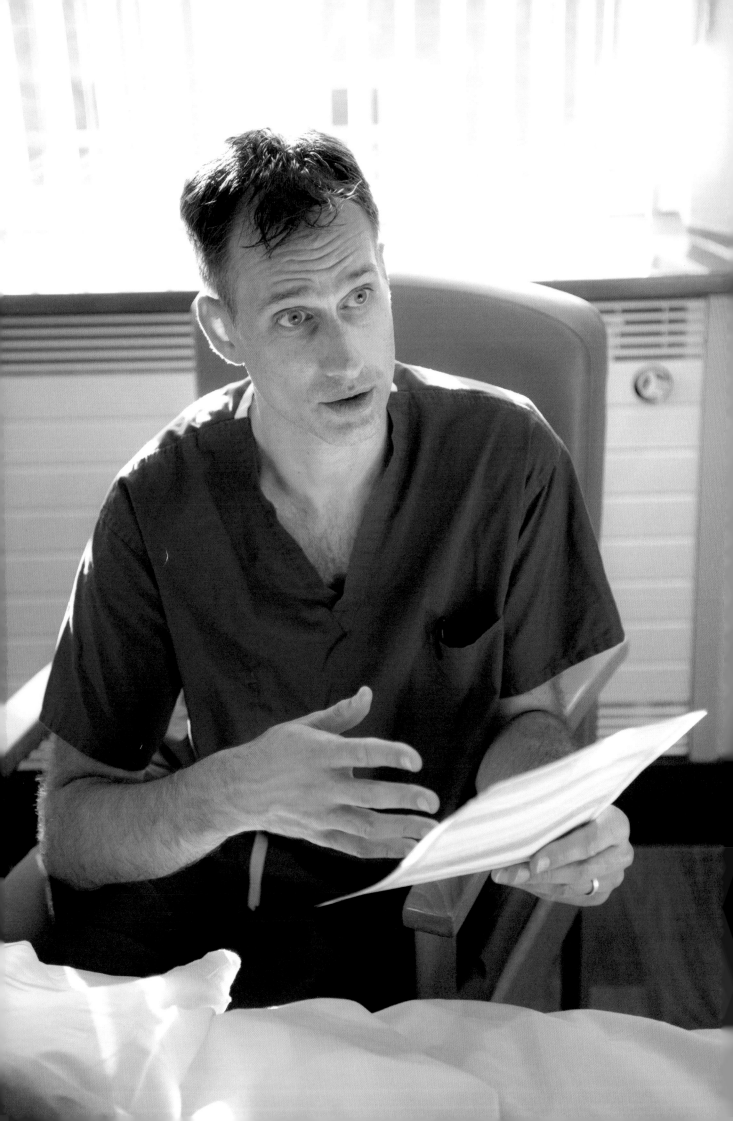

Making decisions about CPR

In this chapter

Ethical and legal principles

Emergency care and treatment plans (including CPR)

Shared decision-making, effective communication and clear documentation

Deciding whether to provide CPR

Deciding to stop CPR

Auditing cardiac arrest and decisions about CPR

The learning outcomes will enable you to:

Consider the ethical and legal principles involved in decision-making about emergency care and treatments including CPR

Participate in shared decision-making to create personalised recommendations for a person's clinical care and treatment in a future emergency in which they are unable to make or express choices

Communicate effectively to elicit patient preferences, and explain what is realistic in terms of their care and treatment

Record clear, relevant information relating to emergency care and treatment plans (including CPR)

Understand when it is reasonable to not to attempt and / or discontinue CPR

and to feel more confident in:

Reaching shared decisions about emergency care and treatments and encourage others to follow best practice in shared decision-making

Introduction

Cardiopulmonary resuscitation (CPR) can be a lifesaving intervention bringing extended, precious life to many. However, it is far from being universally successful and, like any invasive medical treatment, can cause harm. When someone is dying from an irreversible cause, CPR is unlikely to work but can subject them to an undignified death, or even cause suffering and prolong the process of dying. Don't assume that everyone whose heart and breathing stop would consider survival a successful outcome. Prolonging life at all costs is not an appropriate goal of medicine.

Do not attempt CPR (DNACPR) decisions have existed for many years and provide a mechanism to not to attempt CPR when it will not restart the heart or breathing for a sustained period, where the balance of burdens exceeds the benefits, or the patient does not wish to receive CPR. However, CPR is not provided in isolation from other treatments and should always be considered as part of an overall emergency care treatment plan.

The Recommended Summary Plan for Emergency Care and Treatment (ReSPECT) process provides a framework to enable shared decision-making in relation to emergency treatment decisions (including CPR) when the person is unable to participate in decision-making at the time. This chapter summarises the legal and ethical considerations for making such recommendations and describes how to engage patients and their families in shared decision-making.

Ethical and legal framework

Health and care professionals must practice ethically and within the law. Laws relevant to CPR, including those on matters relating to capacity and consent, vary from nation to nation, both outside and within the UK. Detailed guidance is provided in **Decisions relating to cardiopulmonary resuscitation**. The ethical and legal principles that underpin this guidance apply equally to the broader planning approach taken by the ReSPECT process and other emergency care and treatment plans. As an ALS provider you should read and be familiar with that guidance, and be familiar with relevant aspects of the law in the nation where you live and work.

Table 16.1 summarises Beauchamp and Childress' four key principles of medical ethics. Every decision about CPR must be based on a careful assessment of each person's situation at any particular time. These decisions must never be dictated by 'blanket' policies. Individual decisions about CPR must be made with the person, or, where they lack capacity, with those close to them. The courts have made clear that there should be a presumption in favour of involving people in discussions about whether or not CPR will be attempted. This upholds the principle of autonomy and the provisions of the Human Rights Act (1998).

Table 16.1 Summary of Beauchamp and Childress' four key principles of medical ethics

Autonomy	Requires people to be allowed and helped to make their own informed decisions, rather than having decisions made for them. A person with capacity must be adequately informed about the matter to be decided and free from undue pressure in making their decision. Autonomy allows an informed person to make a choice, even if that choice is considered illogical or incorrect by others, including health professionals.
Beneficence	Involves provision of benefit to an individual, while balancing benefit and risks. Commonly this will involve attempting CPR for cardiac arrest. If CPR will offer no benefit or the risks clearly outweigh any likely benefit it will mean not attempting CPR. Beneficence includes also actions that benefit the wider community, such as providing a programme of public access defibrillation.
Non-maleficence	Means doing no harm. CPR should not be attempted in people in whom it will not succeed, where no benefit is likely but there will be a clear risk of doing harm.
Justice	Requires spreading benefits and risks equally within a society. If CPR is provided, it should be available to all who may benefit from it. There should be no discrimination purely on the grounds of factors such as age or disability. Justice does not imply an entitlement to expect or demand CPR for everyone. If limited resources are engaged in attempting CPR on people with no chance of benefit those resources may not be available when needed by others who are likely to benefit.

There are two rare circumstances where it is legally and ethically acceptable to make a CPR decision without discussion with the person or those close to them:

1. Where it is believed that having a conversation with the person will cause physiological or psychological harm to them (Tracey v Cambridge University Hospital).

2. In the case of a person who lacks capacity to make a decision regarding CPR, where it is impracticable or inappropriate to contact those close to them before a decision needs to be made (Winspear v City Hospitals). This would include, for example, emergencies where an individual had lost capacity and there was insufficient time to contact those close to them, or it was not possible to reach them.

Integrating recommendations relating to CPR into overarching emergency care and treatment plans

Research has shown that when DNACPR decisions are made in isolation they lack clarity on the overall goals of treatment. In some cases, this has unintentionally led to fewer invasive medical treatments, reduced observations, less escalation to medical and outreach staff and reductions in even basic nursing care. The integration of decisions relating to CPR in to overarching emergency care and treatment plans has been shown to reduce harms, increase clarity of overall goals of care, improve concordance between patient's wishes and treatments provided and enhance communication between clinicians and the patient. Therefore it is recommended that decisions to provide or not to provide CPR should always be made in the context of an overall plan for emergency care and treatment.

Shared decision-making

Shared decision-making brings together the individual's expertise about themselves and what is important to them and the clinician's knowledge about the benefits and risks of relevant treatments. Many people welcome the opportunity to discuss their wishes about care, treatments and health outcomes, once they realise that the purpose is to plan with them what treatments they would benefit from. Health professionals are not obliged to offer or deliver treatments that they believe to be inappropriate. Even where treatment options are limited, seek to engage patients in shared decision-making using the steps described below.

Making sure the conversation is not just about CPR but about wider goals of care as this can make the conversation less difficult and more useful for both the person and the clinician. The ReSPECT process has been developed to facilitate good conversations and shared decision-making between the person and the health professionals.

Three steps are recommended:

1. Establish what the person thinks are their most relevant health conditions and develop a shared understanding of the prognosis of these conditions. Find out how the person feels about their current environment and state of health and their views about the future.

2. Establish and record what the person thinks would matter most to them (values and fears) if they suddenly became less well, both in their daily lives and in a possible future emergency.

3. Having established what is most important to the person, agree upon and record what interventions may result in the desired outcomes and so are wanted, and which ones have little realistic chance of success, or a high probability of resulting in a feared outcome, and so are unwanted or would not work. This includes but is not limited to a recommendation about CPR.

Specific training in having these sensitive conversations can help health professionals to communicate effectively and to recognise that these conversations are important and are not necessarily difficult. Explore your opportunities for such training as part of your professional development. Requirements for effective communication include providing information in a format that the person can understand and checking that they have understood it. It may be necessary to have more than one conversation to reach a shared understanding and a decision. Offer opportunities for further discussion and be aware that people may change their minds if they wish to.

Don't force conversations on people who don't want them, but don't withhold them from those who do. Whenever possible, they should be undertaken by health professionals who know the person well, but that may not be possible when they are needed by someone with an acute illness or injury and no previous advance plan.

Findings from an evaluation of ReSPECT, funded by the National Institute for Health Research, found that ReSPECT conversations take time for health professionals to do well. Good decisions were characterised by building rapport and trust through:

- exercising medical judgment when recommending certain treatments
- soliciting a person's view about their values and preferences
- taking these into account when making treatment recommendations
- talking a person through the rationale for these recommendations
- ensuring that decisions are understood
- recording how the harms and benefits associated with treatment options were weighed up.

Communication: discussing recommendations with those close to the person

An important component of high-quality care is effective communication with those close to a person (often but not always family members) and keeping them fully informed. You must respect a person's wishes regarding confidentiality, but most people want family members or others close to them to be involved in discussions about treatments such as CPR and to have their support in making these decisions. Whenever possible encourage patients to think about and discuss their wishes in advance with members of their family. Knowing a patient's wishes helps relatives to feel more confident in situations when they are asked what they think a patient would have wanted.

Communication: discussing recommendations when a person lacks capacity

If a person lacks capacity, they can still be involved in decision-making to the limit of their ability. Formal assessment of their capacity should be undertaken and recorded; remember that capacity is decision specific. Assess whether they can understand, retain and weigh up the relevant information (e.g. about attempting CPR) and communicate their wishes to you.

If a person does not have capacity to be involved in the discussions and recommendations being made, then decisions about their treatment, including about CPR, must be made in their best interests.

If (as defined in the Mental Capacity Act 2005 (MCA 2005) which applies in England & Wales) they have made a valid and applicable Advance Decision to Refuse Treatment (ADRT) that refuses CPR "even if their life is at risk" that ADRT is legally binding and must be respected. If a person who lacks capacity has a legal proxy (e.g. an 'attorney for health and welfare') with power to make such decisions on their behalf, that person must be involved in the decision-making process. The courts have stated also that, when considering a decision about CPR for a person who lacks capacity, there is a duty to consult anyone engaged in caring for them or interested in their welfare. In some circumstances the law requires you to involve others. For example, the MCA 2005 requires an Independent Mental Capacity Advocate (IMCA) to speak on behalf of a person who lacks capacity and has no other representatives, guiding a best-interests decision by the senior clinician. The conversation you have with the relative or IMCA should follow the same structure provided above: establish a shared understanding of the person's condition, what is known of their wishes and fears, and what treatments, including CPR, that they would benefit from.

If a person is critically ill and an urgent decision is needed in order to plan the best care for them, that decision should not be delayed if their family or other carers cannot be contacted, or there is not enough time to appoint or contact an IMCA. Make the decision that is in the person's best interests, but also make and record a clear plan to consult their family or others close to them, or to contact an IMCA, at the earliest practicable opportunity. Document the basis for any decision clearly and fully.

Deciding whether or not to provide CPR

When an informed person with capacity refuses CPR as a potential treatment option it should not be attempted. If CPR would not restart the heart and breathing for a sustained period because a person is dying as an inevitable result of underlying disease or a catastrophic health event CPR should not be attempted. A person (or someone representing them) is not entitled to insist on receiving a treatment that is clinically inappropriate. Health professionals are not obliged to offer or deliver treatments that they believe to be inappropriate. Explaining these matters requires sensitive discussion.

The overall responsibility for proper decision-making and planning about emergency care and treatment (including CPR) rests with the senior health professional in charge of the person's care at the time. When making advance plans there should be appropriate consultation with other health professionals involved, as well as appropriate discussion with the person themselves and those close to them.

If a difference of opinion arises between the healthcare team and the person or their representatives this can usually be resolved by careful discussion and explanation. If not, a second clinical opinion must be offered. Seeking a decision by legal authorities may involve delay and uncertainty. Formal legal judgement may be needed if there are irreconcilable differences between the parties. In difficult cases, the senior clinician may wish to seek legal advice from their indemnity provider or other professional organisation.

Recording emergency care and treatment plans (including CPR)

Ensure records include:

- patient identifier information
- whether the patient had mental capacity to be involved in the recommendations which are being recorded
- who was involved in making the recommendations
- patient preferences and priorities for treatment
- how the clinician weighed the potential burdens and benefits of treatment to reach a recommendation
- recommended treatments and those that should not be provided
- whether CPR should be attempted or not.

Recommendations relating to emergency care and treatment (including CPR) should be recorded clearly and using terms that will be understandable to those who may need to act on them. Recommendations should be specific to the relevant treatments and also the setting where they may be applied. Terms such as 'forward based care' lack clarity on treatment goals and have limited relevance when someone is discharged from hospital.

Ensure the record is available immediately if it is needed in a crisis. For example, if such a recommendation is recorded on a paper form, this should be readily available to help an ambulance clinician decide whether to attempt CPR in a person's home. People should be encouraged and helped to make those close to them aware of their wishes and resulting recommendations, and of where to find the record of these.

Various forms have been developed in different places to record people's treatment decisions in advance. RCUK favours the use of a standard document that is used and accepted by all health and care provider organisations, so that it is effective across geographical and organisational boundaries. RCUK supports the use of the ReSPECT process and form: www.respectprocess.org.uk.

Communicating recommendations and the person's wishes

There should be effective verbal communication with all those caring for the person and robust written and/or electronic documentation to ensure that recommendations are known, and the records remain available if the person travels to a different location, however briefly. Within a hospital, that might involve, for example, attending a radiology or physiotherapy department for investigation or treatment. In the community, it might involve, for example, attending a healthcare appointment or going out with or visiting friends or family.

When it is reasonable not to attempt CPR

In cardiac arrest, where immediate treatment is necessary to preserve life, unless an anticipatory decision has been made to not to attempt CPR or there are signs of irreversible death, resuscitation should usually be commenced. This allows those present to obtain sufficient information to determine the appropriateness of continuing resuscitation.

Many out-of-hospital cardiac arrests are attended by ambulance clinicians, who face dilemmas about when CPR will not succeed and when it should be stopped. In general, CPR will be started in out-of-hospital cardiac arrest unless there is a valid ADRT refusing it, or a valid recommendation not to attempt CPR.

Ambulance service guidelines allow trained personnel to refrain from starting CPR in defined situations, for example in people with mortal injuries such as decapitation or hemicorporectomy, known submersion for more than 1.5 h, incineration, rigor mortis and hypostasis or where a person is known to be in the final stages of an advanced and irreversible condition, in which CPR would be both inappropriate and unsuccessful. In such cases, the ambulance clinician may identify that death has occurred but cannot certify the cause of death (which in most countries can be done only by a doctor or coroner).

Similar recognition that death has occurred and is irreversible and a resulting decision not to start CPR may be made by experienced nurses or ambulance clinicians working in the community or in settings that provide care for people who are terminally or chronically ill. Whenever possible, advance recommendations about CPR should be considered as part of advance care planning before they are needed in a crisis.

A recorded recommendation not to attempt CPR means it is not appropriate to start CPR for cardiorespiratory arrest, unless the circumstances of the arrest are not those envisaged when the recommendation was recorded.

Make sure that all other treatment is given in accordance with the person's treatment plan and is of the highest standard. This may include recording physiological observations, and treatments both at home and requiring transfer into hospital.

As an ALS provider, make sure that a properly made and recorded recommendation not to attempt CPR does not (through your actions or those of others) lead to withholding from a person other care or treatment.

Decisions about implanted cardioverter-defibrillators

When a person who is approaching the end of their life has an implanted cardioverter-defibrillator (ICD), a discussion with them about CPR should prompt also a sensitive discussion about whether and when they may wish to have the shock function of their ICD deactivated.

A proportion of people who die with an active ICD in place will receive shocks from the device in the last hours or days of their life. These are usually painful and can be distressing for the patient and for those close to them.

However, it must not be assumed that a recommendation not to attempt CPR automatically warrants deactivation of an ICD. Some people may wish to have prompt treatment from an ICD, but choose not to have CPR for cardiac arrest, which is much more traumatic, would have a lower chance of success and greater risk of harm.

Defining 'success' and 'futility'

Achieving return of spontaneous circulation (ROSC) does not mean that CPR has been successful. A resuscitation attempt can only be regarded as successful if it restores a person to a duration and quality of life that they themselves regard as worth having.

Attempted resuscitation can only be regarded as being truly futile if it has no chance of achieving that outcome.

These statements emphasise the importance, whenever possible, of knowing a person's wishes, fears and beliefs in advance, and ideally documenting them in their own words. Achieving outcomes which are valuable to them, while avoiding those that are feared can be considered a success.

Predicting outcome

Predicting the outcome from CPR for cardiac arrest is far from easy. The outcome is dependent on many factors, including the prior state of health of the person and the times from arrest to starting CPR and attempting defibrillation as well as the time taken to achieve ROSC.

A scoring tool has been developed to predict chances of surviving attempted CPR with a good neurological outcome (Ebell et al.). Using this tool may assist in conversations with a person and those close to them, but it should not be used in isolation, since different people will value different outcomes.

Predictors of non-survival after attempted resuscitation have been published, but do not have sufficient predictive value to be used in general clinical practice in the immediate period after ROSC.

Avoiding discrimination

It is crucial that discussions and decisions are non-discriminatory and, for example, do not deprive people of CPR purely on the grounds of factors such as age or a disability. The age of the person may be considered in the decision-making process but is only a relatively weak independent predictor of outcome. However, many elderly people have significant comorbidity, which influences outcome. Remember also to avoid discriminating by attempting CPR with no realistic chance of benefit on a person, simply because they are younger or because of an assumption that they would want this; opening discussions with people and those close to them can help prevent this.

Deciding to stop CPR

Many resuscitation attempts do not succeed and in those circumstances at some point, a decision has to be made to stop CPR. This decision can be made when continuing CPR will not achieve ROSC, or an outcome that would be valued by the person. Factors influencing the decision will include the person's clinical history and prognosis, the cardiac arrest rhythm that is present, the response or absence of response to initial resuscitation measures, and the duration of the resuscitation attempt.

Do not discontinue resuscitation based on single criteria (e.g. pupil size, CPR duration, end-tidal carbon dioxide value, cardiac standstill on ultrasound, co-morbidities, lactate) as they are not sufficiently reliable in isolation to predict an adverse outcome.

Sometimes during a resuscitation attempt, information becomes available that was not known when CPR was started and indicates that CPR will not succeed or was not wanted. It is appropriate to stop CPR in those circumstances.

In general, CPR should be continued if a shockable rhythm or other potentially reversible cause for cardiac arrest persists. It is accepted that asystole for more than 20 min, in the absence of a reversible cause and with all ALS measures applied, is unlikely to be corrected by further CPR and is a reasonable basis for stopping CPR.

In some countries, including the UK, paramedics may cease a resuscitation attempt in this situation. Their strict protocol requires that conditions that might indicate a remote chance of survival (e.g. hypothermia) are absent, and the presence of asystole must also be established beyond reasonable doubt and documented on an ECG recording.

A decision to stop CPR should be made by the leader of the resuscitation attempt after consultation with other team members. Ultimately, the decision is based on a clinical judgement that further ALS will not restart the heart and breathing.

Special considerations

Certain circumstances at the time of cardiac arrest (e.g. hypothermia) enhance the chances of recovery without neurological damage. In such situations, do not use prognostic criteria (such as asystole persisting for more than 20 min); continue CPR until the reversible problem has been corrected (e.g. re-warming has been achieved).

Withdrawal of other treatment during the post-resuscitation period

It is difficult to predict the clinical and neurological outcome in people who remain unconscious during the first three days after ROSC. In general, other supportive treatment should be continued during this period, after which the prognosis can be assessed and predicted with greater confidence. This topic is covered in more detail in Chapter 13.

Auditing cardiac arrests and decisions about CPR

Every cardiac arrest is best regarded as a critical clinical event, irrespective of the setting. The decisions made and actions taken by those present must be recorded clearly and accurately. Local audit of such events should take place routinely, allowing recognition of good practice and allowing corrective action where system failures have led to poor or absent decision-making or inappropriate responses. Recording all arrests in one of the national databases (in-hospital: National Cardiac Arrest Audit, out-of-hospital: Out-of-hospital Cardiac Arrest Outcomes) will help to identify variation in practice and outcome to try to ensure equality of access to and delivery of treatment.

Health Service Circular 2000/028 states 'NHS Trust chief executives are asked to ensure that appropriate resuscitation policies which respect patients' rights are in place, understood by all relevant staff, and accessible to those who need them, and that such policies are subject to appropriate audit and monitoring arrangements.' As making anticipatory recommendations about emergency care and treatments, including CPR, is an integral part of good clinical care the decision-making process and the documentation of discussions and decisions about these should be audited routinely in all healthcare settings.

Further reading

British Medical Association, Resuscitation Council (UK) and Royal College of Nursing. Decisions relating to cardiopulmonary resuscitation. 3rd Edition, First revision 2016. www.resus. org.uk/library/publications/publication-decisions-relating-cardiopulmonary

Council of Europe. Guide on the decision-making process regarding medical treatment in end-of-life situations. http://www.coe.int/en/web/portal/-/council-of-europe-launches-a-guide-on-the-decision-making-process- regarding-medical-treatment-in-end-of-life-situations

Ebell MH, Jang W, Shen Y, Geocadin RG; Get With the Guidelines–Resuscitation Investigators. Development and validation of the Good Outcome Following Attempted Resuscitation (GO-FAR) score to predict neurologically intact survival after in-hospital cardiopulmonary resuscitation. JAMA Intern Med. 2013 Nov 11;173(20):1872-8.

Fritz Z, Slowther AM, Perkins G. Resuscitation policy should focus on the patient, not the decision. BMJ 2017;356:j813.

General Medical Council. Treatment and care towards the end of life. 2010. www.gmc-uk.org

Hawkes CA, Fritz Z, Deas G, et al. Development of the Recommended Summary Plan for Emergency Care and Treatment (ReSPECT). Resuscitation. 2020 Mar 1;148:98-107.

Mentzelopoulos SD, Couper K, Van de Voorde P, Druwe PM, Blom MT, Perkins GD, Lulic I, Djakow J, Raffay V, Lilja G and Bossaert L. European Resuscitation Council Guidelines 2021: Ethics of resuscitation and end of life decisions Resuscitation. 2021;161.

Perkins GD, Griffiths F, Slowther AM, et al. Do-not-attempt-cardiopulmonary-resuscitation decisions: an evidence synthesis. NIHR Journals Library; 2016 Apr. https://www.journalslibrary.nihr.ac.uk/hsdr/hsdr04110/#/abstract

Perkins GD, Hawkes C, Eli et al. Evaluation of the Recommended Summary Plan for Emergency Care and Treatment. NIHR Journals Library; 2021 https://www.journalslibrary.nihr.ac.uk/programmes/hsdr/151509/#/

Pitcher D, Soar J, Hogg K, et al: the CIED Working Group. Cardiovascular implanted electronic devices in people towards the end of life, during cardiopulmonary resuscitation and after death: guidance from the Resuscitation Council (UK), British Cardiovascular Society and National Council for Palliative Care. Heart 2016;102:A1-A17.

Pitcher D, Fritz Z, Wang M, Spiller, J. Emergency care and resuscitation plans. BMJ 2017;356:j876.

Resuscitation Council UK. British Cardiovascular Society and National Council for Palliative Care. Deactivation of implantable cardioverter- defibrillators towards the end of life. www.resus.org.uk

Resuscitation Council UK. CPR, AEDs and the law. https://www.resus.org.uk/library/publications/publication-cpr-aeds-and-law

The Scottish Government. Adults with Incapacity (Scotland) Act 2000: A short guide to the Act. https://www.legislation.gov.uk/asp/2000/4/contents

UK Government. Mental Capacity Act 2005 Code of Practice. https://www.gov.uk/government/collections/mental-capacity-act-makingdecisions

16: Summary learning

Decisions to provide or not provide CPR should be integrated into overarching emergency treatment plans such as ReSPECT.

Emergency care and treatment plans (including CPR) should be based on a careful assessment of each person's situation at any particular time. Do not apply blanket policies.

The patient (or those close to the patient if they lack capacity) must be consulted when making a decision to not to attempt CPR.

Shared decision-making brings together the individual's expertise about themselves and what is important to them together with the clinician's knowledge about the benefits and risks of relevant treatments.

Establish a shared understanding of prognosis and treatments available, the patients values and fears and use these to agree on an overall treatment plan.

Situations where it is reasonable to not to attempt CPR include where it will not restart the heart and breathing for a sustained period, where the benefits of prolonging life outweigh the potential burdens and risks or where the patient (or legal representative) refuses CPR.

Record recommendations clearly using terms that are understandable to those who may need to act on them. Avoid using terms which lack clarity on treatment goals.

In the event of cardiac arrest, unless an anticipatory decision has been made to not to attempt CPR or there are signs of irreversible death, start resuscitation promptly.

Consider discontinuing CPR if it will not achieve ROSC or an outcome that would be valued by the person. Base decisions on a comprehensive assessment of relevant information. Do not rely on single criteria to predict outcome.

My key take-home messages from this chapter are:

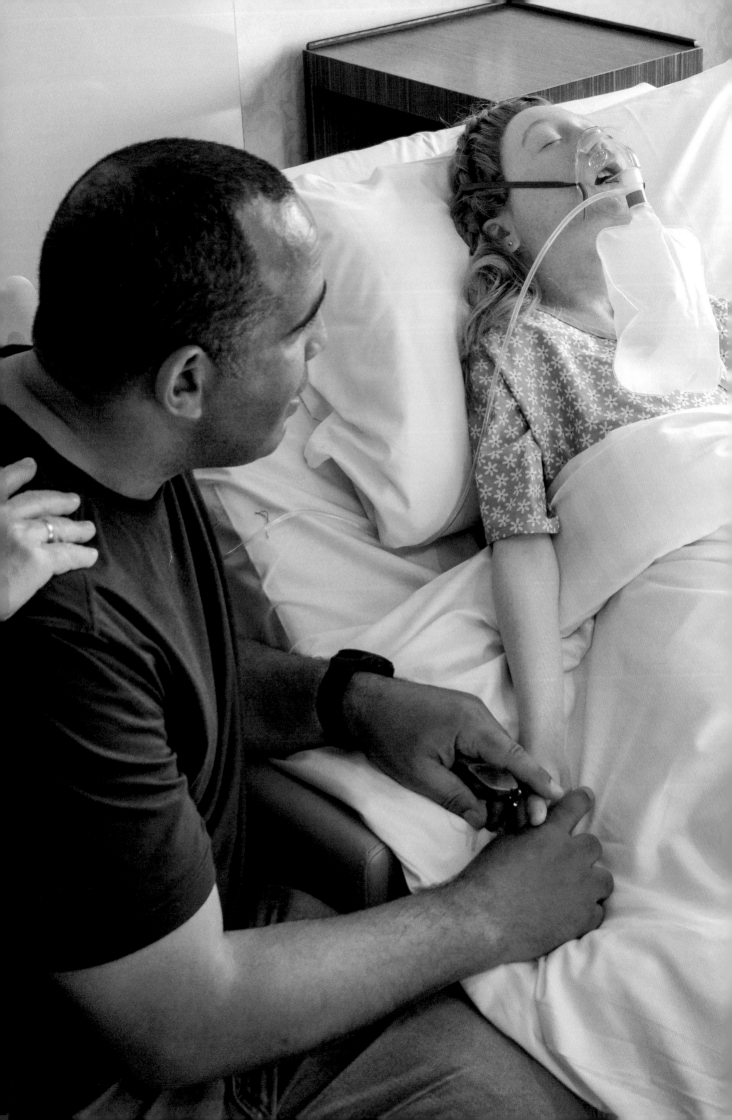

Supporting relatives and teams in resuscitation practice

Throughout this chapter, the term 'relatives' includes close friends/other people important to the patient.

Introduction

In many cases of out-of-hospital cardiac arrest, the person who performs CPR will be a close friend or relative and they may wish to remain with the patient. Many relatives find it more distressing to be separated from their family member during these critical moments than to witness attempts at resuscitation.

In keeping with the move to more open clinical practice, healthcare professionals should take the preferences of patients and relatives into account. If the resuscitation attempt fails, relatives perceive a number of advantages of being present during resuscitation:

- It helps them come to terms with the reality of death, reducing the severity or duration of grief.
- The relative can speak while there is still a chance that the dying person can hear.
- They are not distressed by being separated from a loved one at a time when they feel the need to be present.
- They can see that everything possible was done for the dying person, which helps with their understanding of the reality of the situation.
- They can touch and speak to the deceased while the body is warm.

There are also potential disadvantages to relatives being present:

- The resuscitation attempt may be distressing, particularly if the relatives are not kept informed.
- Relatives may physically or emotionally hinder the staff involved in the resuscitation attempt. Actions or remarks by medical or nursing staff may offend grieving family members.
- Relatives may be disturbed by the memory of events, although evidence indicates that fantasy (about unwitnessed events) is worse than fact (about events that have been seen). The staff should take into account the expectations of the bereaved and their cultural background during and following death.
- Relatives may demonstrate their emotions vocally or physically whilst others may wish to sit quietly or read religious text. The staff must have sufficient insight, knowledge and skills to anticipate individual needs and identify potential problems.

In this chapter

The involvement of relatives and friends

Caring for the recently bereaved

Staff support and debriefing

The learning outcomes will enable you to:

Know how to support relatives witnessing attempted resuscitation

Know how to care for the recently bereaved

Consider the religious and cultural requirements when a patient has died

Consider the legal and practical arrangements following a recent death

> In keeping with the move to more open clinical practice, healthcare professionals should take the preferences of patients and relatives into account

> Relatives perceive a number of advantages of being present during resuscitation

The involvement of relatives and friends

Care and consideration of relatives during resuscitation becomes increasingly important as procedures become more invasive. Support should be provided by an appropriately qualified healthcare professional whose responsibility is to care for family members witnessing cardiopulmonary resuscitation. Adopt the following safeguards:

- Acknowledge the difficulty of the situation. Ensure that they understand that they have a choice of whether or not to be present during resuscitation. Avoid provoking feelings of guilt whatever their decision.

- Explain that they will be looked after whether or not they decide to witness the resuscitation attempt. Ensure that introductions are made and names are known.

- Give a clear explanation of what has happened in terms of the illness or injury and what they can expect to see when they enter the resuscitation area.

- Where possible, hospitals should allow relatives the opportunity to observe attempted resuscitation of their loved one.

- Ensure that relatives understand that they will be able to leave and return at any time, and will always be accompanied.

- Ask relatives not to interfere with the resuscitation process but offer them the opportunity to touch the patient when they are told that it is safe to do so.

- Explain the nature of procedures in simple terms. If resuscitation is unsuccessful, explain why the attempt has been stopped.

- If the patient dies, advise the relatives that there may be a brief interval while equipment is removed, after which they can return to be together in private.

- Offer the relatives time to think about what has happened and the opportunity for further questions.

Caring for the recently bereaved

Caring for the bereaved compassionately will ease the grieving process. Adapt the following considerations to the individual family and their cultural needs:

- early contact with one person, usually an experienced healthcare professional

- provision of a suitable area for relatives to wait (e.g. relatives' room)

- breaking bad news sympathetically and supporting the grief response appropriately

- arranging for relatives to view the body

- religious and pastoral care requirements

- legal and practical arrangements

- follow up and team support.

Early contact with one person

Ideally this should be the person who has supported the relatives during the resuscitation attempt. If the resuscitation attempt was not observed allocate a member of the care team specifically to support the relatives. Communication between the emergency services and the receiving hospital should ensure that the arrival of relatives is anticipated for an out-of-hospital arrest. A warm, friendly and confident greeting will help to establish an open and honest relationship.

Provision of a suitable room

This should provide the appropriate ambience, space and privacy for relatives to ask questions and to express their emotions freely.

Breaking bad news and supporting the grief response

An uncomplicated and honest approach will help avoid mixed messages. The most appropriate person (not necessarily a doctor) should break the bad news to the relatives. It may be more appropriate for the healthcare professional who has been accompanying the relatives to break the news, although relatives may take comfort from talking to a doctor as well and this opportunity should always be offered.

SPIKES Model for Breaking Bad News provides a useful step-wise framework for communication (Table 17.1).

Table 17.1   SPIKES model for breaking bad news (adapted from Baile WF et al. 2000)

S	Setting up	Establish an appropriate setting.
P	Perception	Check the patient or relative's perception of the situation prompting the news regarding the illness or test results.
I	Invitation	Determine the amount of information known or how much information is desired.
K	Knowledge	Know the medical facts and their implication before initiating the conversation.
E	Emotions with empathy	Explore the emotions raised during the conversation and respond with empathy.
S	Summary	Summarise and establish a strategy for support.

Other considerations include to:

- Confirm that you are talking with the correct relatives and establish their relationship to the deceased. Briefly establish what they know and use this as the basis for your communication with them.

- Use tone of voice and non-verbal behaviour to support what you are saying. Use simple words and avoid medical jargon and platitudes that will be meaningless to relatives. Use the word 'dead', 'died' or 'death' so that there is no ambiguity.

- When breaking bad news allow periods of silence for relatives to absorb and think about what they have been told.

- Anticipate the different types of reaction/emotional response you may experience after breaking bad news. Possible responses to grief include acute emotional distress/shock, anger, denial/disbelief, guilt and catatonia.

- An individual's gender, age and cultural background will influence the response to grief. Respect cultural requirements and, where possible, provide written guidelines for individual ethnic groups.

Arranging viewing of the body

Many newly bereaved relatives value the opportunity to view their loved ones. Their experience is likely to be affected by whether the deceased appears in a presentable condition. Advise relatives what to expect before they view the body, particularly if the deceased has suffered any mutilating injuries. People are less concerned about medical devices and equipment than is generally believed. Being in the physical presence of their loved one may help them work through the grieving process. Ensure the opportunity to touch/hold the deceased is given. Staff should accompany relatives during the viewing process and they should remain nearby to offer support or provide information as required.

Religious requirements, legal and practical arrangements

Variations in handling the body and expressions of grief are influenced by a patient's religious convictions. The resuscitation team should take into account the beliefs, values and rituals of the patient and the family. There is an increasing emphasis on the need for care practice to be culturally sensitive, as a way of valuing and respecting the cultural and religious needs of patients. Religious representatives from the patient's denomination or faith are usually available to attend in-hospital. Hospital chaplains/spiritual care teams are a great source of strength and information to families and staff. Prayers, blessings, religious acts and procedure are all important in ensuring that relatives are not distressed further. It is also important to respect the views and wishes of those who have no religious belief.

Legal and practical arrangements following death are equally important. These include:

- notification of the coroner or other appropriate authority

- notification of the patient's family doctor

- organ and tissue donation decisions

- provision of information about what to do in the event of death

- involvement of religious advisors

- adherence to hospital procedure about the return of patients' property and valuables

- information concerning social services that are available

- information concerning post-mortem examination where indicated

- follow-up arrangements for relatives, which may involve long-term counselling

- provision of a telephone contact number for relatives to use and a named staff member who they can call should they have any further questions.

Staff support and debriefing

Witnessing resuscitation can be a traumatic experience for team members. When possible, make arrangements for staff to discuss with the team leader and the rest of the team any issues that may have emerged from the resuscitation event. This can be done individually or as a group and provides a valuable opportunity for reflection. All members of the team are encouraged to participate in debriefing but it should not mandatory. Data-driven, performance-focused debriefing can provide opportunities for feedback, learning and reflection. STOP-5 is a 5 min debrief tool that can be used by resuscitation teams following treatment of a patient (Figure 17.2). Anything discussed in the debrief should be treated as confidential.

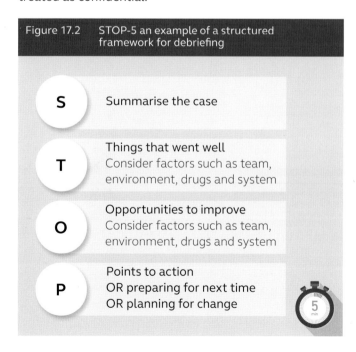

Figure 17.2 STOP-5 an example of a structured framework for debriefing

S Summarise the case

T Things that went well
Consider factors such as team, environment, drugs and system

O Opportunities to improve
Consider factors such as team, environment, drugs and system

P Points to action
OR preparing for next time
OR planning for change

5 min

17: **Summary learning**

Many relatives want the opportunity to be present during the attempted resuscitation of their loved one. This may help the grieving process.

Communication with relatives during resuscitation and after bereavement should be honest, simple, and supportive.

Post-resuscitation debriefing can provide opportunities for feedback, learning and reflection.

My key take-home messages from this chapter are:

Further reading

Baile WF, Buckman R, Lenzi R, Glober G, Beale EA, Kudelka AP. SPIKES—a six-step protocol for delivering bad news: application to the patient with cancer. Oncologist. 2000;5(1):302–311.

Jabre P, Tazarourte K, Azoulay E, et al. Offering the opportunity for family to be present during cardiopulmonary resuscitation: 1-year assessment. Intensive Care Med 2014;40:981–7.

Office for National Statistics Death certification advisory group September 2018, Guidance for Doctors completing medical certificates of cause of death in England & Wales.

Porter J, Cooper S, Sellick K Attitudes, implementation and practice of family presence during Resuscitation (FPDR): A qualitative literature review. International Emergency Nursing 2013;21:26-34.

Scottish Government, What To Do After A Death In Scotland - Practical Advice For Times Of Bereavement - 11th edition Scottish Government 16 Nov 2016.

Watts, J Death, Dying and Bereavement: Issues for practice. Dunedin 2010.

Walker C. "STOP 5: stop for 5 minutes" – our bespoke hot debrief model. 2018. https://www.edinburghemergencymedicine.com/blog/2018/11/1/stop-5-stop-for-5-minutes-our-bespoke-hot-debrief-model.

Drug			
Adrenaline	**Shockable (VF/pVT)**	**Non-Shockable (PEA/Asystole)**	Adrenaline has been the primary sympathomimetic drug for the management of cardiac arrest for 50 years. Its alpha-adrenergic effects cause systemic vasoconstriction, which increases coronary and cerebral perfusion pressures.
	Dose: 1 mg (10 mL 1:10 000 or 1 mL 1:1000) IV	**Dose:** 1 mg (10 mL 1:10 000 or 1 mL 1:1000) IV	
	Given after the 3rd shock once compressions have been resumed	Given as soon as circulatory access is obtained	The beta-adrenergic actions of adrenaline (inotropic, chronotropic) may increase coronary and cerebral blood flow, but concomitant increases in myocardial oxygen consumption and ectopic ventricular arrhythmias (particularly in the presence of acidaemia), transient hypoxaemia because of pulmonary arteriovenous shunting, impaired microcirculation, and increased post-cardiac arrest myocardial dysfunction may offset these benefits.
	Repeated every 3–5 min (alternate loops)	Repeated every 3–5 min (alternate cycles)	
	Given without interrupting chest compressions	Given without interrupting chest compressions	
			Use of adrenaline increases ROSC and the number of survivors with either a favourable or a poor neurological outcome. The potential benefit may be greater when adrenaline is given early for cardiac arrest with a non-shockable rhythm.
Amiodarone	**Shockable (VF/pVT)**	**Non-Shockable (PEA/Asystole)**	Amiodarone is a membrane-stabilising anti-arrhythmic drug that increases the duration of the action potential and refractory period in atrial and ventricular myocardium.
	Dose: 300 mg bolus IV diluted in 5% dextrose (or other suitable solvent) to a volume of 20 mL	Not indicated for PEA or asystole	
			Atrioventricular conduction is slowed, and a similar effect is seen with accessory pathways.
	Given during chest compressions after three defibrillation attempts		Amiodarone has a mild negative inotropic action and causes peripheral vasodilation through non-competitive alpha-blocking effects.
	Further dose of 150 mg if VF/pVT persists after five defibrillation attempts		Amiodarone may improve short-term survival especially when it is given early after onset of cardiac arrest.
			Amiodarone should be flushed with 0.9% sodium chloride or 5% dextrose.
Calcium	**Dose:** 10 mL 10% calcium chloride (contains 6.8 mmol Ca²⁺) or 30 mL 10% calcium gluconate IV	Calcium plays a vital role in the cellular mechanisms underlying myocardial contraction. High plasma concentrations achieved after injection may be harmful to the ischaemic myocardium and may impair cerebral recovery. Do not give calcium solutions and sodium bicarbonate simultaneously by the same route.	
	[10 mL 10% calcium gluconate contains 2.2 mmol Ca²⁺]		
	Indication: PEA caused specifically by hyperkalaemia, hypocalcaemia or overdose of calcium channel blocking drugs.		
Sodium bicarbonate	**Dose:** 50 mmol (50 mL of an 8.4% solution) IV	Cardiac arrest results in combined respiratory and metabolic acidosis as pulmonary gas exchange ceases and cellular metabolism becomes anaerobic.	
	Routine use not recommended.	The best treatment of acidaemia in cardiac arrest is chest compression; some additional benefit is gained by ventilation.	
	Consider sodium bicarbonate in shockable and non-shockable rhythms for	Bicarbonate causes generation of carbon dioxide, which diffuses rapidly into cells. This has the following effects:	
	• cardiac arrest associated with hyperkalaemia	• it exacerbates intracellular acidosis	
	• tricyclic overdose.	• it produces a negative inotropic effect on ischaemic myocardium	
	Repeat the dose as necessary, but use acid-base analysis to guide therapy.	• it presents a large, osmotically-active sodium load to an already compromised circulation and brain	
		• it produces a shift to the left in the oxygen dissociation curve, further inhibiting release of oxygen to the tissues.	
		Do not give calcium solutions and sodium bicarbonate simultaneously by the same route.	
Fluids	Infuse fluids rapidly if hypovolaemia is suspected.		
	Use 0.9% sodium chloride or Hartmann's solution, or blood for major haemorrhage.		
	Avoid dextrose, which is redistributed away from the intravascular space rapidly and causes hyperglycaemia, which may worsen neurological outcome and survival after cardiac arrest.		
	Avoid the routine infusion of large volumes of fluid in the absence of evidence of hypovolaemia.		

Drug		
Fibrinolytics	A number of drug regimens have been described for use during CPR and the best regimen is uncertain.	Fibrinolytic therapy should not be used routinely in cardiac arrest.
	Options include:	Consider fibrinolytic therapy when cardiac arrest is caused by proven or suspected acute pulmonary embolus.
	Tenecteplase 500–600 mcg kg⁻¹ IV bolus	If a fibrinolytic drug is given in these circumstances, consider performing CPR for at least 60–90 min before termination of resuscitation attempts.
	Alteplase 50 mg IV bolus if cardiac arrest with known or suspected PE. Consider a further bolus dose of 50 mg IV during a prolonged CPR attempt (e.g. 30 min after the first dose).	Ongoing CPR is not a contraindication to fibrinolysis.

Drug	Indication	Dose	
Adenosine	Paroxysmal SVT	6 mg IV bolus If unsuccessful, give a further rapid bolus of 12 mg after a 1–2 min interval. Give a third dose of 12 or 18 mg after a further 1–2 min interval.	Adenosine is a naturally occurring purine nucleotide. It blocks transmission through the AV node but has little effect on other myocardial cells or conduction pathways. It has an extremely short half-life of 10–15 s and, therefore, is given as a rapid bolus into a fast running intravenous infusion or followed by a rapid saline flush. Warn patients of transient unpleasant side effects; in particular, nausea, flushing, and chest discomfort. When using an 18 mg IV bolus dose consider the individual patient's ability to tolerate the side effects of adenosine. Apparent lack of response to adenosine will be more likely if the bolus is given too slowly or into a peripheral vein.
Adrenaline	Bradycardia (alternative to external pacing)	2–10 mcg min^{-1}	An adrenaline infusion is indicated also for bradycardia associated with adverse signs and/or risk of asystole, which has not responded to atropine, if external pacing is unavailable or unsuccessful.
	Anaphylaxis	0.5 mg IM for anaphylaxis and repeated every 5 min (Chapter 12) 50 mcg IV bolus dose titrated to effect whilst awaiting infusion to be readied (Chapter 12)	
Amiodarone	Control of haemodynamically stable monomorphic VT, polymorphic VT and wide-complex tachycardia of uncertain origin (caution in long QT syndromes) To control a rapid ventricular rate caused by accessory pathway conduction in pre-excited atrial arrhythmias (e.g. atrial fibrillation (AF)) and/or achieve chemical cardioversion After unsuccessful electrical cardioversion, to achieve chemical cardioversion or to increase the likelihood of further electrical cardioversion succeeding	300 mg IV over 10–60 min (depending on haemodynamic stability of patient) Followed an infusion of 900 mg over 24 h	Intravenous amiodarone has effects on sodium, potassium and calcium channels as well as alpha- and beta-adrenergic blocking properties. In patients with severely impaired heart function, intravenous amiodarone is preferable to other anti-arrhythmic drugs for atrial and ventricular tachyarrhythmias. Major adverse effects (caused by the solvent, not the active drug) are hypotension and bradycardia, which can be minimised by slowing the rate of drug infusion. Whenever possible, intravenous amiodarone should be given via a central venous catheter; it causes thrombophlebitis when infused into a peripheral vein, but in an emergency it can be injected into a large peripheral vein.
Aspirin	Acute coronary syndromes	300 mg orally, crushed or chewed, as soon as possible	Aspirin improves the prognosis of patients with acute coronary syndromes, significantly reducing cardiovascular death. The efficacy of aspirin is achieved by anti-platelet activity and preventing early platelet thrombus formation
Atropine	Sinus, atrial, or nodal bradycardia or AV block, when the haemodynamic condition of the patient is unstable because of the bradycardia.	Repeated doses to maximum of 3 mg	Atropine antagonises the action of the parasympathetic neurotransmitter acetylcholine at muscarinic receptors. Therefore, it blocks the effect of the vagus nerve on both the sinoatrial (SA) node and the AV node, increasing sinus automaticity and facilitating AV node conduction. Side effects of atropine are dose-related (blurred vision, dry mouth and urinary retention). It can cause acute confusion, particularly in elderly patients. Asystole during cardiac arrest is usually caused by primary myocardial pathology rather than excessive vagal tone and there is no evidence that routine use of atropine is beneficial in the treatment of asystole or PEA.

Drug	Indication	Dose	
Beta-blockers	Narrow-complex regular tachycardias by vagal manoeuvres or adenosine in patients with preserved ventricular function To control rate in atrial AF and atrial flutter when ventricular function is preserved.	Atenolol 5 mg IV over 5 min, repeated if necessary after 10 min Metoprolol (beta-1) 2.5 mg IV at 5 min intervals to a total of 15 mg Propranolol (beta-1 and beta-2 effects) 100 mcg kg^{-1} IV slowly in three equal doses at 2–3 min intervals Esmolol Short-acting (half-life of 2–9 min) beta-1 selective beta-blocker IV loading dose of 500 mcg kg^{-1} over 1 min followed by an infusion of 50–200 mcg kg^{-1} min^{-1}	Beta-blocking drugs reduce the effects of circulating catecholamines and decrease heart rate and blood pressure. They also have cardioprotective effects for patients with acute coronary syndromes. Side effects of beta blockade include bradycardia, AV conduction delay, hypotension and bronchospasm. Contraindications to the use of beta-adrenoceptor blocking drugs include second- or third-degree heart block and hypotension. They should be used with extreme caution in severe congestive heart failure and lung disease associated with bronchospasm.
Verapamil	Stable regular narrow-complex tachycardias uncontrolled or unconverted by vagal manoeuvres or adenosine. To control ventricular rate in patients with AF or atrial flutter and preserved ventricular function when the duration of the arrhythmia is less than 48 h.	2.5–5 mg IV given over 2 min In the absence of a therapeutic response or induced adverse event, give repeated doses of 5–10 mg every 15–30 min to a maximum of 20 mg	Verapamil is a calcium channel blocking drug that slows conduction and increases refractoriness in the AV node. These actions may terminate re-entrant arrhythmias and control the ventricular response rate in patients with atrial tachycardias (including AF and atrial flutter). Intravenous verapamil should be given only to patients with narrow-complex paroxysmal SVT or arrhythmias known with certainty to be of supraventricular origin. Giving calcium channel blockers to a patient with ventricular tachycardia may cause cardiovascular collapse. Verapamil may decrease myocardial contractility and critically reduce cardiac output in patients with severe LV dysfunction.
Digoxin	Atrial fibrillation with fast ventricular response	250–500 mcg IV over 30 min	Digoxin is a cardiac glycoside that slows ventricular rate by increasing vagal tone, decreasing sympathetic activity by suppression of baroreceptors, and prolonging AV node refractory period.
Vasopressors and inotropes	Hypotension in the absence of hypovolaemia Cardiogenic shock	Noradrenaline 0.05–1 mcg kg^{-1} min^{-1} Dobutamine 5–20 mcg kg^{-1} min^{-1}	Noradrenaline, with or without dobutamine, and fluid is usually the most effective treatment for the myocardial dysfunction and inflammatory response that occurs after cardiac arrest. Noradrenaline is a potent vasoconstrictor but also has a positive inotropic effect. Noradrenaline is indicated in the post-resuscitation period when hypotension and poor cardiac output cause reduced tissue perfusion. Dobutamine is often the positive inotropic drug of choice in the post-resuscitation period. Its beta agonist activity also causes vasodilation and an increase in heart rate. Dobutamine is indicated when poor cardiac output and hypotension cause significantly reduced tissue perfusion. It is useful particularly when pulmonary oedema is present and hypotension prevents the use of other vasodilators.
Magnesium	Polymorphic ventricular tachycardia (torsade de pointes) Digoxin toxicity	Dose: 2 g IV over 10 min May be repeated once if necessary Correction of hypomagnesaemia	Magnesium facilitates neurochemical transmission; it decreases acetylcholine release and reduces the sensitivity of the motor endplate.